CHALLENGING MEDICAL ETHICS

Volume 2

PATIENTS IN DANGER
The Dark Side of Medical Ethics

CHALLENGING MEDICAL ETHICS

Volume 2
Patients in Danger: the Dark Side of Medical Ethics

ISBN-10: 0 9552840 0 7   **ISBN-13:** 978 0 9552840 0 7

Published by Enterprise House, Northampton, UK.
Printed by Pegasus Print, Northampton, UK.

Please address orders and enquiries about this book to:
PO Box 341, Enterprise House,
Northampton NN3 2WZ.

This book addresses a controversial and sensitive aspect of medical
practice. The publisher, editor and distributors can take no responsibility
for any actions or omissions that result from the content of this publication,
or of any references cited therein. All doctors and nurses have a
responsibility to respect human life, and should at all times act in their
patient's best interest.

CHALLENGING MEDICAL ETHICS

Volume 2

PATIENTS IN DANGER
The Dark Side of Medical Ethics

Compiled and edited by Gillian Craig.

The weight of this sad time we must obey
Speak what we feel, not what we ought to say
The oldest hath borne most. We that are young
Shall never see so much, nor live so long.

(Shakespeare. King Lear. Act 1V, Scene 111)

Acknowledgements

Dr Gillian Craig is indebted to many people for permission to use their copyright material in this volume, including:

- BMJ Books for extracts from 'Withholding and withdrawing life-prolonging medical treatment'.
- Peter Brookes for permission to use his cartoon from The Times of Jan.6th 1999.
- The Centre for Bioethics and Public Policy for articles from Ethics and Medicine.
- Jonathan Chamberlain for quotes from his book about Stevie.
- Maggie Craig for allowing me to print some of her teaching material.
- Dr Anthony Cole, Chairman, Medical Ethics Alliance.
- Joni Eareckson for permission to quote from her books.
- Nursing Times for quotes from "No regrets" by Mark Gould © Nursing Times 1999.
- Oxford University Press for quotes from "A Preface to Paradise Lost."
- Rutherford House, Edinburgh for a quote from Dying without Dignity.
- Bishop Mark Santer, for his address to the BMA in 1994.
- Wesley J.Smith for generous provision of his copyright material from the USA.
- Taylor and Francis Ltd for copyright material from Brain Injury.
- The American Medical Association, for quotes from the Journal of the American Association.
- Parliamentary material is reproduced with the permission of the Controller of HMSO on behalf of Parliament.
- The Baha'i Chair For World Peace. University of Maryland for quotes from a paper by David Cadnam.
- The Catholic Herald for quotes from two articles published on Sept 29th 2000.
- The Catholic Medical Quarterly for 'Respect for Life' and PEG paper by Craig.
- The Church Times for quotes from a review by John Habgood.
- The Daily Mail, for articles by Nick Hopkins, Ann Kent & Cardinal Winning.
- Telegraph Group Limited for permission to reprint editorials and other material from The Daily Telegraph and quotes from The Sunday Telegraph.
- The Most Reverend and Right Honourable John Habgood, for permission to quote from 'Being a Person' (Hodder and Stoughton).
- The General Medical Council for quotes from their Guidelines of 2002.
- The Medical Ethics Alliance for permission to reprint their guidelines.
- The National Review Inc. 215 Lexington Avenue, New York, NY10016 for permission to reprint articles by Wesley J Smith.
- The Royal College of Paediatrics and Child Health for permission to quote from their framework of 1997 and May 2004.

- The Vatican for an address by Pope John Paul II
- Times Newspapers Limited for several articles published on Jan 6th 1999.
- Pamela Vack, for sending me her book 'Facing The Lion.'
- Dr Michael Wilks for permission to quote comments he made on the radio.

Note. Permission to use copyright material has been sought by the editor with care. If any copyright has been breached inadvertently, please contact the editor and the matter will be rectified at the first opportunity. All material is presented for educational purposes to promote debate and advance understanding of moral, ethical, legal, medical and social issues. We believe that this constitutes a 'fair use' of copyright material in keeping with copyright law in the USA and the UK.

Special thanks go to my publisher, the late Stuart Peel of Fairway Folio, who had the courage to take on a task that others found too daunting. Sadly he died before completing the project. Enterprise House of Northampton took over and published this volume with technical support from Pegasus Print.

This book in brief outline

Food and water are essential for life, so those who withhold food or water are, in effect depriving a person of life. Yet some years ago, judges in their wisdom, decided that food and water, given by means of a tube, is medical treatment that can be withheld if the patient is permanently unconscious. Now patients with lesser degrees of brain damage are at risk of having tube feeding withdrawn with the result that they will die. Many people feel that this is morally wrong. Yet when politicians and economists want to limit the cost of health care matters of morality may carry little weight. Consequently battle lines have been drawn between those who consider all human life to be sacred and those who do not. This book explores the complex moral, social and legal dilemmas that may arise when life-prolonging measures such as tube feeding are withheld or withdrawn.

Contributors

Sarah Boseley *The Guardian*.

Professor David Cadnam, Chairman of Prince of Wales Foundation 1999-2001.

Jonathan Chamberlain, author of *Wordjazz for Stevie*.

Dr Gillian Craig, formerly Consultant Geriatrician, Northampton, UK.

Maggie Craig. Specialist teacher, Cambridgeshire, UK.

Dr Anthony Cole, Chairman, Medical Ethics Alliance.

Dr Anthony Daniels *The Sunday Telegraph*.

Christine Doyle *The Daily Telegraph*.

Richard C.Eyer, Assistant Professor of Philosophy, Concordia University, Wisconsin.

Mark Gould *The Nursing Times*.

Professor Sir John Grimley Evans, Oxford University.

John Habgood, former Archbishop of York and member of the House of Lord's Select Committee on Medical Ethics 1993/94.

Nick Hopkins *Daily Mail*.

Michael Horsnell *The Times*.

Ann Kent *Daily Mail*.

Dominic Lawson, when Editor of *The Sunday Telegraph*.

Ann Lesley *Daily Mail*.

C. Ben Mitchell, Editor *Ethics and Medicine*.

Richard Neuhaus. The Institute of Religion & Public Life, New York.

His Holiness Pope John Paul II.

Mrs Ann Rogers of Northamptonshire, UK.

Joshua Rozenberg, Legal Correspondent, *The Daily Telegraph*.

Mark Santer, formerly Bishop of Birmingham, England.

Wesley J.Smith, Author and Attorney, California, USA.

Dr Thomas Stuttaford, Medical Correspondent, *The Times*.

Jean Ware, Director of Special Education, St Patrick's College, Dublin.

Dr Michael Wilks, Chairman, Medical Ethics Committee of the British Medical Association.

The late Cardinal Thomas Winning, Roman Catholic Archbishop of Glasgow.

Katherine Wright, formerly a member of the House of Commons Library staff.

Professor John Wyatt, Neonatal Paediatrician, University College Hospital, London.

Contents

Part 3

Children Matter

Part 4

Old People Matter

Preface

Some years ago in 1994, I posed the question "Has palliative medicine gone too far?" The question provoked an intense debate about the ethical use of artificial hydration in people who are terminally ill. In this book the debate widens to include decisions to withhold or withdraw life-prolonging measures such as the provision of food and water from patients who are not terminally ill, but whose lives depend on sustenance given by means such as tube feeding. Thus the debate moves into very controversial territory and spans a wide range of attitudes to 'end-of-life' decisions in medicine. Many people are deeply disturbed by prevailing trends in medical ethics and warn of euthanasia by stealth, of euthanasia 'in the guise of palliative care.'

Knowledge can be used for good or ill. It is no secret that human beings need food and water- without sustenance we die. Yet how far should doctors go in using technology to provide food and water to those who need assistance such as tube feeding? Is this a medical matter at all? If it is, do doctors have the right to withhold sustenance from those who lack self-awareness, or are mentally incapacitated? If it is not, who is to make such decisions- the next of kin, an economist, a social worker, a priest, a politician, a lawyer? Should such decisions be made at all? Is it ever right to allow another human being to die of dehydration or starvation if something can be done about it? Where do we draw the line?

Despite an outcry from people who find it morally repulsive to withhold food and fluids from fellow human beings under any circumstances, the practice has gained momentum. Opinion in the developed world has become polarised with the emergence of two groups holding widely different and incompatible views. The debate has become a battleground between those who feel that all human life is sacred, and those who do not. This book explores some of these difficult issues, which are so crucial to the medical profession, their patients, and society.

This book has evolved over the past decade for it includes essays that I wrote from time to time to record events as they unfolded in the UK from 1994 onwards. Some of these are published for the first time in this book. Others have been published in professional journals. A few have been circulated privately to stimulate debate and inform key individuals when the time seemed appropriate. I have also voiced concern in professional circles and responded to consultation papers that came to my notice. Latterly the stakes have risen because whistle blowers receive short shrift. Nevertheless, the faithful few fight on, for the integrity of the medical profession and the safety of our patients is as stake.

The first chapter of the book is about artificial hydration, and whether it should be considered as medical treatment or not, this being a crucial issue in law. Subsequent chapters focus on a consultation document issued by the British Medical Association in 1998, and controversial guidelines that emerged from the BMA in 1999. Then in August 2002 the General Medical Council (GMC) issued their equally controversial guidance on withholding and withdrawing life-prolonging medical treatment. Those who purport to speak for the medical profession in the UK have taken the dangerous step of condoning the withdrawal of hydration and nutrition from some patients who are not necessarily dying. Several attempts have been made to protect patients through Parliament, but all have failed to date. A recent survey indicated that about 200,000 patients died in the UK in 2004 having had treatment withdrawn. Medicine has become dangerously death-orientated.

The second part of the book describes what has been happening in the USA, seen through the eyes of Americans who have kindly allowed me to reprint their work. It is clear that events in medical ethics in the UK tend to follow those in the USA with a lag period of a few years. We may yet have time to slow the pace of change, but this could prove difficult, for with the passage of the Mental Capacity Act of 2005, the British Parliament moved our medical practice a step closer to the American pattern. Before long we too will have legally binding advance directives, and proxy health care decision makers. We too may see protracted legal battles to save the lives of mentally incapacitated people who are at risk of having life-prolonging medical treatment or tube feeding withdrawn.

The final chapters of the book include some case reports to bring the ethical dilemmas to life. Patients of all ages are at risk for we live in a society that is rather intolerant of disability. The causes of ageism in medicine are analysed from the perspective of a Consultant Geriatrician. Some brave people find life worthwhile and precious despite severe neurological disability, but others find it all too much and want to die. Dedicated special needs teachers are finding ways to communicate with children with learning disabilities. Some parents find their lives enriched by such children, but others struggle to cope.

Secular society may find the right to die appealing, when life becomes too challenging, but people of faith oppose euthanasia on the grounds that all human life is sacred. The battle between opposing factions is proving long and hard.

I hope that this book will be helpful to those who are involved in difficult personal decisions at the end of life. I hope it will also make those in authority realise that patients need to be protected in law. Those who want to refuse treatment are entitled to do so, but those who want to be treated and to receive food and water until they die also have a right to be heard.

I thank all who have published my work, supplied me with information, or shared their concerns with me over the years. I pay tribute to journalists who have brought matters to the attention of the public and thank all who have allowed me to reprint copyright material. I hope that through the efforts of many people, this book will help to protect vulnerable patients and turn back the tide of death.

Gillian Craig, Northampton UK, December 2005.

Part 1

The Debate in Great Britain

Withholding treatment from people
who are not dying

Setting the Scene

In a hospital in the North of England in 1993, a young man is in bed, apparently unconscious. He opens his eyes from time to time, but this is only a reflex action. He can breathe normally but needs to be tube fed. His parents sit quietly watching him. Football regalia surround them, memories of happier times. Three years before, the man was a spectator supporting his team, but he was crushed and unable to breathe as the crowd surged forward to congratulate the winning players. He suffered severe brain damage, from lack of oxygen, on that fateful day at the Hillsborough Stadium. Many fans died in the crush, but Tony Bland survived and was taken to hospital. Eventually it became clear that he was in a permanent vegetative state, from which it was unlikely he would ever recover.

His parents visited frequently for three years, hoping against hope. Finally they felt it would be best for Tony to be allowed to die. They wanted to lay him to rest and get on with their own lives. But the doctors said "No". They could not stop feeding him for that would be murder. What was to be done?

Enter the Official Solicitor, who represents the interests of people with mental incapacity. After some debate the case goes to the High Court. Eventually the highest court in the land becomes involved.

Enter the Law Lords. They decree, after careful deliberation, that tube feeding is medical treatment, a form of life support that can be stopped in this particular case with their permission. So Tony Bland died, and with his death the protective wall of English Law became fatally weakened and "misshapen".

Before long the Lord Advocate in Scotland decided that a woman in "near PVS" could die, and so the movement to withhold artificial nutrition and hydration gained momentum.

Introduction

Treatment limiting decisions achieved prominence in the United Kingdom (UK) with the case of Tony Bland, an Englishman with a permanent vegetative state (PVS), who died when hydration and food, given via a tube, was withdrawn.[1] Now the spotlight has moved to other people with long-term physical and mental illnesses that are disabling but not necessarily fatal. Many of these people are elderly and suffer from strokes, dementia or other degenerative diseases. Others have brain injury due to accidents or infections. Some are born with disabilities and never enjoy a normal life.

Many such unfortunate people have some degree of mental incapacity or infirmity but are cared for lovingly by their family, or in nursing homes or other institutions. Their quality of life may be poor as judged by normal standards, but they are nevertheless people and entitled to the full protection of the law. That protection can no longer be guaranteed.

Doctors are often faced with difficult questions about how far to go in prolonging life by measures such as tube feeding. Sometimes their views differ from those of the family. Insensitive handling can have adverse emotional effects on dissenting relatives. The whole issue of who decides, and makes the final judgement is now under intense discussion by the medical profession, lawyers and society as a whole. Medical ethics is moving into dangerous territory.

Anglican and Roman Catholic Bishops made a valuable contribution to medical ethics in 1993, when they stated some important guiding principles on the distinction between killing and letting die. They said...

> "Doctors do not have an overriding obligation to prolong life by all available means. The Declaration on Euthanasia in 1980 by the Sacred Congregation for the Doctrine of the Faith proposes the notion that treatment for a dying patient should be proportionate to the therapeutic effect to be expected, and should not be disproportionately painful, intrusive, risky or costly in the circumstances. Treatment may therefore be withheld or withdrawn. This is an area of fine judgement. Such decisions should be made collaboratively and by more than one medical person. They should be guided by the principle that a pattern of care should never be adopted with the intention, purpose or aim of terminating the life, or bringing about the death of a patient. Death, if it ensues, will have resulted from the underlying condition which required medical intervention, not as a direct consequence of the decision to withhold or withdraw treatment. It is possible however, to envisage cases where withholding or withdrawing treatment might be morally equivalent to murder."[2]

The Bishops recognised "the complexity of the issue of artificial hydration and the associated medical regimes", but felt that there could be no blanket permission to withdraw nutrition and hydration from PVS patients or those in a similar situation. At the very least, every person's needs and rights must be dealt with on a case by case basis.[3]

The important question of whether artificial hydration and nutrition (ANH) should be regarded as medical treatment is discussed in some detail in the first chapter of this book, the issue being considered from various aspects- Christian, ethical, legal, medical and purely practical. The author shares the view of the House of Lords' Select Committee on Medical Ethics of 1993/94, for their Lordships found it impossible to make a firm ruling. Food and fluids, by whatever means they are given, are best regarded as a basic human need. Their Lordship's comments on treatment-limiting decisions are appended.

Treatment – limiting decisions
Conclusions of the House of Lords' Select Committee on Medical Ethics[4]

Paragraph 251. The issue of treatment-limiting decisions is crucial to many of the concerns which our witnesses raised with us. For most practical purposes we do not discern any significant ethical difference between those decisions which involve discontinuing a treatment already begun and those which involve not starting a treatment. To make such a distinction could result in patients being subjected to the continuation of unnecessary and burdensome procedures simply because they had been started previously; or it could restrict a doctor's freedom to do everything possible for the patient in an emergency or when diagnosis is uncertain. We do not therefore distinguish between withholding and withdrawal of treatment, in our discussion of treatment-limiting decisions. However, we acknowledge that, in the case of neonates particularly, the withdrawal of treatment becomes harder as time passes, as more love and commitment are invested in the child as an individual.

252. All our witnesses agreed that there is a point at which the duty to try to save a patient's life is exhausted, and at which treatment may be inappropriate. But this is not a point which can be readily defined, since it must be identified in the light of each patient's individual condition and circumstances. Obviously it is inappropriate to give treatment which is futile in the sense that it fails to achieve the hoped for physical result. Indeed to continue a treatment in such circumstances could be irresponsible. A decision not to do so will rarely be controversial.

253. In other cases, a decision to limit treatment may depend on the balance between the burdens which the treatment will impose and the benefits that it is likely to produce. Competent patients can often, with medical advice and after full discussion, make such decisions themselves, perhaps for example foregoing the possibility of a few extra weeks of life because the possible side effects of the proposed treatment might necessitate being in hospital rather than at home. Such a decision is made on the basis of the quality rather than the length of life, but few would dispute the right of the patient to choose in that way.

254. Controversy arises when treatment-limiting decisions based on the balance of burdens and benefits must be made in respect of incompetent patients. The spectre of one individual judging the quality of life of another gives rise to potent fears. But such decisions, however difficult, must be made if incompetent patients are not to be subjected to the aggressive over-treatment to which competent patients would rightly object.

255. Treatment-limiting decisions in respect of an incompetent patient should be taken jointly by all those involved in his or her care, including the whole health-care team and the family or other people closest to the patient. Their guiding principle should be that a treatment may be judged inappropriate if it will add nothing to the patient's well-being as a person.

In most cases full discussion will ultimately lead to agreement on what treatment is appropriate or inappropriate. Where agreement cannot be reached after adequate discussion and time for reflection, provision should be made for a party to the decision-making to apply for a decision from the new forum which we have recommended.

256. Some people may suggest that clearer guidance is needed as to the circumstances in which treatment may be judged inappropriate. But we are not satisfied that this is either possible or desirable. Such a judgement must be made in relation to the condition, circumstances and values of the individual patient. Such matters cannot be defined or legislated for and consensus must be developed on a case-by-case basis, inching forwards as best we can. For these reasons we do not favour legislation... We are confident that, in making treatment-limiting decisions, doctors who act responsibly, in the way we have described, have adequate protection under existing law.

257. Nor do we think it helpful to attempt a firm distinction between treatment and personal care, implying that the former may be limited and the latter not. The two are part of a continuum, and such boundary as there is between them shifts as practice evolves and particularly as the wider role of nursing develops. This boundary is one which the courts were required to define in the case of Tony Bland, and that gave rise to much debate about whether nutrition and hydration, even when given by invasive methods, may ever be regarded as a treatment which in certain circumstances it may be inappropriate to initiate or continue. This question has caused us great difficulty, with some members of the committee taking one view and some another, and we have not been able to reach a conclusion. But where we are agreed is in judging that the question need not, indeed should not, usually be asked. In the case of Tony Bland, it might well have been decided long before application was made to the court that treatment with antibiotics was inappropriate, given that recovery from the inevitable complications of infection could add nothing to his well-being as a person. We consider that, had Tony Bland's health-care team and family been in agreement on this course, it would have been ethically and practically appropriate for such treatment to have been discontinued. Because of his established pvs there was no duty to strive to preserve his life by medical means. We consider that progressive development and ultimate acceptance of the notion that some treatment is inappropriate should make it unnecessary to consider the withdrawal of nutrition and hydration, except in circumstances where its administration is in itself evidently burdensome to the patient.

Report of House of Lords Select Committee on Medical Ethics.
© *HMSO London 1994.*

References

1. Airedale NHS Trust v Bland [1993] 1 All ER.
2. A Joint Submission from the Church of England House of Bishops and the Roman Catholic Bishops' Conference of England and Wales to the House of Lord's Select Committee on Medical Ethics. 1993. Paragraph 15.
3. Ibid. Para 16.
4. Report of the House of Lords' Select Committee on Medical Ethics. *HMSO* 1994.

Note. Parliamentary material from the Report of the House of Lords' Select Committee on Medical Ethics is reproduced with the permission of the Controller of HMSO on behalf of Parliament.

Chapter 1

Artificial Hydration and Nutrition.
Medical Treatment or Basic Human Need?

Author Gillian Craig

Introduction

Is artificial hydration and nutrition a medical treatment or a basic human need? A great deal hinges in law and medicine on the answer to the question – because doctors are allowed to discontinue medical treatment if they deem it to be futile.

For the purposes of this discussion I will define artificial hydration and nutrition as fluid and nourishment taken into the body by some means other than a voluntary act of swallowing.

There is a general ill-defined feeling in the field of medical ethics, that hydration cannot be equated with treatment such as antibiotics, tablets for epilepsy, or tablets to control the rhythm of the heart. What is the reason for this? In this paper I attempt to explore these issues.

Water is a fundamental necessity for all forms of life in the plant and animal kingdom. A few plants are specially adapted to survive in dry conditions and some humans, such as the Bushmen of the Kalahari desert are capable of surviving for longer than the rest of us without water. However, every cell of the human body requires a constant solution of salts and water in order to function. Claude Bernard - a great French physiologist - called this the *milieu interieur*. Without this stable internal environment, innumerable incredibly complex and marvellous biochemical transactions that underpin life, cannot take place. Without salt and water each cell shrinks and collapses and the body eventually dies. The outward signs of this cellular collapse can be seen as hollowing of the eyes, a haggard look, a dry tongue, and looseness and lack of turgor of the skin. In a plant there will be wilting, as every gardener knows. So quite clearly, water is essential for life - it sustains life.

In medicine, decisions about hydration and nutrition give power over life and death. Awesome power! Should such responsibility remain in the hands of one profession, or should it be shared more widely? The advent of artificial hydration and nutrition has created new and difficult ethical dilemmas for society that should be approached with wisdom and humility by all concerned.

One of the major problems facing western society is to decide at what stage efforts to preserve life by giving food and drink artificially, should cease. In the United Kingdom, the church, the legal profession, the medical profession, and Parliament, have been trying to address these difficult matters for a number of years, without reaching a consensus.

The Christian perspective

People have understood that food and drink are essential for life since time immemorial. A psalmist, writing in Old Testament times, many centuries before the Birth of Christ, wrote –

"My strength is dried up like a potsherd: and my tongue cleaveth to my jaws;
and thou has brought me into the dust of death."[1]

Later, in New Testament times, it was considered a matter of basic etiquette and morality to give food and water to strangers and those who are hungry or thirsty.[2] Christians are expected to minister to the least of our brethren in this way. Therefore in a Christian society, people with dementia, learning difficulties, or physical incapacity and frailty, should be cared for. Albert Schweitzer spoke of "reverence for life"; but our secular society is more likely to think in terms of the quality of life, and to be rather dismissive of those whose quality of life seems to be poor. We have become wary of supporting life regardless of the quality.

Anglican Bishops from all over the world met in London in 1998 for the Lambeth Conference. Towards the end of their deliberations they attempted to decide how to define euthanasia, and how to distinguish this from a death that occurred by means "consonant with the Christian faith". The proposed resolution condoned "withholding, withdrawing, declining, terminating, excessive medical treatment or intervention in enabling a person to die with dignity". The Bishop of Singapore, the Rt. Rev. Moses Tay, who was once a hospital doctor, opposed the resolution, saying "Basic nutrition and hydration is not part of medical treatment in the normal sense. Giving food and water is a basic act of Christian charity. Withdrawing food and drink is the equivalent of starving a person to death. It is cruel. It is killing". The debate was adjourned without reaching a conclusion.[3] This was hardly surprising – the Conference was not the best venue to discuss such complex ethical issues.

I have referred to the helpful guiding principles stated in 1993 by Anglican and Roman Catholic Bishops (*see page 1 of this book*). They continue to bring a Christian perspective into debates in the House of Lords. But some clergy are less helpful. Those who lack scientific training may shudder at the thought of drips and tube feeding. In addition a belief in an after-life can reduce the imperative to strive to stay in this world. If Heaven awaits death may be seen as a welcome release from suffering. Nevertheless the timing of death should be left to the wisdom of God, for "The foolishness of God is wiser than the wisdom of men".[4]

An ethical perspective

In the UK, the House of Lord's Select Committee on Medical Ethics considered the ethics of treatment limiting decisions in 1993, at the time of the Bland case. They failed to reach a consensus on the question of whether nutrition and hydration could ever be regarded as medical treatment, even when given by invasive means. Some members of the committee took one view, others another. They commented:

". . . we do not think it helpful to attempt a firm distinction between treatment
and personal care, implying that the former may be limited and the latter
not. The two are part of a continuum . . ."[5]

Table 1   The feeding cascade or continuum

*Items marked * are currently defined as artificial nutrition*

Oral food and drink
Minced/puréed food and drink
Thickened and fortified drinks
Special drinking cups/straws/syringe
* Nasogastric tube feeding
* Fine bore nasogastric tube feeding
* Percutaneous endoscopic gastrostomy (PEG)
* Total parenteral nutrition

Let us consider that continuum for a moment (*see Table 1*). We show friendship, care and concern by inviting people to share a meal with us. With increasing frailty, some people find eating and drinking more difficult and may need to be fed by a member of their family, a carer or a nurse. Various ploys are used to make eating and drinking easier – for example – special drinking cups and straws. The use of thickened drinks or puréed food may be helpful for those who choke on solids. It is only a short step logically, from being given a drink through a straw, to being given a drink through a tube that goes further down into the stomach. Yet the psychological and aesthetic consequences of this step are enormous. As soon as tube-feeding is suggested, ethical dilemmas arise. Warning bells ring. People start to wonder whether they should be doing this. Some murmur darkly about "the technological imperative", others label the intervention intrusive or meddlesome. Yet such intervention can be life-saving. Some medical or nursing knowledge is needed for the introduction of a naso-gastric tube and specialist skills are required for the insertion of a tube through the abdominal wall (a percutaneous endoscopic gastrostomy or PEG). Therefore most people would regard the insertion of a PEG as a medical procedure, but once inserted the management of a PEG is not difficult.

Food and fluid given via a tube sustains life; it does not cure illness and therefore strictly speaking it cannot be regarded as treatment. (Similarly the provision of dentures is a dental procedure but the use of the dentures is a natural function of eating). So why do we get so concerned about feeding tubes and artificial hydration? I am inclined to think that it is not so much the technological intrusion that bothers us, but concern about the quality of the life that is maintained by this means. Over-aggressive attempts to prolong life artificially, regardless of the quality, are as worrying as premature cessation of feeding. So where should society draw the line? At what stage should efforts to prolong life cease? Who decides?

The legal perspective

In the case of Tony Bland, the Englishman with a permanent vegetative state, the House of Lords in their ruling decided that artificial nutrition and hydration (ANH) was medical treatment – a form of life support – that could be withdrawn with permission from an appropriate court. According to one commentator "there was apparently overwhelming evidence at the time that this was the consensus view of medical opinion in England and the USA. The Court were therefore bound to find as a fact, but not as a matter of law, that medical opinion regards feeding and hydration by means of a tube, as medical treatment. However, since the decision in the Bland case it has become apparent that there is not a consensus on this matter".[6] The Irish Medical Council for example, takes a different view as does the Medical Ethics Alliance.

If ANH is merely a medical life support system like mechanical ventilation or renal dialysis, why do we need to refer to the courts at all? Other forms of life-support are stopped without reference to the courts. If the courts are involved routinely they could be swamped by cases relating to the withdrawal of ANH. The practical problems would be immense.

Resort to the legal profession has been seen as a safeguard to protect the interests of patients and doctors when patients are mentally incapacitated and unable to decide such matters for themselves. However judges sometimes question their role in matters that seem essentially ethical in nature.[7] Some judges have proved so exceedingly reluctant to make rulings in difficult medical cases that they have been accused of abdicating responsibility. As Melanie Phillips of the Sunday Times put it - "Who are we to decide these great issues?" they cry. "Leave it to the doctors. Leave it to Parliament. Leave judgement to anyone but us."[8] The result, said Melanie Phillips is that they refuse to apply fundamental principles laid down in law.[8]

In one case in 1999 a High Court Judge refused to make an order to ensure that life-saving treatment would not be withdrawn from a 12 year old severely disabled boy, David Glass. The remedy of a judicial review said Judge Scott Baker, was "too blunt a tool" for the "sensitive and ongoing problem raised by the case".[9] The case eventually went to the European Court of Human Rights where the judges took a more robust view.

There is, in fact, a growing realization that the provision of food and water whether orally or by other means, is not a medical life-support system akin to mechanical ventilation or renal dialysis. It does come into a rather different category. Controversial decisions about the provision or non-provision of ANH to mentally incapacitated patients do require scrutiny by a Judge. Such decisions should not be left to doctors, lawyers or families acting on their own. Men of wisdom and humility realize that there are times when "We need the distilled ethical experience of the race to guide us . . .".[10]

Judges in the UK had an excellent opportunity to influence events in a positive way when, in 2004, they were called upon to consider the legality of professional guidelines issued by the General Medical Council (GMC). A judicial inquiry into the case of Leslie Burke brought the issue of withholding ANH to the attention of the legal profession and the public.[11] The Burke case was a golden opportunity to call a halt to some dubious practices that have evolved in our hospitals in the wake of the judgement in the case of Airedale NHS Trust v Bland. Unfortunately, as will be explained later in this book, the golden opportunity was lost.

Who decides? The Law Commission's proposals
In 1998 the Lord Chancellor's Department in London issued a consultation paper "Who decides? Making decisions on behalf of mentally incapacitated adults."[12]

This addressed issues such as withholding or withdrawing tube feeding and hydration from mentally incapacitated adults, with the result that they would die of dehydration. It also raised the issue of whether advance directives should be made legally binding in the UK. Both these questions have immensely important implications for the future practice of medicine in the UK.

The Law Commission's proposals now enshrined in the Mental Capacity Act allow for proxy decision making in matters such as the non-provision of ANH. The Act received the Royal Assent following a stormy passage through Parliament in April 2005 and is expected to reach the statute book in 2007. Under the terms of the Act difficult "life or death" medical decisions in mentally capacitated people may be taken by legally authorized proxy-decision makers, who will be empowered to over rule the advice of doctors. Advance directives that indicate a wish *not* to be treated will be legally binding, but there is no provision in the Act to ensure that the wishes of those who want to receive ANH will be respected. Some people who have studied the Act carefully predict that its implementation could cause public revulsion and demands for active euthanasia by a lethal injection rather than a slow death from dehydration or starvation. Yet public attitudes to the Act appear to be equally divided between those who oppose the legislation and those who support it. Many people remain unaware of the serious implications or are suffering from 'consultation fatigue'. As the late Cardinal Winning predicted in 1997, the nation appears to be " sleepwalking towards disaster."

A medical perspective

The Bland case raised serious questions about the legality of many areas of medical practice. When it comes to ANH it is illogical to give maximum protection to people in PVS, and to give minimal protection to less incapacitated people who are sensate.[13] In the UK and other countries, many sensate patients are having ANH withheld and withdrawn with the result that they die. Professional guidelines have proved to be of little value in practice. Cases of concern do not get the attention they deserve, whistle blowers risk serious damage to their professional careers and members of the public who do not qualify for legal aid have little access to justice.

The British Medical Association (BMA) Medical Ethics Committee issued an important consultation paper in July 1998, at a time when most people were on holiday. The paper touched on many crucial matters but shed little light on grey areas of medical practice. [14] The paper was mainly about treatment limiting decisions in chronically disabled people, with strokes or dementia, who are not, strictly speaking, terminally ill. The BMA posed, but failed to answer the crucial question about hydration, namely- *"On what grounds might a valid distinction be made between artificial nutrition and hydration and other life-prolonging treatments?"* I will now address that question.

Life-prolonging treatment

Under this heading one might include the following:
- Antibiotics for the cure of life-threatening infections.
- Insulin and/or tablets, for diabetes.
- Cortisol replacement therapy in deficiency states.

- Thyroid hormone therapy in myxoedema.
- Medication to support muscle function in myasthenia gravis.
- Tracheostomy in airways obstruction.
- Mechanical ventilation in respiratory failure.
- Kidney dialysis in renal failure.
- Total parenteral nutrition in intestinal failure.
- Percutaneous endoscopic gastrostomy.
- Chemotherapy for cancer, leukaemia etc.
- Organ transplants.
- Cardiac pacemakers and artificial valves.
- Artificial hydration in fluid deficiency states.
- Vitamin supplements and food in malnutrition.
- Blood transfusions for bleeding etc.

In the main, these varied treatments cure or relieve specific diseases or hormonal deficiency states, or take over the functions of specific organs, parts of organs or body systems. In contrast, artificial hydration and nutrition supports all systems and all organs. It supplies essential fluid and nutrients to every cell in the body and so is far more than 'medical treatment'. Food, water and oxygen are the only resources that the body has to obtain from outside sources. They are truly basic human needs.

Artificial hydration as a life-support system

Water is essential for the survival of every cell in the body. If a person cannot drink, within a week or so their circulation will fail, their kidneys will fail and they will die, irrespective of whether their heart, brain and kidneys are capable of working normally. Fluid therefore supports the life of the whole body, without the need for machinery, such as mechanical ventilators or kidney machines.

One could argue that a supply of oxygen and normal kidneys are also essential for the survival of every cell in the body, and no one would dispute that. Mechanical ventilation supports the function of breathing in patients whose lungs are failing. Normal kidneys are needed to eliminate waste chemicals from the body, to prevent a lethal build up of potassium for example. Kidney dialysis machines can be used to take over from the kidney in patients whose kidneys have failed.

It is fair to say that respiratory failure and kidney failure are just as lethal as dehydration, but the support systems needed are highly technical and complex in comparison to artificial hydration and nutrition The patient on a respirator has to be connected to a complex and bulky machine via a tube into the wind pipe and may need to be sedated to prevent distress. The machine requires servicing and electricity to keep it going and the patient's life is dependent on the machine every minute of the day.

A person on a kidney dialysis regime requires a minor operation to give permanent access to a vein in their arm. This enables them to be connected up to the kidney machine two or three times a week for several hours, while their blood circulates through the machine and is cleared of impurities. Blood tests are required to monitor progress, and skilled medical supervision is needed. A few people cope with their own dialysis and have machines at home, but others travel to special hospital units for their treatment.

A feeding tube is child's play in comparison to other forms of life support. It is simple, cheap, rarely causes side effects, and does not require a power supply or skilled supervision. The only requirements after insertion of a feeding tube are proprietary food supplies and water at normal meal times, and a suitably trained carer. Modern percutaneous gastrostomy tubes (PEGS) for children are unobtrusive and do not restrict normal activities in any way.

Far more people worldwide are likely to need a feeding tube or artificial hydration at some stage in their life than will ever need a respirator or kidney machine. Far more people die of dehydration for one reason or another than ever die of respiratory or renal failure. Life saving fluid replacement should be available to all who need it, and can benefit from it.

The distinction between killing and letting die

This distinction is an important one in medicine, but it can become somewhat blurred. Ethicists consider that there are cases where letting die is morally equivalent to killing.[15] Doctors working in the hospice movement in the UK have always stated that they are opposed to active euthanasia, but they argue that it is essential for them to be allowed to let patients die.

In their evidence to the House of Lords Select Committee in 1993, the National Council for Hospice and Specialist Palliative Care Services commented:

> "It is essential to point out that medical treatment is never withdrawn – all patients are entitled to measures to improve their comfort . . . It is only life-sustaining and life-prolonging measures which should be withheld or withdrawn if the competent patient refuses them, or it is reasonably certain that the benefits of their use are outweighed by the burdens and harms they impose, or that the quality of life provided would be unacceptably poor."[16]

Thus, if your aim is to let your patient die, a life-sustaining intervention such as a drip becomes, at a stroke, in the twinkling of an eye, not 'medical treatment', not a basic human need, not a moral necessity, but a "measure".

If we look at a dictionary definition of "treatment" it is *"The application of remedies with the object of effecting a cure"*. This being so, artificial hydration given with the object of sustaining life is not strictly speaking treatment, but artificial hydration given with the aim of curing existing dehydration, would be. Similarly, food or nourishing solutions given down a feeding tube with the object of maintaining nutrition would not, strictly speaking, be treatment - whereas food given to relieve malnutrition would be. This may seem semantic, but it is important to define terms carefully and accurately.

The NHS End of Life Programme.

In 1997 palliative care specialists recognised that the hospice model of care could not be neatly extrapolated to other patient groups [17]. Two years later hospice doctors were careful to stress that their experience did not extend "to care of patients in a PVS, nor to those with long-term disabling physical or mental illnesses which may be non-fatal, or fatal only after a period of many years." [14] But things are changing. An extensive NHS End of Life Programme is now under way in the UK led by palliative care consultants and the Department of Health. The palliative care approach is to be extended to patients with a wide range of conditions [18]. The elderly in residential and nursing homes will receive special attention in the hope that symptom control will be improved and the number admitted to hospital to die will be reduced. While this may be laudable in some respects, there is a risk that some patients who would benefit from active treatment will not receive it. I hope therefore that palliative carers will liaise with colleagues trained in geriatric medicine for the benefit of their patients.

A practical perspective

Food growing, gathering and preparation is an essential activity for human society. Communal effort is needed to ensure that food is available to all. Individual effort is involved in eating the food and drink prepared. You cannot force feed a person who does not want to eat or drink, unless that person is under age and likely to die of malnutrition (e.g. in cases of anorexia nervosa). Therefore if a competent adult wishes to refuse food and drink that is their responsibility, unless they are suffering from depression with suicidal ideas. If the person concerned has made a valid advance directive that should be respected.

If a child is unable to eat, it is the responsibility of an adult to assist. If the child is unable to swallow, tube feeding should be carefully considered. Many disabled children are fed in this way. If a competent adult is unable to eat or drink and wishes to live, it is the responsibility of others to ensure that food and fluids are given if humanly possible, and this may involve tube feeding with the patient's consent. In the case of mentally incompetent adults who are unable to make such decisions for themselves, others have to decide for them. Hence the Lord Chancellor's paper "Who decides?"- which led to the draft Mental Incapacity Bill of 2002 [19] which was later renamed the Mental Capacity Bill. Quality of life questions, such as the level of consciousness, and issues of 'personhood' may come into play. Factors such as the nature of the underlying pathology and prognosis are crucial. Time must be allowed for careful consideration of all such factors. Irrevocable life and death decisions should never be made in haste.

In conclusion

It is not possible to make a firm ruling and say that all artificial hydration and nutrition is medical treatment. Food and fluids, by whatever means they are given are best regarded as a basic human need. The Catholic view as restated by Pope John Paul II in March 2004 is unequivocal on this point [20]. However there may come a stage for some patients, when it is agreed by all concerned that to initiate or continue tube feeding is burdensome, inappropriate, and futile.

Decisions about the risks and benefits of tube feeding do require some medical input and knowledge of the patient's condition, but the techniques required to *provide* sustenance do not alter the fact that the food and water provided remain food and water, and *not primarily treatment*.

References

1   The Bible. Authorised King James Version. Psalm 22; verse 15.
2   ibid. St Matthew, Chapter 25, verses 34-46.
3   Combe V. Support for 'dying with dignity". *Daily Telegraph*, London August 7th, 1998; p.4.
4   St Paul. First letter to the Corinthians, Chapter 2, verse 25. The Bible.
5   House of Lords Select Committee. Report on Medical Ethics. *HMSO*. 1994; Para. 257
6   Gerard Wright Q.C. Section 1(a) in 'Who Decides?' *Medical Education Trust* PO Box 174317, London, SW3 4WJ. 1998.
7   The Rt Hon. Dame Elizabeth Butler-Sloss. 'Who is to judge?' The role of the judiciary in ethical issues'. The 14th Eric Symes Memorial Lecture at Westminster Abbey, May 1999.
8   Phillips M. Hospital doctors learn how to kill, while the law-makers look the other way. *Sunday Times* 28th March 1999.
9   Shaw T. Mother loses battle over care for disabled son. *The Daily Telegraph*. 23rd April 1999, p.8.
10 Austin Baker J. Moral good and evil. Chapter 4, p.101 in "The Foolishness of God". *Collins*. Fontana Books, 1975.
11 Queen's Bench Division. R (Burke) v General Medical Council before Mr Justice Munby. Judgement July 31st 2004. *The Times*, (Tabloid version) p62, August 6th 2004.
12 Who decides? Making decisions on behalf of mentally incapacitated adults. Lord Chancellor's Department. Family Division. London. January, 1998.
13 Craig GM. On withholding artificial nutrition and hydration from sedated terminally ill patients. The debate continues. *Journal of Medical Ethics* 1996; **22**; 147-153.
14 Withdrawing and withholding treatment. Consultation paper from BMA Medical Ethics Committee. *BMA*, London, July, 1999.
15 Gillon R., Euthanasia, withholding life-prolonging treatment, and moral differences between killing and letting die. *Journal of Medical Ethics*. 1988; **1**: 115-117.
16 Key Ethical Issues in Palliative Care. Occasional Paper 3. *National Council for Hospice and Specialist Palliative Care Services*. London, 1993, p. 7.
17 Corner J and Dunlop R. New approaches to care. p289 in New Themes in Palliative Care. Ed. Clark D, Hockley J and Ahmedzai S. *Open University Press* 1997.
18 Ellershaw JE, Murphy D. The Liverpool Care Pathway (LCP) influencing the UK agenda on care of the dying. *International Journal of Palliative Nursing*. 2005; **11.3**:132-134.
19 Report of the House of Lords and House of Commons Joint Committee on the draft Mental Incapacity Bill. Session 2002-2003. *The Stationary Office Ltd.* November 2003.
20 Pope John Paul II. Address given in Rome, March 20th 2004. International Congress on "Life sustaining treatments and vegetative state: scientific advances & ethical dilemmas" (*See chapter 15 of this book*).

Chapter 2

To Die Or Not To Die?
That Is The Question

Author Gillian Craig

Introduction

Many years ago in 1977, Dr Jack Dominion said "The real corruption of our age is disposable relationships." Nowadays the real corruption is disposable people. This is not a new problem. Jews were disposable in the holocaust of Nazi Germany, as were people with mental deficiency and other disabilities. The danger now is that the lessons of the holocaust have not been learnt by all western countries. We risk losing our integrity as human beings for the sake of short-term economic gains, and the pursuit of utilitarian philosophical ideals. We live in a world where economists view the early death of elderly people as advantageous[1] and where hard-pressed doctors see the elderly uncured as troublesome 'bed-blockers'. Some clergy raise questions about the validity of life for people with dementia[2] while others strive to communicate with such people, and listen to their fading voice.[3]

Some bioethicists argue that human dignity and the right to live should be dependent on qualities such as self-awareness and rational thinking. This dangerous line of thought is now creeping into clinical decision making disguised as 'absence of personhood'. In a recent booklet on ethical and legal aspects of clinical hydration and nutritional support, the concept of absence of personhood appears in the context of some severe stroke patients, and patients in the terminal stages of dementia. Absence of personhood, say the authors, can be regarded as close to the vegetative state.[4] This statement paves the way to withdrawal of treatment with the approval of the courts. Society should pause and think long and hard before going further down that road.

I dislike the concept of lack of personhood. All patients however disabled mentally or physically, should be treated as human beings. The decision whether to hydrate and feed them should depend on other issues, such as the burdens and benefits of intervention, not on whether they can be written off as people. Even severely demented or deeply unconscious patients have a residual spark of humanity.

The situation at present in the United Kingdom is that patients who are insensate with a permanent vegetative state (PVS) can have their tube feeding discontinued only following a court order. Ironically other patients, who may well be sentient, have their nutrition and fluids stopped by doctors without reference to the courts. In practice, doctors have to make such decisions about the long-term management of patients quite often, and it would be totally impracticable for all such decisions to be referred to the courts. Clearly it is illogical to have safeguards for patients with PVS and no safeguards for less seriously incapacitated people.

The BMA Consultation Paper. "Withdrawing and withholding treatment"

This consultation developed as a response to expressions of concern and requests for advice from many doctors. The Medical Ethics Committee of the British Medical Association (BMA) launched a consultation paper in July 1998 and invited comments over a period of three months.[5] The results of their deliberations were published in June 1999. This time scale may prove to have been over-optimistic, given the nature of the fundamental ethical problems that were addressed. The comments that follow relate to the consultation paper only.

The BMA excluded from their remit discussion about treatment limitation in people for whom death is thought to be imminent, who might benefit from treatment for only a matter of days or weeks. They took the view that withdrawal of treatment from such patients does not raise the same ethical and legal difficulties as withdrawal of treatment that would prolong life for much longer. However, the shorter time scale in the dying does not eliminate the legal and ethical dilemmas.[6] The BMA mentioned that there is broad concern about the 'double effect' argument and wondered whether it should, or could be replaced. Some brief comments about sedation in the dying were also made.[7]

The main purpose of the consultation paper was to obtain views, and thereafter produce workable guidelines on treatment limitation in patients who are seriously mentally incapacitated by brain damage of one sort or another. The consultation therefore linked with the Law Commission draft Mental Incapacity Bill, as discussed in the Lord Chancellor's Green Paper *Who decides?*[8] The BMA were addressing the issue 'How do doctors decide?'

Serious mental incapacity can be caused by birth injury, or may arise in later life as a result of severe strokes, meningitis, head injuries, or prolonged asphyxia. Some affected people may survive in a debilitated state for many years, and some are kept alive by long-term artificial nutrition and hydration (ANH) via tube feeding. The BMA consultation considered treatment limitation in such people, the main issue being whether or not to withhold or withdraw ANH.

The main aims of the BMA Medical Ethics Committee, as set out in the consultation paper were to identify the main factors that clinicians currently take into account, to stimulate debate about how problematic cases should be resolved, and to seek views as to whether there are clear categories of 'problematic cases' in which a court order would be desirable.[9]

The underlying objective of the debate was '…the elaboration of clear guidelines for some practices which appear to be little discussed such as the withdrawal of nutrition and hydration from severely impaired stroke patients…*and* non-treatment decisions made for handicapped babies and young people'.[10] In raising these issues for debate the BMA Medical Ethics Committee 'would not wish to create the impression that it is facilitating or encouraging non-treatment decisions'. That however was the impression given to many people!

At one point the Ethics Committee professed to be somewhat uncertain about the current pattern of medical practice saying ' Best practice regarding some unfortunately common conditions remain uncodified…'[11]

16

What exactly do they mean by this strange word 'uncodified'? Is it to be interpreted as unlawful, unprincipled, lacking a code of conduct? All these interpretations could be valid. The judgment in the Bland case has highlighted areas of medical practice that do not stand up to legal scrutiny. The medical and legal professions are now trying to sort out the medico-legal morass and reach some kind of consensus. The Chairman of the BMA Medical Ethics Committee has now advised doctors that decisions about withdrawing nutrition and hydration from patients who are not dying should be taken "only with great care and with legal advice."[12]

There is undoubtedly a problem with regard to non-treatment decisions in patients suffering from severe strokes and profound dementia. 'In this type of case decisions... appear currently...to be made by patients' relatives and the health care team' observed the BMA. [11] Note the slight element of doubt about precisely who is responsible for clinical decision-making. This may seem surprising, but perhaps it suited the BMA to fudge this issue. Ultimately however, the Consultant has responsibility for clinical decisions in hospital practice, and the General Practitioner in the community. Sometimes but by no means always, difficult decisions are shared with relatives. In specialties such as geriatrics, psychogeriatrics and palliative care, a multidisciplinary team may be involved. Even so the senior doctor has considerable influence and carries ultimate responsibility for decisions made. When treatment-limiting decisions are made in the privacy of a patient's home, or in small community hospitals or nursing homes, decisions may be made by one doctor and no questions asked. Hence the need for safeguards such as a second specialist opinion, for the patient.

A doctor's attitude to ethical and social problems will be determined largely by personal experience and upbringing, coloured by the approach of those who influenced him/her during undergraduate or post-graduate training. Multidisciplinary case conferences are a relatively new innovation, and medical ethics has only recently been introduced into the core curriculum of budding doctors. Some doctors are still extremely isolated professionally and may have little opportunity to discover how colleagues approach complex ethical and social problems. Built into the professional psyche and medical etiquette, is reluctance to intervene in another doctor's case, except on request. So doctors may be unaware that down the road, or in another county, colleagues have a rather different approach.

The scatter gun approach

Many difficult questions on which the BMA sought views or made comments, were scattered throughout the consultation paper – some examples are listed below. In the final section of the consultation paper the questions were gathered together into eighteen short paragraphs on which the BMA invited views. Anyone who managed to struggle through the paper and submit views before the deadline deserved a medal! Much more time was needed for discussion.

Some questions posed

- Where are the main gaps in UK guidance relating to patients with PVS or near PVS?[13]
- Where does responsibility for death lie when a doctor omits any life-prolonging treatment?[13]
- Are dilemmas caused by patients having difficulty articulating their intentions or wishes regarding treatment common?[13]
- Should difficult cases be reviewed by an ethics committee?[11]
- On what grounds might a valid distinction be made between artificial nutrition and hydration and other life-prolonging treatments?[11]
- Should there be some special safeguards regarding the withholding or withdrawal of artificial hydration and nutrition, and if so, what? [11]
- Should it always be essential to seek a specialist second opinion about the likelihood of recovery…prior to considering withdrawal of nutrition? [11]
- Have health professionals developed protocols for assessing 'best interest' in complex cases?[11]
- Should the 'double effect' doctrine be replaced? [7]

Key issues

At one point in the consultation paper, on the subject of PVS, the BMA stated that 'the patient does not suffer pain as a result of withdrawal of food and fluids.'[14] This is a contentious statement and depends on the interpretation of the word pain. Patients with PVS become restless when dying of dehydration, and the restlessness may be an indication of distress due to thirst. Thirst can persist unless the hypothalamic thirst centre has been destroyed by brain damage.[15]

The BMA also stated that:

> ' Withdrawing or withholding food and fluids may also be considered for other patients following the wide publicity given to cases involving PVS. Many health professionals feel anxious about the future development of this option.'

This of course, was what the whole consultation was about! The BMA leadership must have known perfectly well that some doctors were already withholding or withdrawing ANH from severe stroke patients and people with advanced dementia. Now the time had come to justify this practice, bring it out of the shadows and push medical ethics further down the slippery slope in the wake of the Bland judgement. Underlying BMA thought, and perhaps driving the agenda were cost-saving considerations. So doctors and nurses had good cause to be anxious! Their anxiety proved to be justified.

The BMA Medical Ethics Committee quoted from an earlier BMA publication to the effect that:

' efforts to prolong life may be regarded as intrusive in circumstances where the patient's capacity to experience life and relate to others is severely impaired or non-existent.'[16]

They appreciated however that:

' medicine is not a precise science. Frequently a balance between benefit and harm cannot be confidently predicted. In each clinical circumstance, the doctor must make a careful and conscientious judgement, recognizing the elusiveness of absolute certainty regarding the consequences of the decision.'

These superficially benign statements require close scrutiny and qualification. Most would agree that where the patient's capacity to relate to others is non-existent, provided that the situation is irreversible and untreatable (as in PVS) - then efforts to prolong life may be inappropriate. However, if the patient's capacity to experience life and relate to others is 'severely impaired' rather than non-existent, the situation is rather different. One would need to know much more about the level of impairment and the patient's circumstances before giving an opinion.

'Intrusive' is not a word that enters into normal medical parlance. It can have various meanings, such as an unwelcome addition, or (in law) 'illegal entry upon or appropriation of the property of another'. We need to be quite clear about definitions if such words are to be used in a medical context.

Medicine may not be a precise science, but doctors are well placed to understand the practical problems of prolonging life in each clinical situation. In the context of ANH the main issue is whether the patient would find the means of administration of food and fluids an undue burden. Would the person be harmed by the technical procedures involved? Would they rather be dead than tube fed? As to the benefits, the judgement is whether life itself is of any benefit to the individual concerned. Balancing benefit and harm can be exceedingly difficult and subjective. Careful and conscientious clinical assessment is vital.

The BMA make too much of the elusiveness of certainty. There can be no uncertainty about the consequences of withholding ANH – the end result will be death. Whether this can be regarded as a benefit or a harm, will depend upon whose opinion is sought. Therefore the interests of patients must continue to be protected by the Courts.

The BMA state that 'Terms such as 'quality of life' are problematic because of the perjorative implication that they may convey that some lives are less valid '[17]. Nevertheless they admit that the concept underlies much of the discussion and decision-making at the end of life. They consider whether an individual's ability to interact and relate to other people is a key indicator of their quality of life. Finally, we are told that in their response to the Lord Chancellor's consultation paper *Who Decides?* the BMA expressed the view that the important factor making withdrawal of artificial hydration and nutrition ethically acceptable is 'the loss of specific and definable neurological pathways leading to permanent loss of sensitivity to external stimuli and difficulty in swallowing.' So the patient as a person is forgotten and we are back to basic pathology and practical problems!

The fundamental question

The fundamental question that the BMA and others are struggling to address is what is the underlying value of life? At what point does severe brain damage or devastating illness make life itself purposeless? Is there a point at which the medical profession and relatives can agree that meaningful life has ended and that attempts to prolong life should cease?

Many people would consider that meaningful life has ended for a person in a permanent vegetative state, assuming of course that the diagnosis is correct. Yet even when people can no longer communicate or relate to those around them, they can be valued and loved by those who care for them. Moreover, who are we to say that there is absolutely no possibility of awareness, no residual spark of humanity? Can anyone see another person's thoughts or dream their dreams? Can anyone detect the soul?

Some relatives need to continue to care for loved ones, even when the person's self-awareness has ceased. To disrupt such a relationship by insisting that all care must end, can be psychologically damaging to the relative. So each case must be addressed in a sympathetic manner. There can be no hard and fast rules.

We must not be too ready to dismiss those with dementia, for even in the later stages, they may retain, like Iris Murdoch 'some still inviolate region' of themselves.[19] Eventually however, there may come a time when they cease to drink and cannot be persuaded to do so. Most people would consider artificial hydration inappropriate at this stage and death a merciful release. Decisions in patients with severe strokes or brain damage from other cerebral insult, are much more complex, and patients need very careful skilled assessment. Those with communication problems may find the situation extremely frustrating. We must not give up on them too soon. One patient whose response was limited to blinking and jaw and eye movements, evolved a system of communication by blinking. On the night of the Bland decision he blinked "Don't you bloody put me down as well". The following June he won £50 on the Derby, just by signalling![20]

We are already on a slippery slope. Patients with PVS are now expendable, as are some with 'near PVS'. Attempts to drag patients with dementia and severe strokes into this category are already discernable. Such attempts should be resisted otherwise humanity will slide headlong into the abyss. A palliative medicine physician once voiced his fears as follows- "If ever our hospices or hospitals become places where patient's lives are terminated, I believe that prospective patients will enter them much more anxious and fearful about what their doctor is actually going to do to them. Medical care will then have started down a totally new road, which will lead very literally to destruction." [21]

It is not too late to turn back, but sadly there are subversive forces at work in society that condone euthanasia by omission and seek to bring about a change in the law to permit active euthanasia.[22] In 1996 a geriatrician Dr C.A Crowther[23], responding to a particularly blatant example of this in the British Medical Journal[24], drew attention to Pope John Paul II's letter Evangelium Vitae, which upholds the value of human life, and exposes the prevailing 'culture of death' in which we are immersed [25]. Robert Balfour, a Consultant Obstetrician [26] also responded. He quoted Dr Everett Koop, a former Surgeon General in the USA who predicted a euthanasia programme for various categories of citizens and pleaded "Let it never be said by historians…that there was no outcry from the medical profession." [27]

The guidelines that emerged following the BMA consultation caused alarm and consternation in some quarters. Attempts were made in Parliament to protect patients, but the legislation proposed lacked the necessary support. Physician-assisted suicide is now on the agenda. Patients are in serious danger.

References

1. Patrick D.L, Beresford S.A.A, Ehreth J. et al. Interpreting excess mortality in a prevention trial for older adults. *International Journal of Epidemiology* 1995;**24:No.3** (Suppl.1), p.S27-S33.
2. Anon. Quoted by Goldsmith M. Dementia, a challenge to Christian Theology and Pastoral Care. Page 111-135 in 'Spirituality and Ageing.' *Jessica Kingsley* 1999.
3. Goldsmith M. Hearing the voice of people with dementia. *Jessica Kingsley* 1996.
4. Lennard Jones J.E. Ethical and Legal Aspects of Clinical Hydration and Nutritional Support. A report for the *British Association for Parenteral and Enteral Nutrition*. 1999.
5. Withdrawing and Withholding Treatment: A Consultation Paper from the BMA Medical Ethics Committee. *BMA* London July 1998.
6. Craig G.M. On withholding artificial hydration and nutrition from terminally ill sedated patients. The debate continues. *Journal of Medical Ethics* 1996;**22**: 147-153.
7. As reference 5 above, paragraph 2.7.
8. The Lord Chancellor's Green Paper 'Who Decides'? Making decisions on behalf of mentally incapacitated adults. *HMSO*, London, December 1997.
9. As reference 5 above, paragraph 1.3.
10. Ibid at paragraph 2.4.
11. Ibid at paragraph 2.2.
12. Wilks M. quoted by Horsnell M. in 'Police investigate more backdoor euthanasia'. *The Times* January 28th 1999, p.8, col.5.
13. As reference 5 above at paragraph 2.1.
14. Ibid at paragraph 2.3.
15. McCullagh P. Thirst in relation to withdrawal of hydration. *Catholic Medical Quarterly* 1996; **XL VI**: p. 5-12.
16. Medical Ethics Today: Its Practice and Philosophy. *BMA* 1993;p.165. Quoted in reference 5 above at paragraph 2.93.
17. As reference 5 above at paragraph 2.9.7.
18. BMA response to the Lord Chancellor's Green Paper 'Who Decides? Making decisions on behalf of Mentally Incapacitated Adults'. *HMSO* London, 1998.
19. Bayley J. "I was alone with Iris when she died- her death was so peaceful". *The Daily Telegraph*. March 1st, 1999; p.14-15.

20. Dulake M. The Persistent Vegetative State. In 'A Time to Die' 1997. *C.B.P.P* 53 Romney Street, London SW1P 3RF.
21. Smith A. in 'Death without Dignity.' Ed.Cameron N. © *Rutherford House*, Edinburgh 1990.
22. Craig G.M. Paradise Lost: the devolution of medical practice. Guest Editorial, *Ethics and Medicine* 2000;Vol **16:1**: 1-3.
23. Crowther C.A. Letter to *British Medical Journal* 1996;**313**:227.
24. Roberts J., Kjeilstrand C., 'Jack Kevorkian: A Medical Hero' *British Medical Journal* 1996; **312**:1434.
25. Pope John Paul 11. 'Evangelium Vitae.' London. *Catholic Truth Society*, 1995.
26. Balfour R. Letter to *British Medical Journal* 1996; **313**:228.
27. Schneffer P.A., Everett Koop C. 'Whatever happened to the human race?' *Marshall Morgan and Scott*, London 1980.

Further reading

Habgood J. "Being a Person". *Hodder and Stoughton,* London, 1998.

Chapter 3

The Times Takes Up The Debate

The front page headline in *The Times* of January 6th 1999 read: Police check hospitals over "backdoor euthanasia". Journalist Michael Horsnell drew the issue of sedation without hydration to the attention of the public in the context of a disturbing number of deaths of elderly patients in general hospitals and psychogeriatric hospitals in the UK. His article ran as follows:

Police check hospitals for "backdoor euthanasia"
by Michael Horsnell.

The deaths of at least 50 hospital patients around Britain are being investigated by police and health officials amid allegations of a creeping tide of backdoor euthanasia.

Seven separate inquiries are looking into claims that doctors have withheld intravenous drips from dehydrated patients, often while they were under sedation, and left them to die of thirst. The patients involved were suffering from strokes, asthma, other common medical conditions and dementia. At least five hospitals in Derby, Surrey, Kent and Sussex- are at the centre of police inquiries as a result of relative's complaints or nurse' whistle-blowing, while others have been referred to the General Medical Council and health authorities.

The Crown Prosecution Service will soon decide whether to prosecute in two important cases in which doctors have been accused of manslaughter due to criminal negligence. In the most serious of these police are investigating 40 deaths at the Kingsway Hospital in Derby, where nurses complained that dementia sufferers on a psycho-geriatric ward were starved and dehydrated until they became so weak that they died of infections.

The inquiry was launched in November 1997 after junior nurses complained, and papers relating to patients at the hospital between 1993 and 1997 are expected to be sent to the CPS in the spring.

In general, the practice of denying nutrition and fluids to patients believed to be entering the final phase of a terminal illness is defended as "helping nature to take its course." But some doctors condemn it as involuntary euthanasia.

The cases of patients in a persistent vegetative state (PVS), such as the Hillsborough disaster victim Tony Bland, must be referred to the courts. But a grey ethical area allows doctors to "exercise their clinical judgement" in other cases.

Sources in the medical profession suggest that some may be using their discretion to keep patients quiet and acquiescent on the wards. Some who have had a momentary choking fit, for example, have then been put on a nil-by-mouth regime and left to dehydrate.

Dr Gillian Craig, a retired consultant geriatrician from Northampton, has told the Royal College of Physicians that water and food are basic human needs that should not be regarded as treatment that a doctor may give or withhold. "Sadly there are times when sedation without hydration seems tantamount to euthanasia.

"This strengthens the hand of those who are pressing to legalise physician-assisted-suicide. Good palliative medicine is a major defence against euthanasia, but please heed my warning. Sedation without hydration has enormous potential for misuse. I would like to see this regime consigned to the dustbin of history.

"Attention to hydration is not merely an option, it should be a basic part of good medicine."

Another case being considered by the CPS concerns the death of an 81-year old woman who was admitted to hospital in Surrey in May 1997 for treatment of constipation and a urinary infection. Her health was otherwise good. She was denied intravenous fluids despite the pleading of relatives.

At one stage a hospital crash team, called at her daughter's insistence by a doctor previously unconnected with the case, carried out emergency measures that required cutting into her neck and groin arteries to insert fluid lines. But septicaemia and multi-organ failure had set in. Her daughter said: "This was not a dying patient when she was admitted. In fact she was a relatively healthy lady, full of fun, with a relatively common problem. Six days later she was on her deathbed as a direct result of dehydration. I had literally begged them with my hands pressed together in supplication to rehydrate her."

The issue of withholding or withdrawing treatment has been taken up by the British Medical Association in a huge consultation exercise and the association's medical ethics committee hopes to produce practical guidelines when it is complete.

The consultation paper, Withdrawing and Withholding Treatment, asks whether food and drink might be withdrawn from patients such as severely impaired stroke victims as well as those in a persistent vegetative state.

But Dr Craig said: "This is already happening with no regulation whatsoever. Moreover, the BMA are clearly aware of this...."

Some doctors are concerned about the distress dehydration can cause even in PVS patients. Dr Anthony Cole, a consultant paediatrician at Worcester Royal Infirmary and chairman of a Roman Catholic ethics committee said: "There is some evidence that, if the base of the brain is intact, patients will experience thirst even if the higher functions have been lost. Death from dehydration is painful and unacceptable."

Copyright Times Newspapers Ltd. Jan.6th 1999.

The Times medical correspondent Dr Stuttaford drew attention to differing attitudes to euthanasia between older and younger doctors saying:

Shifting views on euthanasia
by Dr Thomas Stuttaford

Forty years ago, when I was a junior house doctor, the ethics that determined our care of the elderly and the terminally ill were well understood. We didn't need a High Court decision, welcome as the recent one (that of Annie Lindsell) has been to allow us to use adequate doses of analgesia to control pain, albeit that the side effects might shorten the patient's life. However, even if we didn't strive officiously to keep patients alive by overtreating those whose lives had become a misery, we did nothing to shorten life deliberately when the only objective was the early death of the patient. Older doctors are shocked at the idea of deliberately dehydrating patients.

All doctors realise that there are patients who are unlikely to make a good recovery but are likely to survive. A problem is that, whereas to a young doctor the quality of life of these patients may seem so low as to be not worth keeping, most of the patients are very grateful for what life they have. Research has shown that the criteria considered to warrant euthanasia by people who believe in it when they are young and active become much more stringent once the person questioned is older and nearer death.

If fluids are withdrawn death is inevitable from dehydration within days. If the patient is conscious the only way of saving them the discomfort, pain and restlessness that would precede their death is to tranquillise them, even if the sedatives prescribed will further hasten their end. If the same sedatives were given as one massive dose nobody would have any doubts that this was euthanasia; and even if they were given in smaller doses over a period of time, the end result is the same.

It is ironical that before a life-support machine can be turned off in the case of someone who, for instance has suffered an irremediable head injury, the procedures that have to be fulfilled are exhaustive, and the decision is taken at the highest level.

If, on the other hand, fluids are withheld so that the patient will surely die, this may be at the behest of junior staff.

Relative Trust
Leading article The Times January 6th 1999

Doctors today need to be as expert in medical ethics as anatomy. Fine judgements about the balance between relieving pain and preserving life are among the most difficult they have to face. Confronted with an elderly man who writhes in agony, a doctor may well find it necessary to sedate him. Some doctors, however, are accused today of seeing sedation as more than just a temporary relief from pain.

Patients' children have noticed that their parents have suffered from dehydration after sedation, and then died from an infection. The cry has been raised that doctors are allowing "backdoor euthanasia". Physicians argue that they have simply been trying to relieve suffering. As we report, there is a disturbing trend of these cases in Britain's hospitals. A thorough investigation of these deaths and clear guidance for doctors on the use of sedatives is essential if the medical profession is to avoid accusations of allowing doctors to play God with their patients.

While doctors treating patients in a persistent vegetative state must refer their case to the courts before switching off any life support system or denying them food or water, doctors whose patients have common illnesses are left to "exercise their clinical judgement". Some, it seems, sedate their patients and deprive them of food and water – allegedly without the patient's authorisation or that of his or her family. If a patient dies, the death certificate will state that the cause of death was the underlying medical condition, not dehydration. This lack of regulation and transparency must be addressed.

The British Medical Association is currently consulting its members on the guidelines surrounding this practice. It should recommend greater clarity on the way doctors make decisions about a patient's treatment, and how they communicate their decision to the patient or his family. If doctors are expected to refer a case of a patient in a persistent vegetative state to the courts, why should they not be expected to do the same for other patients?

Yet this debate must not obscure the more crucial question. Why were the doctors sedating their patients? There appear to be a multitude of reasons depending on the specific circumstances. Whatever the case, the BMA should decide whether it is ethically right to help nature take its course.

Copyright Times Newspapers Ltd. Jan.6th 1999.

The Times coverage of January 1999 included a cartoon by Peter Brookes, showing an aged and terrified Britannia lying in a hospital bed, while two politicians – the French president Jacques Chirac and the German Chancellor Gerhard Schroder – in the guise of doctors, offered her a "Euro" to do her a power of good. The politicians' actions were not entirely altruistic – they had their reasons for removing the patient from the scene. The cartoon was prescient for it encapsulated the concept of geronticide for political and economic gain.

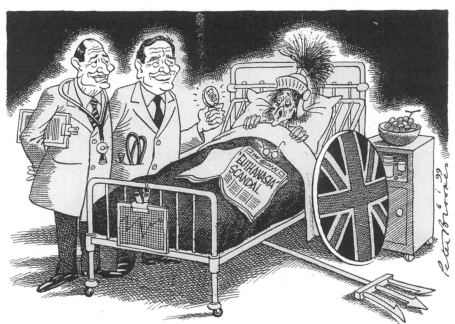

"TAKE THIS... IT'LL DO YOU A POWER OF GOOD..."

Sedation without hydration as depicted by Peter Brookes.
Reproduced with permission.
Copyright Times Newspapers Limited. January 6th 1999.

* * *

Further articles appeared in *The Times* as more allegations of "backdoor euthanasia" emerged. Within weeks Dr Michael Wilks, chairman of the medical ethics committee of the British Medical Association, admitted to journalist Michael Horsnell that some doctors may be acting outside the law. Writing in *The Times* of January 28th 1999, Michael Horsnell quoted Dr Wilks as saying:

> "There may be cases where best interest judgements and full clinical assessments have not been adequate." Dr Wilks advised doctors that decisions about withdrawing nutrition or hydration from patients who are not dying should be taken "only with great care and with legal advice…It appears to us that the law is so unclear that doctors would be well advised to have recourse to the courts before they withdraw hydration. I am speaking of patients with, say Alzheimer's or those who have serious strokes. We feel doctors withholding hydration are outside the law even though their intentions were no doubt made in the best interest of the patient as they saw it."

All copyright material is reprinted with permission from Times Newspapers Limited and the journalists concerned.

Update and Progress Reports

The situation as seen by Dr Craig in December 2005.

On sedation without hydration

Thoughts on the ethical use of sedation, artificial hydration and nutrition in the terminally ill and dying have clarified over the years as a result of debate within the medical profession. The story of that debate is documented in "No Water-No Life: Hydration in the Dying." [1] That book shows how exceedingly difficult it has been to convince palliative carers that attention to hydration is a basic part of good medicine. This is especially worrying because palliative carers in the UK are expanding their activities in the community through the NHS End-of-Life Programme. One can only hope that they will work closely with colleagues experienced in other disciplines, especially geriatric medicine, so that patients are given the best possible care.

Thanks to articles in *The Times* and other national newspapers the dangers of sedation without hydration are now more widely recognised by the British public. Relatives are learning to ask awkward questions, and doctors are learning to listen and explain. In the USA doctors now advise that palliative sedation must be explained to the patient or surrogate, to the family, and to the health care team. [2]

Professional guidance on the use of palliative sedation was published in the *Journal of the American Medical Association* in October 2005. The American authors Dr Lo and Dr Rubenfeld were careful to distinguish between palliative sedation, correctly used, and euthanasia. They argue that palliative sedation may be justified as a last resort in the following circumstances: 1) For dying patients if intolerable symptoms cannot be relieved in any other way. 2) The intention must be "to relieve symptoms, not shorten life, otherwise the physician's action cannot be logically distinguished from euthanasia, which is illegal in the United States and highly controversial ethically." 3) The patient should be moribund, i.e. "at the point of death, in a dying state or close to death" so that survival is unlikely to be significantly shortened. [2]

In the USA doctors also use sedation to suppress symptoms of hunger and thirst in patients, such as serious stroke cases, or patients in PVS, who have had life-prolonging artificial hydration and nutrition (ANH) withheld or withdrawn.

In the Netherlands where euthanasia is permitted, the Dutch Attorney General has called for the legal controls on euthanasia to be extended to "terminal sedation" as well, but the Dutch Medical Association would prefer to rely on guidelines. [3] In one survey an estimated 10% of all deaths in the Netherlands in the year 2001 were preceded by sedation without ANH, often with the explicit intention of hastening death. [4] Thus terminal sedation remains a danger zone in medical ethics.

Outcome of investigations into deaths at Kingsway Hospital

As noted in *The Times* of January 6th 1999, the police investigated 40 deaths on a pyschogeriatric ward at Kingsway Hospital Derby. Following their investigation the police passed the files over to Crown Prosecution Service (CPS). The CPS concluded that no charges should be brought and the cases were passed to Mr Peter Ashworth, the Coroner for Derby and South Derbyshire.

Mr Ashworth sent the records of 23 patients to the clinical director of elderly people's services in an NHS Trust in Bedfordshire for her opinion. According to an article in *The Sunday Times* of February 8th 2004, the clinical director concluded that 11 of the deaths "may have been speeded up." Mr Ashworth realised that an inquest might raise issues that were not within his jurisdiction to consider, so, since he considered the matter so serious he wrote to the Department of Health to ask that the inquest be superseded by a judicial inquiry to investigate practices at the hospital. The Department offered to hold a confidential inquiry after the inquest, but relatives and the coroner wanted a full public inquiry.[5]

Inquests were eventually held in January 2005, responsibility being delegated to the Deputy Coroner a retired High Court Judge, Sir Richard Rougier. In his introductory comments on January 18th 2005 Sir Richard Rougier took the view that whatever the reasons behind the decision to withdraw food, the underlying illnesses played "an inexorable progress" in the patients' deaths.[6] Having heard all the evidence Sir Richard Rougier concluded that the deaths were due to natural causes.[7]

Solicitors acting for seven of the families issued a statement that mentioned that the Deputy Coroner had raised concerns about practices on Rowsley ward and the way in which the ward was run. The solicitors said: "…It is important that these concerns are now addressed by the Strategic Health Authority and the Department of Health, so that other families do not have to go through the anxiety that these families have been through." [6] No information is available on the nature of the concerns raised. The ward has now been closed, and Kingsway Hospital is scheduled for closure.

References

1. "No Water-No Life: Hydration in the Dying." Ed Craig GM. 2005. *Fairway Folio*. ISBN 0 9545445 3 6.
2. Lo B, Rubenfeld G. Palliative sedation in dying patients. "We turn to it when everything else hasn't worked." *Journal of the American Medical Association*. Oct. 12th 2005; Vol. 294 No.12: 1810-1815. "Copyrighted 2005, American Medical Association. All Rights Reserved." Quoted with permission.
3. Sheldon T. Dutch doctors choose sedation rather than euthanasia. *British Medical Journal* online. August 14th 2004, p329-368.
4. Rietjens J, van der Heide A, Vragging AM et al. Physician reports of terminal sedation without hydration or nutrition for patients nearing death in the Netherlands. *Annals of Internal Medicine* 2004, **141**: 3; 178-186.
5. Rogers L. Coroner seeks inquiry into 'mass euthanasia' at hospital. *The Sunday Times*, February 8th 2004.
6. Britten N. *The Daily Telegraph*, January 19th 2005, page 9.
7. Elderly patients died of natural causes. http://alexanderharris.co.uk. © Alexander Harris 2005.

Chapter 4

BMA Guidelines For Decision Making:
A Critical Appraisal

Author Gillian Craig

The British Medical Association (BMA) guidelines on "Withholding and Withdrawing Life-prolonging Medical Treatment"[1] were published on June 23rd. 1999, in advance of the annual representatives meeting in July, and so without the general approval of BMA members.

The guidelines state that an important factor in making treatment-limiting decisions is whether the person is thought to be aware of his or her environment or own existence by, for example:-

1. being able to interact with others.
2. being aware of his or her own existence and having an ability to take pleasure in the fact of that existence.
3. having the ability to achieve some purposeful or self-directed action, or achieve some goal of importance to him or herself.

If any one of these abilities can be achieved, say the BMA, then life-prolonging treatment may be a benefit. If none can be achieved, then 'treatment' is unlikely to be a benefit and may be discontinued, according to the BMA.

The initial response from the public and the press was unfavourable. Journalists arriving at the press conference found a figure of death 'the grim reaper' standing outside BMA House, as aggrieved relatives made their point. The *Daily Telegraph* published an editorial 'Doctors as Killers'[2]. In *The Times* the science editor noted that "by choosing self-awareness as one of the signs that a patient is alive and deserves treatment, the BMA has plunged into one of the oldest philosophical disputes of all"[3]. Many people were deeply offended by the suggestion that doctors should deny life-prolonging treatment and withhold food and water from people who lack self-awareness.

Dr Anthony Daniels wrote a scathing article in the *Sunday Telegraph* saying:

"Life unworthy of life: it was with precisely this phrase that the Nazis justified the slaughter of the mentally ill and the handicapped... The terminally unconscious patient is not just a tissue culture on a much larger scale, and cannot be treated as such by anyone of minimal sensibility. The fact is, we can only behave well towards each other if we reverence human life and treat it as if it were sacred, whether or not we have any religious beliefs . . .. To treat such a patient without due respect offends us in the same way as the desecration of a grave offends us. It is an offence against the value and significance of human life."[4]

However Dr Daniels conceded that "perhaps" the refusal of food and fluid to a patient "may not always" represent an outrage to human dignity.

Ann Leslie of the *Daily Mail* found the assumptions in the BMA report

"astounding, appalling and deeply disturbing. Under the guise of being compassionate, sensible, and in line with occasional current - but often unadmitted – practice, the report seeks to clarify the ethical issues facing doctors today. It is seductive, appealing stuff, but deeply dangerous".[5]

Professor Raanon Gillon, a highly respected medical ethicist represented the BMA at the press conference. He was reported by journalists to have said that "staying alive is no good unless it means a flourishing life". The choice of the word 'flourishing' was unfortunate.

"But what exactly is a flourishing life?" asked Dr Daniels – "and who is to judge?" He added, "It seems that we are, for if the report's recommendations were implemented, doctors would be enjoined on their own authority to overrule, wherever necessary, the relatives who wish to keep such patients alive." [4]

Ask any geriatrician whether their patients are flourishing and the answer will almost certainly be negative. Our patients are more often at the withering and fading stage of life – but that does not mean to say that they are not valued human beings, with a right to be alive, and a desire to live.

The doctors' dilemma is to make correct and compassionate decisions about those cases where withholding life-prolonging treatment may truly seem to be in the patient's best interests. This might indeed include some desperately disabled stroke patients, and people in the terminal stages of dementia, or Creutzfelt-Jacob disease for example. Life in such people may hold no pleasure, and their self-awareness may be reduced. This does not however, give doctors the right to kill them.

The BMA criteria for self-awareness are problematical

The media outcry was fully justified for the BMA criteria for self-awareness are open to serious criticism. For example a person's level of interaction may be heavily dependent on the communication skills of others, and sometimes on the level of technological support available. Stephen Hawking, the brilliant mathematician, is totally dependent on a computer for verbal communication. Some patients can only communicate by blinking, or by some other limited movement. One severely disabled child was taught to choose music by hitting a knob with his forehead. One particular song gave him enormous pleasure and he 'asked for it' time and time again. This was his only form of communication and interaction with the outside world.[6]

It may be extremely difficult for an observer to know whether a severely disabled person is aware of his own existence, or whether his/her thoughts are pleasant. A fleeting smile may be the only indication of inner happiness. Achieving goals may be unrealistic for many disabled people who are entirely dependent on others. Milton, in his blindness came to recognize that "They also serve who only stand and wait". Disability and old age force many people to exist and endure - and to be alive, rather than to achieve goals in life. It is enough *to be* alive.

Treatment-limiting decisions

Part 3C of the BMA guidance of June 1999 refers to treatment-limiting decisions for children or adults who lack the ability to make decisions or communicate. The BMA stress that decisions should be based on the best available clinical evidence, and should take account of relevant guidelines. Some of these are referred to in the notes, but important guidelines on the ethical use of artificial hydration in patients who are terminally ill, issued by the National Council for Hospice and Specialist Palliative Care Services in July 1997 are not mentioned in the BMA guidance.

Paragraph 17.3 of the BMA guidance states that:
> "where treatment is unable to achieve its intended clinical goal, or the patient's imminent death is inevitable, active treatment may provide no benefit and may be withheld or withdrawn".

Comment. This statement is contentious. Attention to hydration *may* provide benefit even when death is imminent.

Paragraph 17.4 states:
> "Except where the patient's imminent death is inevitable, a decision to withhold or withdraw all treatment is likely to be inappropriate and potentially unlawful..."

Comment. The BMA were clearly aware that the guidance they issued was legally dubious, so why did they issue it? They must have known that they had supporters in the Department of Health. "Forget the law" is the message conveyed to doctors, "Carry on regardless until someone stops you, but cover yourselves by taking additional procedural safeguards when withholding artificial hydration and nutrition (ANH) in case you are challenged. And of course take legal advice!"

Wise doctors will consult their medical defence advisors. Dissenting relatives should also seek legal advice if time permits. If the patient is mentally incapacitated and has not made a valid advance directive the Official Solicitor should be consulted before any irrevocable decisions are taken. When the Mental Capacity Act reaches the statute books, proxy health care decision makers will enter the equation. For the time being the legal situation remains unclear.

Paragraph 17.7 states "Where there is reasonable doubt about its potential for benefit, treatment should be provided for a trial period with a subsequent prearranged review . . . etc."

Paragraph 17.8 stresses the need for time, care, resources, and a multidisciplinary team approach to assess the patient's condition, "including, where appropriate, the patients potential for self-awareness..."

Paragraph 17.10 states "The benefits, risks and burdens of the treatment in the particular case should be assessed."

Paragraph 19.1 makes it clear that the 'overriding purpose or objective' should be to ensure that treatment which is not in the patient's best interests, is avoided.

Ethical factors to be taken into account

See section 18 of the guidelines. Decisions should be made on the basis of what is right and in the 'best interest' for each individual patient. The BMA list the type of factors that should be taken into consideration. These include the patient's level of self-awareness, the likelihood of severe or unmanageable pain or suffering, the likelihood of improvement if treatment is provided, the invasiveness of treatment and the effectiveness of treatment. The BMA stress the importance of involving the whole health care team, and people close to the patient when the patient is not able to take part in discussions.

Comment. The whole question of benefit and best interest needs much wider public and professional debate. To withhold treatment solely with the intention of shortening life is unlawful in the UK.

On consulting relatives and others close to the patient

Paragraph 18.3 contains a lot of valuable information and insight. However, the BMA make it absolutely clear that the final decision rests with the clinician in charge of the patient's case.

Comment. This view was not well received by the media . . . "withdrawing food from those who would otherwise survive, requires examination on a case by case basis - and not by doctors alone" said *The Daily Telegraph* [2]. The situation will change under the terms of Mental Capacity Act for advance directives are to become legally binding and proxy health care decision makers may be involved.

Para 18.4 refers to the possibility of serious conflict within the health care team, or between the health care team and those close to the patient. It is suggested that attempts should be made to resolve this through discussion, informal conflict resolution mechanisms or by obtaining a further independent opinion. In rare cases a legal review will be needed.

Comment. Cases reported in this book demonstrate how far short of ideal, are the present arrangements for conflict resolution in the UK. The BMA report will do nothing to improve this situation.

Withholding artificial nutrition and hydration (ANH)

The BMA case relies heavily on the view that ANH can be classified as medical treatment. They concede however "that many people perceive there to be an important distinction between this and other treatments". They overlook the fact, discussed earlier in this book, that some people do not regard ANH as medical treatment at all, but see it as a basic human need. If this argument is accepted it is not in a doctor's remit to withhold ANH unless the means of administration is in itself too great a burden for the patient. Bearing in mind people's differing perceptions of ANH, and the legal uncertainty, the BMA recommend additional procedural safeguards that should be followed before ANH is withheld or withdrawn from patients whose death is not imminent and whose wishes are not known. They stress that particular care should be taken when making decisions to withhold ANH from patients who have suffered severe strokes, or have severe dementia.

Additional procedural safeguards

These are set out in Part 3D, paragraph 22. In essence they specify that

> • *All such proposals should be subject to a formal clinical review by a senior clinician who is not part of the treating team.*

Comment. For common conditions where the patient is in a nursing home, the BMA suggest that the 'senior clinician' could be a general practitioner. In saying this, the BMA lost a good opportunity to increase the level of expertise available to the frail elderly in the community. Moreover, as a *Daily Mail* journalist noted, the 'senior clinician' could be drawn from the ranks of those who favour euthanasia [5]. There is concern that it will be only a matter of time before ANH is withdrawn 'on demand' as happened with abortion. As *The Daily Telegraph* editorial noted: "once adopted by the medical profession, procedures too often become commonplace" [2]. This prediction seems to be supported by the fact that the General Medical Council in their guidance of August 2002 suggest that the 'senior clinician' could be a nurse.

> • *Legal advice should continue to be sought in England, Wales and Northern Ireland if the patient is in PVS, or a state closely resembling PVS.*
> • *All cases where ANH is withheld or withdrawn should be reviewed at a local level (after the event), to ensure that procedures and guidelines were followed.*
> • *Anonymised information should be available to the Secretary of State on request and, where applicable, to the "Commission for Health Improvement".*

The Commission for Health Improvement.

The BMA suggested that this untried Commission, with a name that sounds like a figment of George Orwell's imagination, should take over responsibility for monitoring "patterns of ethical decision making" in these controversial areas. How macabre that *deaths* due to the withdrawal of hydration and nutrition should be monitored by a Commission for *Health* Improvement! Who are these people I asked myself? Where are they? To whom do they report? Are their conclusions to be published and if so where? Will there be an inquiry into deaths following terminal sedation?

It transpired that the Commission for Health Improvement (CHI or CHIMP) did not exist when the guidelines were published. It came into being in April 2000. Way back in 1997, the British Government proposed to create this new statutory body, "to provide independent scrutiny of local efforts to improve quality and to help to address serious problems . . ." in the NHS [7]. Basically it was intended that CHI would inspect local clinical governance arrangements [8].

The plan was that CHI would investigate as follows:

> "Where local action is not able to resolve serious or persistent problems, the Commission will be able to intervene on the direction of the Secretary of State, or by invitation from Primary Care Groups (i.e. GPs), Health Authorities and NHS Trusts . . . The Commission will have a membership drawn from the professions, NHS, academic and patient representatives . . . The Commission will not replace mainstream NHS performance assessment and management, but will complement and reinforce these processes . . . The Commission's findings will be reported to the Trust concerned, and shared with the appropriate Health Authority or NHS Executive Regional Office. A summary will be made public . . ." [7]

Thus the Commission had a wide remit to 'spot check' anything from the handling of complaints to the treatment of coronary heart disease. It could also undertake an agreed programme of systematic service reviews. There was inevitably concern that the Commission would become yet another ineffective cog in the bureaucratic machine. Any plans that were made for a national monitoring system were overtaken by devolution in Scotland and Wales. CHI had no specific remit to monitor deaths due to withdrawal of artificial hydration at a national level, and no other body was given this role.

CHI ceased to exist in 2003. A new body the *'Commission for Healthcare Audit and Inspection'* was formed by the Health and Social Care (Community Health and Standards) Act 2003 and came into being on April 1st 2004. It is generally known as *The Healthcare Commission*. This Commission has many duties in England, including the consideration of unresolved complaints about NHS, and investigation of serious failures in the provision of healthcare.

Critical incident reporting systems. Government documents on clinical governance specifically mention the need for critical incident reporting systems.[9] I would say that a death due to withdrawal of hydration and nutrition is, at the very least, a critical incident. Dehydration should be recorded on the death certificate as a factor contributing to death. There should be a statutory obligation for doctors to report all such deaths to the Coroner. Unless this is done, there is a grave danger that such deaths will go undetected, which is perhaps the intention.

The need for a confidential inquiry into the use of parenteral sedation without hydration in terminal care has not been taken up by the BMA or the Department of Health. Eyes have they, and they see not!

Legal aspects

The guidance given by the BMA goes far beyond the limits of what is currently accepted in law in the UK. In England, Wales and Northern Ireland all requests to withdraw artificial hydration and nutrition from patients in a permanent vegetative state have to be subject to judicial approval. The same should apply to all patients who are mentally incompetent, or lacking in self-awareness, or aware but unable for any reason to make their views known. The BMA guidance throws out a clear challenge to the legal profession and Parliament. It is in effect inciting doctors to exploit the law, as laid down at the time of the Bland case, and to extend the judgement to many categories of patient who do not have PVS. This comes as no surprise, since it is only relatively recently that medical practice in this grey area has been called into question. The Bland case judgement set a dangerous precedent that has weakened English criminal law, leaving it open to attack.

There is concern that the BMA has been unduly influenced by people who are trying to campaign for euthanasia and physician-assisted suicide. The danger, of course, is that some unscrupulous doctors and managers who wish to clear their beds of troublesome elderly bed-blockers, will welcome the guidance. General practitioners supervising medical care in nursing homes could also find themselves under pressure from relatives, who do not wish to see their inheritance dissipated by nursing home fees. There must be rigorous safeguards to protect our most vulnerable patients from such people. I am not convinced that a second opinion from a supposedly senior clinician, will suffice.

The medical profession may gain the impression that those who follow the BMA guidelines will be protected, if challenged in a court. This may not be the case, for the guidance does not represent a consensus view even within the profession, and it has not received public support. The guidance does however have the support of the Department of Health. In recent years two serious attempts to protect patients by parliamentary means have failed. I refer to the Medical Treatment (Prevention of Euthanasia) Bill of 1999/2000 and the Patient Protection Bill of 2003.

Several English Members of Parliament noted the BMA report with concern, and called on the Secretary of State to circulate all hospitals and health-care workers to emphasise that the guidelines do not represent legal guidelines, and should not be adopted.[10] In Scotland, the newly devolved Government chose not to legislate on these issues because there was no public consensus.

Public disapproval

I have already referred to the unfavourable media response to the guidelines. Important religious leaders in the UK also expressed regret and concern.

The Chief Rabbi, Professor Jonathan Sachs, urged medical experts and religious leaders of all persuasions to call for the recognition of the sanctity of life. He also appealed to politicians, regardless of political affiliation, to exert their influence to curb a disturbing trend towards the legalisation of euthanasia.[11]

Rabbi Rapoport, a member of the Chief Rabbi's Cabinet commented:

"If the BMA's recommendation were to be implemented, it would endow the doctor with a position beyond his or her remit, that of supreme moral arbiter. It would also undermine the role of the patient's close family in such crucial decisions. The most disturbing facet of these suggestions is that they represent a shift from a value system in which human life is considered sacrosanct, to one in which its value is relative and subjective . . . we believe that life is sacred. It is a gift of God and may only be taken by Him. The withdrawal of food and water from patients, for whatever motive, is at odds with this value, so long central to Western civilisation. It is wrong in itself, and a disturbing erosion of a fundamental moral and religious principle."

When questioned about the quality of human life without the capacity to engage in anything meaningful, and the burden to family, medical institutions and society, Rabbi Rapoport added:

"There is only one meaning to 'death with dignity' and that is death after a dignified life, surrounded by caring people. Unfortunately, severe deterioration of the human faculties is often part of the challenge of old age . . .. Ultimately, the test of our humanity is our ability to face our fate and that of those close to us with courage, humility and dedication; not to hasten death because dying has become burdensome. It is the duty of religious leaders and physicians to preserve this conviction in the conscience of humanity."[11]

His Grace the late Cardinal Thomas Winning, Roman Catholic Archbishop of Glasgow, and President of the Bishops' Conference of Scotland, said:

"The new BMA guidelines are both sinister and worrying. They will cause very sincere anxiety among thousands of patients and their families. There can be no justification for starving and dehydrating people to death. That this should happen in NHS hospitals with the full approval of the BMA is almost beyond belief. In essence these guidelines give doctors the power of life and death over stroke victims, accident victims, the elderly and those with Alzheimer's disease. I would urge all people of good will, whatever their religious or philosophical background, to seriously consider the implications of these guidelines. If they are allowed to develop without challenge, then every one of us will be the losers."[12]

The Muslim Council of Britain, Medical and Health Committee that covers all major Islamic medical associations in Britain expressed strong disapproval of the guidelines. A spokesman said:

"The withholding of food and fluids from patients with the object and intention of bringing life to an end is morally unacceptable. In Islamic teaching the power to give and take life rests entirely with Almighty God, and the doctor's role is purely to sustain life and let it run its own course, whilst doing everything to remove pain and suffering."

The Medical Ethics Alliance. A coalition of concerned doctors alarmed by the BMA guidance formed the Medical Ethics Alliance (MEA). The MEA includes the Guild of Catholic Doctors, the Muslim Council of Britain medical and health committee, and three non-religious pro-life medical groups. Nurses are also welcome to join. The MEA therefore represents several thousand health care professionals who argue that food and fluids should not be withheld from terminally ill patients, except when it is 'inappropriate' or 'burdensome' to the patient.[13] The BMA used a procedural device to avoid a vote on a motion to this effect at their annual representatives' meeting in July 1999. The MEA later issued their own guidance that is reprinted in Chapter 6 of this book.

Wider aspects of the BMA guidance

Public attention following publication of the guidelines focused mainly on withdrawal of artificial hydration and nutrition. However, the guidelines cover much more than this. They cover for example cessation of chemotherapy in some children. In fact, the guidance in general is intended to cover the withdrawal of any form of life-prolonging treatment. This was not made absolutely clear. The BMA tend to refer to the withdrawal/withholding of 'active treatment (including artificial hydration and nutrition)', without being more specific. Ventilatory support is mentioned at one point, insulin at another, antibiotics somewhere else. Cardiopulmonary resuscitation, chemotherapy and dialysis all receive passing mention only. Yet the range of ethical problems created by limitation of any one of these life-prolonging treatments will be enormous. The BMA made no attempt to address these problems in any depth.

The information in Part 3C relates to decisions to withhold or withdraw any form of life-prolonging treatment, including artificial hydration and nutrition. The additional procedural safeguards recommended in Part 3D relate to withholding or withdrawing artificial hydration and nutrition only. The BMA considered the issues in broad and general terms only. They wisely stressed that evaluation must be undertaken on a case-to-case basis. No hard and fast rules can be made to guide doctors through the medical and moral minefields.

We do of course, have to draw a line somewhere in these difficult matters, especially where the use of artificial hydration and nutrition are concerned. To go to extreme lengths to provide ANH, even when the means of administration is clearly burdensome to the patient, would be wrong. The result could be wards full of tube-fed, distressed and demented or unconscious patients - a truly nightmare scenario. In their efforts to avoid such a scenario, the BMA and their advisers have taken treatment attenuation to dangerous extremes. Withholding and withdrawing treatment may merge, all too easily into medical negligence that results in death. These guidelines put at risk the lives of countless people whose lives may depend on artificial hydration and nutrition. Society must ensure that all vulnerable people are protected and treated appropriately.

Professor John Keown, a lawyer well known for his work in the field of euthanasia considers that the BMA guidelines should be withdrawn.[14]

The euthanasia question.

The BMA have tried very hard to argue that withholding artificial hydration and nutrition, and life-prolonging treatment does not amount to euthanasia. The public have not been persuaded. Perceptive people detect a disturbing trend towards acceptance of euthanasia by those who purport to speak for the medical profession in the UK. It is significant that Professor Sheila McLean, the Director of the Institute of Law and Ethics in Glasgow, a leading advocate of assisted suicide, was a member of the small working group that prepared the guidance for the BMA. Writing in the Journal of Medical Ethics in 1996, she argued for . . .

1. "a legislative framework which concedes that there is no absolute commitment to the sanctity of all life and . . .
2. "guidelines, based on principle, which can point the decision-makers to a consistent, accountable and transparent decision."[15]

The BMA guidelines appear to be the outcome.

McLean and Britton have produced a template for an assisted suicide act.[16] Pressure groups in favour of voluntary euthanasia in Britain are said to feel that in the present climate, legalisation of assisted suicide is a more attainable goal than euthanasia legislation.[16,17] In due course the BMA arranged a conference on assisted suicide. Meanwhile the Royal College of Physicians of London and the Royal College of General Practitioners hosted a combined working party on euthanasia, and tried to decide whether euthanasia can be morally justified under certain circumstances.

The official BMA policy as stated in 1997 noted that "there is a wide spectrum of views about the issues of physician-assisted suicide and euthanasia and strongly opposes any changes in the law for the time being". In 2005, by somewhat dubious means, the BMA shifted its official position on assisted suicide and adopted a neutral position.

The BMA appear to be following in the footsteps of the Royal Dutch Medical Association who, in 1997, produced a position paper on end of life decisions in incompetent patients. The Dutch paper was about decisions to withhold or withdraw life-prolonging treatment in neonates, psychogeriatric patients and comatose patients, according to information in the British Medical Journal [18]. There is evidence that 44% of the deaths of mentally disabled people in institutions in Holland are the result of euthanasia, which is often carried out without their consent. Those who campaign for euthanasia in the UK should be warned by events in Holland, but they turn a blind eye. Regrettably, attempts to change the law in the UK to permit assisted suicide continue to be made in Parliament.

In conclusion

It is sad that a professional body like the BMA should have produced guidelines that have provoked such strong disapproval from so many people. One cannot help wondering whether the BMA has been hijacked by pressure groups who favour euthanasia, or by politicians who are worried by the financial burden of an ageing society.[19] Setting aside such thoughts, the guidelines may be seen as a serious, but flawed attempt to rationalize and regulate a difficult and sensitive area of medical practice.

The guidelines have some good features. Decisions to withhold artificial hydration and nutrition should no longer be made by one doctor. Doctors will be less reluctant to start tube-feeding, if they know that they can stop it later if continued treatment is inappropriate or burdensome to the patient. The profession intends to monitor decisions to withhold artificial hydration and nutrition, but arrangements for this need to be clarified.

On balance I fear that the guidelines will do more harm than good. They do not extricate doctors from the medico-legal morass that resulted from the Bland judgement. They represent 'a body of opinion' that may carry some weight in court, but the evidence on which this opinion is based has not been made public. The guidelines do more to protect doctors than to protect their vulnerable patients.

Readers will search the guidelines in vain for signs of the gentleness, wisdom and humanity that are essential if these difficult issues are to be resolved without undue distress to all concerned. I fear that the end result may be to increase public concern, and reduce public trust in the medical profession.

Doctors have no overriding obligation to prolong life by all available means,[20] but they do have an obligation to honour their position of trust within society, and to respect the law of the land. There will undoubtedly be cases where withholding or withdrawing treatment or artificial hydration or nutrition will be morally equivalent to murder. When such cases come to light they should be dealt with firmly. All human beings, whether mentally incapacitated or not, should receive equal protection under the law.

References

1   'Withholding and Withdrawing Life-Prolonging Medical Treatment'. Guidance for decision making. © *BMJ Books* 1999.

2   Editorial 'Doctors as killers'. *The Daily Telegraph*, London. 24th June 1999. p. 27.

3   Hawkes N. 'Sanctity of life tests mettle of philosophers'. *The Times*. 24th June 1999, p.13 col. 1-3.

4   Daniels, A. 'When do you say a life isn't worth living?' *Sunday Telegraph*. 27th June, 1999.

5   Leslie Ann. Saturday Essay. *Daily Mail*. 26th June, 1999.

6   Craig, M. M. Personal communication, 1999.

7   Department of Health. A First Class Service: Quality in the new NHS. London: Department of Health, 1998 (Health Service Circular: HSC (98) 113).

8   Donaldson L. Clinical governance - medical practice in a new era. *The Journal of the MDU*. 1999; **15**: 7-9.

9   Lee R. Clinical governance and risk management. *The Journal of the MDU*. 1999; **15**: 9-12

10 Winterton N and others. Withdrawal of food and fluids from patients. Parliamentary Motion No. 773 as recorded in Notices of Motions: No. 117. 5th July 1999.

11 Office of the Chief Rabbi. Press release. Proposed BMA Guidelines on life-prolonging medical treatment. 5th July 1999.

12 The late Cardinal T J Winning. Views expressed in July 1999.

13 Coppen L. BMA members challenge 'Sinister' guidelines on the dying. *The Catholic Herald*. July 9th, 1999; p.3, cols 1-8.

14 Keown J. Euthanasia, Ethics and Public Policy. Page 259. *Cambridge University Press*, 2002.

15 McLean S. End-of-life decisions and the law. (Guest Editorial) *Journal of Medical Ethics*. 1996; **22**: 261-262.

16 McLean S. Britton A. Sometimes a small victory. Glasgow Institute of Law and Ethics in Medicine, 1996.

17 Churchill, L. R, King N. M. P. Physician assisted suicide, euthanasia, or withdrawal of treatment (Editorial). *British Medical Journal*. 1997; **315**: 137-138.

18 van der Maas P. J. End of life decisions in mentally disabled people (Editorial). *British Medical Journal*. 1997; **314**: 73.

19. Doughty S. Too costly to be kept alive. *Daily Mail* Feb 5th 2005, pp 1 and 6. (The views of John Reed when Secretary of State for Health.)

20. A Joint Submission from the Church of England House of Bishops and the Roman Catholic Bishop's Conference of England and Wales to the House of Lord's Select Committee on Medical Ethics. 1993.Para.15. *HMSO*.

Chapter 5

The Debate Reaches Parliament At Westminster

This chapter, compiled by Gillian Craig, includes copyright material from several sources, as indicated in the text.

THE MEDICAL TREATMENT
(PREVENTION OF EUTHANASIA) BILL

In December 1999 Mrs Ann Winterton Member of Parliament (MP), announced the Medical Treatment (Prevention of Euthanasia) Bill. This was co-sponsored by Dr Brian Iddon MP. The text of the Bill as released in January 2000 was as follows:

A BILL to prohibit the withdrawal or withholding of medical treatment, or the withdrawal or withholding of sustenance, with the intention of causing the death of the patient, and for connected purposes.

BE IT ENACTED by the Queen's most Excellent Majesty, by and with the advice and consent of the Lords Spiritual and Temporal, and the Commons, in this present Parliament assembled, and by the authority of the same, as follows:-

1. It shall be unlawful for any person responsible for the care of a patient to withdraw or withhold from the patient medical treatment or sustenance if his purpose or one of his purposes in doing so is to hasten or otherwise cause the death of the patient.

2. In this Act:
    "medical treatment" means any medical or surgical treatment, including the administration of drugs or the use of any mechanical or other apparatus for the provision or support of ventilation or of any other bodily function;
    "patient" means a person suffering from mental or physical illness or disability;
    "sustenance" means the provision of nutrition or hydration, howsoever delivered.

3. (1) This Act may be cited as the Medical Treatment (Prevention of Euthanasia) Act 2000.
    (2) This Act shall come into force at the end of the month beginning with the day on which this Act is passed.
    (3) This Act extends to England, Wales and Northern Ireland only.

Footnote:

The text of this Bill and the typographical arrangement of the text are Parliamentary copyright. This material is reproduced with the permission of the Controller of HMSO on behalf of Parliament.

Comments from Mrs Ann Winterton MP

The following article by Mrs Ann Winterton was published in *The Daily Telegraph* on January 27th 2000. [1]

We must stop murdering the old and infirm

"A recent statement in the newsletter of the Voluntary Euthanasia Society of Scotland shows how we are sliding towards the practice of euthanasia. An article by Professor Sheila McLean tells us: "My suspicion is that the routes taken by the courts have been tailored so that they cannot be seen as endorsing voluntary euthanasia…Yet arguably the conclusion must be that the courts are endorsing a form of non-voluntary euthanasia."

This is significant because Prof McLean- an academic lawyer- was an important contributor to the BMA guidelines on withholding and withdrawing life-prolonging medical treatment.

The BMA insists vehemently that it is opposed to euthanasia and that its guidelines do not seek to extend any such practice, but the guidelines do seek to widen the categories of cases from which treatment (including assisted feeding) could be withdrawn, with the clear intention of ending the lives of patients who are not dying. In other words the BMA guidelines extend the cases to which they could apply what Prof McLean describes as "non-voluntary euthanasia".

I have introduced the Medical Treatment (Prevention of Euthanasia) Bill to halt the slide towards the acceptance and practice of euthanasia, by making it clear to doctors that they cannot intentionally bring about the death of their patients by act or omission. The Bill will be debated in the House of Commons tomorrow.

The Daily Telegraph recently publicised a number of cases in which it was alleged that many elderly patients were being denied appropriate medication and food and fluid in hospitals.

While the cases highlighted differed from those in which assisted food and fluid were deliberately withdrawn with the aim of ending the lives of patients who are not dying, they reveal a growing lack of respect and value for the aged and those with disabilities.

Statements from the BMA in which it claims to recommend only the withdrawal of "useless" or "futile" treatment, foster this attitude. As the Muslim Council of Britain has pointed out, it is not the treatment that is futile, it is that the BMA regards the patients as futile.

Food and fluid (however delivered) is basic nursing care, a basic human right; the only reason for doctors to define it as "treatment" is to enable them to end the lives of patients whose existence they regard as "futile" or "useless". This is a very dangerous ethos for society to accept.

My Bill is short, clear and focused, and pursues one simple objective – restoring the integrity of the principle of the law of murder, which was weakened by the Tony Bland judgement.

Although many were originally sympathetic to the Bland ruling (not realising that it resulted in him dying from dehydration and starvation), it nevertheless created a loophole that the euthanasia lobby and the BMA have persistently sought to widen.

Euthanasia is now being introduced via the backdoor – or as Prof McLean so aptly put it: we have a policy that endorses "a form of non-voluntary euthanasia".

In drafting the Bill, we were anxious not to require doctors "officiously to keep alive" dying patients; not to deter doctors from giving patients adequate palliative care, even though this might shorten their lives; and not to require doctors to give genuinely futile treatment.

The Bill concentrates on the "purpose" of the doctor in withdrawing or withholding medical treatment or food or fluid. If the doctor's treatment is to relieve suffering- to stop treatment that is too burdensome or that is futile for the health of the patient- then the doctor is acting lawfully.

If, however, his purpose is to end or to shorten the life of his patient, that is unlawful homicide. That was always the case until the Bland judgement left our law "misshapen" (as one Law Lord described it).

The BMA opposes my Bill, claiming it would "diminish consideration" of a patient's interests and "make worthless" a patient's valid refusal of treatment.

This is untrue. The Bill would not diminish the law's requirement, or the doctor's responsibility and right to consider the best interests, beliefs, views and desires of patients.

The Bill would do nothing except forbid the doctor to pursue a purpose of killing or hastening the death of the patient by withdrawing or withholding treatment with that purpose.

The law has always forbidden doctors from giving medicines intended to kill or hasten death. That in no way diminishes the doctor's duty and right to consider the patient's best interests, beliefs etc., when deciding what treatment to give.

I am no "vitalist" who believes that we must prolong life whatever the circumstances. Death is an event for which we should prepare and to which we should move forwards with confidence and security, not fear of our doctors and their motives.

Many individuals and doctors have contacted me to tell me of their experiences. I have received backing from leaders of many Christian denominations, the Chief Rabbi and prominent leaders among the Muslim community. The Government and the BMA must not be allowed to turn a blind eye to what is happening in hospitals today, and my Bill should have their support tomorrow."

Comments from the British Medical Association

1. Comments from Dr Michael Wilks

On December 9th 1999, shortly after Ann Winterton announced the Bill, Dr Michael Wilks, Chairman of the Medical Ethics Committee of the BMA spoke on BBC Radio 5 Live. When granting Dr Craig permission to quote him Dr Wilks stressed that the BMA Medical Ethics Committee shared his views. The following comments are printed with permission. © Wilks M. 1999.

> "What I think Mrs Winterton is objecting to is our recent advice about withdrawing or withholding treatment in patients who have grossly incapacitating and static illnesses like advanced dementia or severe incapacitating strokes- where over a long period of time it becomes clear that continuing treatment is not a benefit to the patient. In those circumstances we have considered whether doctors might ethically and properly remove treatment.

> "We are not talking about the terminal phase of an illness, we are talking about a group of patients with varying conditions characterised by long term severe incapacity- a kind of vegetative state- where you are simply not communicating and your intellectual function is grossly impaired or absent..." said Wilks. His view was that if doctors concluded that there was absolutely no prospect of any recovery whatsoever, it was appropriate to consider whether treatment had become a burden.

> "By withdrawing artificial hydration and nutrition, and it is no use pretending otherwise, death will result. But in law, and it is a very important point of law, a doctor who intends to cause a death as a primary intent of withdrawing treatment is acting illegally." said Dr Wilks. He continued:

> "A doctor who says 'I no longer think that this treatment is of benefit so I'm going to withdraw it'- (after a long period of discussion and debate) is not acting illegally. If a patient as a consequence of that decision comes to an early end that is not the intention of the doctor. The doctor is compassionately deciding that treatment is of no further benefit." [2]

A comment from Dr Craig

Dr Wilks presented the issue of the withdrawal of life-sustaining food and water as a compassionate medical decision, and evaded the issue of euthanasia. In 1999 the BMA maintained that they were opposed to euthanasia, but they condoned actions that many considered to be euthanasia by omission. The arguments they used to maintain this stance were unconvincing.

With respect to the Bland judgment, Dr Wilks said: "...in withdrawing artificial hydration and nutrition the doctors did not intend Tony Bland to die, they intended to no longer burden Tony Bland with treatment that was burdensome." However as Price noted in a legal journal in 1997 - "In Bland, Lords Lowry and Browne-Wilkinson both specifically commented that the physicians involved possessed the requisite intention to kill." [3]. It could be said that those who asked that Tony Bland's sustenance be discontinued and those who granted their request were accomplices in his death.

Ask yourself the question "What precisely was the burden from which Tony Bland was released? In what way was his treatment burdensome?" A person with a permanent vegetative state will not be aware of a naso-gastric tube or a percutaneous gastrostomy tube, nor will they be aware of their dependent state, or of the thoughts of grieving relatives. Let there be no misunderstanding- the judgement removed from the state the financial burden of care.

The situation of patients with severe dementia or devastating strokes is somewhat different. For those with residual awareness tube feeding may indeed prove to be somewhat burdensome. Lawyers who drafted the Medical Treatment (Prevention of Euthanasia) Bill recognised this fact, but saw no need to spell it out in words of one syllable. The wording of the Bill was crystal clear to its advocates, but it suited the purpose of opponents to create difficulties.

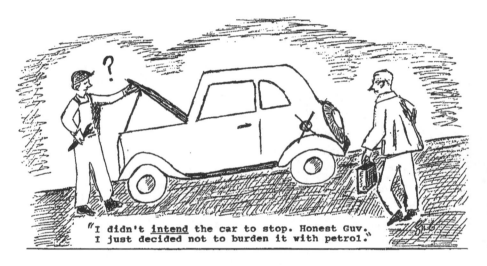

"I didn't **intend** the car to stop. Honest Guv. I just decided not to burden it with petrol."

2. *The Chairman of the Council of the BMA, Dr Ian Bogle wrote to every MP to urge them to vote against the Medical Treatment (Prevention of Euthanasia) Bill.*

Dr Bogle drew attention to the guidance issued by the BMA in 1999 and stated that it was supported by the Royal College of Nursing, the Ethics Committee of the Royal College of Physicians and that of the Royal College of General Practitioners, by the Alzheimer's Society and the Association for Palliative Medicine of Great Britain. Copies of his letter were widely available outside Parliament.

Dr Bogle argued that the Bill would diminish consideration of the patient's best interests, (such as the individuals own moral values, religious or cultural beliefs, views of their own aim or purpose in life, as well as the degree and type of medical treatment they want). The Bill would also "make worthless any valid refusal by restricting the law to have regard only for the 'purpose of one of his purposes' of the doctor (Clause 1)". The BMA guidance was "emphatically not about euthanasia to which the BMA remains firmly opposed." The guidance was intended to help doctors make compassionate decisions about "patients who are likely to live weeks, months, or possibly years if treatment is provided, but who without treatment will, or may die earlier." If enacted, the Bill would "confuse an already complex process, result in poor patient care, and remove patient autonomy." [4]

3. The BMA's interpretation of the Bill was refuted by Finnis, Keown and McColl.
John Finnis, Professor of Law and Legal Philosophy at Oxford University, with Dr John Keown, then lecturer in law at Cambridge University, and Lord McColl, Professor of Surgery at Guy's Hospital, London wrote a memo to all MPs to assure them that the Bill:

❑   Would in no way diminish the law's requirement, and the doctor's responsibility and right, to take into account the best interests, values, beliefs, views and desires of patients.

❑   Would do nothing except prohibit the doctor from pursuing a purpose of killing or hastening the death of the patient by withdrawing or withholding treatment.

❑   Under the terms of the Bill a doctor who withdrew treatment to respect the valid wishes of a competent patient, or on the grounds that treatment was medically futile or too burdensome for the patient, would be acting lawfully.

❑   The BMA's hasty interpretation of the Bill was "completely wrong" and should be ignored, they said. [5]

Despite this assurance many MPs remained convinced that the Bill would make it difficult for doctors to take patient's views into consideration. Some imagined that patients would be "force fed" or transfused against their wishes, although under common law this would constitute an assault.

A briefing paper for MPs.

MPs had access to a briefing paper on the Bill, written by Katherine Wright who was at that time a member of the social policy section of the House of Commons Library. Her paper, which gave unbiased background information of a philosophical nature on ethical issues, was available to the public on the Parliamentary web site.[6] The paper as a whole covered the background to the Bill, case law, the BMA guidance, the Government's intentions as to future law reform, and some ethical issues. The section on ethical issues, reprinted with permission, can be found later in this chapter. In it the author "attempts to summarise some of the possible ethical approaches to the issue of withholding treatment, and to discuss the extent to which current case law is in sympathy with them."

The paper starts with a brief description of three approaches to ethics:
1.   Utilitarian – focus on the *outcomes* of moral decisions
2.   Right's based – which begs the question a) what is a right and b) what if rights conflict?
3.   Duty based – which brings in moral absolutes, religious beliefs, and concerns about the sanctity of life.
Wright notes that conflict can arise between the sanctity of life and personal autonomy. She quotes the views of the Church of England House of Bishops and

the Roman Catholic Bishop's Conference of England and Wales in their submission to the House of Lords Committee on Medical Ethics in 1993.[7]

In the final section of the paper Wright defines some terms that crop up rather often in medical ethics. Terms such as "best interests", "burdensome" "futility" and "justice".[8]

Comments from opponents and supporters of the Bill

The Medical Treatment (Prevention of Euthanasia) Bill did not have the support of the Government. In the weeks leading up to its Second Reading in the House of Commons, opponents and supporters of the Bill engaged the attention of MPs.

The Department of Health saw no need for the Bill, reflected the views of the BMA and reminded MPs in a briefing note that the intentional taking of life is already unlawful throughout the UK under the laws of homicide. There was concern in Government circles about possible effects of the Bill on patient autonomy-concern that those who drafted the Bill refuted.

The Church of England Board of Social Responsibility sat on the fence. While supporting the Bill in principle, they were concerned that it might lead to defensive medicine. They preferred "to encourage purity of motive in all health care practitioners, and then leave them free to make the decisions at the work face, where they belong." [9]

The Office of the Chief Rabbi issued a statement supporting the Bill. The statement read:

"One of the critical tests of a society is how it protects the vulnerable, defends the defenceless and cares for those dependent on the care of others. These principles, at the moral core of the Judeo-Christian tradition, have been throughout Western Civilisation powerful safeguards of the dignity of the individual and the sanctity of life.

"These are currently at risk. The proposal to permit doctors to withdraw treatment, including nutrition and hydration, from the dying and the chronically ill creates the possibility of what may be, in effect, non-voluntary euthanasia. Not only is this unacceptable to our great religious and moral traditions; it also represents to a great many people, a potentially fearful erosion of our duty to protect life, regardless as to its quality or future longevity. Indeed it puts at risk the bond of trust between the public and the medical profession. That trust is based on the premise that though the judgement of a doctor is to be valued on the question of which treatment to pursue, he or she is not empowered to terminate life, if only by omission."[10]

The Medical and Health Committee of the Muslim Council of Britain wrote to every MP and said:

"As practising doctors we would assure you that the profession is fully aware of the difference between withdrawing or withholding treatment (including food and fluid) with the purpose of killing a patient, and withdrawing treatment which is futile or burdensome, while knowing that this will or may, shorten life of a patient....As every doctor is fully aware, there is only one possible result from denying patients food and fluid (by whatever means) and that is death by starvation and dehydration."[11]

The Catholic Bishops' Conference of England and Wales gave strong support to the Bill, which they said, "Fully accords with the Catholic Church's ethical teaching on euthanasia". They considered the Bill to be "timely and necessary".[12]

Second Reading of the Bill: House of Commons, January 28th 2000

The Second Reading of the Bill engendered some good debate. A full report can be found in Hansard.[13]

Mrs Winterton stressed that the purpose of the Bill was to call a halt to what had become the slide towards the acceptance and practice of euthanasia. She referred to international euthanasia bodies who have promoted the idea of withdrawing assisted feeding from profoundly disabled people as a first step to achieving euthanasia.

Sir Paul Beresford who is on the Board of Dental Protection, part of the Medical Protection Society Limited, stated that the society "has deep concerns as to the simplicity of the Bill and foresees the potential of double jeopardy for doctors."[14] David Pinnick QC writing in *The Times* in May 2000, suggested that politics should be left out of the double jeopardy debate.[15] Pinnick explained that "The double jeopardy rule has been part of the common law since the 12th century, preventing the State from seeking to retry a defendant who has already been acquitted of the offence." Similar rulings apply in the USA, but according to Pinnick "an absolute double jeopardy rule is not required by fundamental human rights." The Law Commission was considering the circumstances under which double jeopardy could be overridden in the UK.

George Galloway MP described euthanasia as "the ultimate capitalist policy." He argued that "The deliberate fostering of the sense that old people, disabled people and chronically sick people would be better away is a profoundly unethical, un Christian idea. It comes from those who believe that our only real purpose is to work, to earn and to be individuals when we are strong. It is the weak, vulnerable and those not able to speak for themselves who hon. Members have to speak for and protect." [16]

Jim Dobbin MP criticised the BMA guidance and suggested that "the BMA is confused and requires the guidance of the law to protect its members interests." He stated that not only was the medical profession split on the BMA guidelines, but "in addition not all members of the BMA medical ethics committee, which published the guidelines, were in agreement on the final version." [17]

Sir Nicholas Lyell MP, who is a lawyer, was also critical of the BMA guidance which he said "makes life very difficult for doctors" and "raises genuine fears that medical treatment will be withheld when it should not be..."[18]

Dr Evan Harris, a medical practitioner who is MP for Oxford, is a member of the Parliamentary Group for Doctor Assisted Dying, and a member of the BMA Medical Ethics Committee. He spoke up for the BMA guidelines[19] and mentioned that the Under Secretary of State for Health in the House of Lords had said they were a welcome addition to the debate. Dr Harris spoke of constituents who were afraid of having their lives prolonged at all costs. He argued that patients must be safeguarded from the prolongation of life when that is no longer in their interest. He regarded the Bland case as a safeguard, not a loophole, in the law.[20] However it was noted during the debate that the Government does not intend the Bland decision to become enshrined in statute law.

Some of the most revealing and chilling remarks came from Dr Harris, who wanted to see liberalisation of the law on voluntary euthanasia, with adequate safeguards. Having stated that the BMA remains fundamentally opposed to euthanasia he added "However, there is a utilitarian argument, which claims that, ethically, an act of omission is the same as an act of commission, and that only the end result matters." That remark has serious implications for the frail elderly. In the context of suffering Dr Harris said- " I believe that if the patient wants the suffering to be ended, doctors should be allowed to do that, with appropriate safeguards, by an act of commission as well as acts of omission. If dying is burdensome, doctors should not be forced to make that death drawn out." [21]

Yvette Cooper, then Parliamentary Under-Secretary of State for Health (now working in the Lord Chancellor's Department) noted the choice of the word "purpose" as opposed to "intent". She was unclear how the Bill would fit in with existing criminal laws relating to murder and manslaughter, based on the concept of primary intention. She feared that the Bill would be unworkable in practice, and for this reason the Government was unable to support it. [22]

Dr Liam Fox MP hoped that the Government would not use procedure or their Parliamentary majority to kill the Bill, for he said "The difference between right and wrong is not part of the democratic process, but part of a much higher order." It was a vital moral issue that crossed the party political divide.[23]

Some MPs while supporting the Bill in principle did not want to reverse the Bland judgment. The problem that faces Parliament now is how to prevent escalation of that judgment into widespread euthanasia by omission.

The Bill gained its Second Reading and passed to the committee stage by a vote of 113 for and 2 against. Minor amendments only were made in the committee stage; most people saved their amendments and used them to waste valuable time later.

The Report Stage

When the Bill returned for debate at the Report Stage on April 14th 2000 eighty amendments were tabled by MPs, many of whom claimed to be opposed to euthanasia. Some amendments were ruled out of order, but five new clauses were debated in the limited time available. Opinion was divided as to whether the consent of the Attorney General or the Director of Public Prosecutions should be required before prosecution. MPs were told that the Law Commission had already discussed the consent requirement with regard to the prosecution of doctors for manslaughter, and had concluded that no class of person deserved more protection than another. Nevertheless several MPs with medical connections were concerned to protect the interests of doctors. One spoke at length on all five new clauses and was accused of filibustering, i.e. deliberately wasting time.

One proposed new clause imposing severe restrictions on publicity was in line with Article 6 of the Human Rights Act, but Dr Brand MP felt that once the evidence had been produced to warrant prosecution, that prosecution should be conducted in public.[24] Another new clause would have taken the issue out of the criminal realm into the area of civil wrongs such as negligence or nuisance,[25] but Mrs Winterton felt that liability in tort was "completely inadequate."[26] Yvette Cooper noted that the new clauses would provide hurdles for private prosecutions under the Bill, which she understood was exactly what the proposers of the clauses had in mind. Yet the Law Commission view was that a private prosecution fulfils an extremely useful function, and consent should only be circumscribed where an offence may involve national security, or have some international element.[27]

The debate strayed far from the central precept of the Bill, prompting Ann Winterton to comment that "a legal cat's cradle" had been created.[28] Finally she rose and called for a Closure Motion to end the debate. This required a minimum of 100 "Aye" votes. In the event there were 96 "Aye" votes for closure and 10 against, so the debate continued until time ran out.

After the vote one MP asked whether the government would continue to think about whether it is acceptable to kill patients by starvation- that being at the heart of the matter. Yvette Cooper replied that the Bill had raised "important and weighty matters, and the Government will continue to consider them". She could give no time scale for any amendments or additions to the law.[29] Thus the Medical Treatment (Prevention of Euthanasia) Bill died. The debate was adjourned and no further time for it was found in a busy legislative programme. Matters such as fox hunting took precedence!

The Government position in July 2000

Some months after the demise of "The Medical Treatment (Euthanasia Prevention) Bill" Mr John Denham who was at that time Minister of State in the Department of Health wrote a letter that stated the Government position quite clearly. The letter, dated July 7th 2000, was forwarded to Dr Craig as a formal reply to her letters of concern to MPs and to the Prime Minister. The substance of the letter from John Denham read as follows:

"The Government considers euthanasia to mean the intentional taking of life albeit at the person's request or for a merciful motive. As the Government has repeatedly made clear, euthanasia is unlawful in the United Kingdom and will remain so. Such a deliberate act cannot be justified. When a patient is in hospital there is no doubt that the person's doctor owes that patient a duty of care, and that certainly includes a requirement not intentionally to kill the patient by any means, either by a positive action or by an omission. That said, case law on withholding and withdrawal of treatment, which is sometimes described as an omission, is a complicated area.

"I am aware that public opinion is deeply divided on the subject of the withdrawal of treatment. Although some believe that in circumstances such as those of Mr Tony Bland withdrawal of treatment would constitute euthanasia, others (including our courts) would disagree. A doctor can only have a duty to offer treatment that would actually be of benefit to the patient.

"I am also aware that some believe that mere existence, even in a permanently unconscious state, constitutes a benefit; equally strongly, others believe this not to be the case. In the Bland judgement the courts concluded that there could be no absolute obligation to prolong a patient's life by all available means; rather the test must be whether it is in the best interests of the patient, taking into account all the circumstances, for life-prolonging medical treatment to be continued. If it is not in the best interests of the patient the doctor has no duty (or authority) to provide the treatment. Hence failure to provide it cannot be unlawful, even if as a result the patient dies of his or her illness.

"At present, the (common) law is based firmly in the *rights of the patient* to consent to, or refuse, medical treatment. When the patient is not capable of making his or her own treatment decision, the *best interests of the patient* is the key issue in deciding what is lawful or unlawful. However, this Bill would instead make a *doctor's "purpose or one of his purposes"*, in deciding whether to withhold or withdraw treatment, the key issue. Such a shift in focus from 'patient's best interests' to 'doctors purposes' would be a radical change in the law. Further the lack of clarity about the meaning of "purpose of one of his purposes" means that the present draft would be unworkable in practice, creating uncertainty for both patients and health professionals.

"The British Medical Association, the Royal College of Nursing, Age Concern, the Alzheimer's Society and the National Council for Hospice and Specialist Palliative Care Services have all expressed serious concerns about the potential impact of the Bill on the quality of care which can be provided to patients.

"These are important and sensitive issues. I recognise that many people have sincere and deeply held views about the matters raised in this Bill. But the Government does not believe that the approach that has been adopted meets either the aims of the Bill or the needs of patients.

"With regard to BMA guidelines on *Withholding and Withdrawing Life-Prolonging Medical Treatment,* these are aimed to assist clinicians by identifying the range of clinical, ethical and legal factors which need to be considered in making decisions on withdrawing and withholding medical treatment. They also advise on potential procedures, including consulting the health care team and seeking a second opinion where appropriate, which may assist in ensuring a high quality of decision-making in this difficult and sensitive area. The guidelines recognise the need for appropriate safeguards. But these are, of course, only guidelines and doctors and others responsible for the care of patients must consider each case individually in the light of the law and of other relevant information."

Letter signed *John Denham*

In Conclusion

Almost a year after the demise of the Medical Treatment (Prevention of Euthanasia) Bill in Parliament, a committee chaired by Judge Stephen Tumim under the auspices of the Royal College of Physicians of London and the Royal College of General Practitioners issued a position statement on medical treatment at the end of life. Reporting in March 2001, they took the view that the intent behind a "therapeutic decision" was a central issue for debate within the profession and within society.[30]

The Law Commission have been trying to define what level of intent should be required for a murder conviction, which suggests that some basic changes in English Criminal Law are under consideration. Those who value human life should be sober and vigilant, for the sad truth is that some patients these days appear to have no right to life in the eyes of the law. In the opinion of Judge Butler Sloss "the intervention of the High Court remains a proper safeguard" in cases of PVS but in her view decisions to withdraw treatment in such cases does not breach the right to life under Article 2 or Article 3 of the European Convention on Human Rights.[31] It remains to be seen whether Judges in Strasbourg will agree with this interpretation of the law.

There are undoubtedly times when "therapeutic decisions" are made and treatment withheld, with the deliberate intention of shortening life. Parliament and the legal profession should recognise this fact and take action to protect patients, but there is little reason to believe that they will do so. All the evidence suggests that behind a smokescreen of official denial, the drive for euthanasia legislation in the UK will continue. Meanwhile the process of treatment withdrawal gathers momentum, no longer secretly behind closed doors, but openly, with the support of the British Medical Association, the General Medical Council, and Parliament.

References

1. Winterton A. We must stop murdering the old and infirm. *The Daily Telegraph* January 17th 2000, p28, cols 3-6. © Telegraph Group Limited.
2. Wilks M. BBC Radio 5 Live. December 9th 1999. Quoted with speaker's permission.
3. Price D. Euthanasia, pain relief and double effect. *Legal Studies*, 1997: **17:2**, p339.
4. Bogle I.G. Letter to MPs. January 21st 2000. Widely circulated to members of the public.
5. Finnis J, Keown J. and McColl. (Memo) The BMA's mistaken response. Quoted by Winterton and Dobbin. *Hansard* **343**, No 35, p694, p695 and p699.
6. Wright K. Medical Treatment (Prevention of Euthanasia) Bill House of Commons Library Research Paper No 00/8, Jan 24th 2000. Section on ethics p22-27. © House of Commons Library.
7. A Joint Submission from the Church of England House of Bishops and Roman Catholic Bishops' Conference to the House of Lords' Select Committee on Medical Ethics. 1993. Paragraph 10.
8. Abstracted from reference 6 above.

9. See ref 5 above, p32.
10. *Right to Life News*. Issue 4, April 2000.
11. As ref.10. Issue 4, April 2000.
12. See ref 5 above p.31.
13. Official Report. *Hansard*.343 No 35.January 28th 2000.
14. Ibid p.689.
15. Pannick D. Let's leave politics out of the double jeopardy debate. *The Times*, Law p9 col 1-5. May 23rd 2000.
16. As 13 above, *Hansard*, January 28th 2000 p.709-711.
17. Ibid p.699.
18. Ibid p.713.
19. Ibid p.734-735
20. Ibid p.738
21. Ibid p.742
22. Ibid p.743-749
23. Ibid p750.
24. Official report, *Hansard* **348** No85, April 14th. 2000 p630.
25. Ibid p 632-637
26. Ibid p 637
27. Ibid p640
28. Note. A cat's cradle refers to a child's game in which a simple circle of string is twisted into a tangle resembling a cat's cradle.
29. As ref 24, p648.
30. Medical Treatment at the end of life. A position statement. *Clinical Medicine,* 2001;**1**: 115-117.
31. Butler-Sloss E. Withholding and withdrawing life-prolonging treatment. Lecture for the General Medical Council. Given to an invited audience in London. Friday July 20th 2001.

Acknowledgment

Parliamentary copyright material from *Hansard* is reproduced with the permission of the Controller of Her Majesty's Stationery Office on behalf of Parliament.

Ethical Issues

Author Katherine Wright

Taken from a House of Commons Library Research Paper No 00/8. Jan 24th 2000.
On the Medical Treatment (Prevention of Euthanasia) Bill and related matters.

Introduction

Ethical approaches to these issues vary widely, and the fact that a particular approach has been enshrined in case law does not necessarily mean that it is therefore in accordance with ethical codes. This section of the paper will attempt to summarise some of the possible ethical approaches to the issue of withholding treatment, and discuss the extent to which current case law is in sympathy with them. Inevitably it will be very brief.

Utilitarian approaches to ethics focus on the *outcomes* of moral decisions. The *intentions* behind certain decisions are therefore deemed to be morally irrelevant. Put very simply, an action is ethically right under a utilitarian system of ethics if the result is a net increase in "utility" (measured in a variety of ways, such as the total amount of happiness, or prosperity, or lack of unhappiness, in a particular society). Thus, if the measure of utility is the happiness of the population, then end-of-life decisions will be ethical, or not, depending on the extent to which they increase, or decrease that happiness. If it could be demonstrated that the current legal position causes a significant level of anxiety in the older population, fearing that they will not receive the treatment they need or want, then utilitarians would regard it as unethical since it decreases utility. If, on the other hand, people have a greater fear of being subjected to treatment that they believe that they will *not* want at the end of their lives, then the current legal position would be regarded as ethical. One significant feature of utilitarian philosophy is that it takes no account of the individual, except in so far as this affects the utility of the whole. It could therefore be argued that if withdrawing treatment from patients in PVS would release large cost savings which could treat others more conscious of the benefit, then it would be ethical from this perspective to do so.

Very few people, apart from philosophers, adhere to a purely utilitarian approach to ethics. However, the idea that, other things being equal, it is right to maximise the total good is widespread; for example in the approach to healthcare spending that argues that funding should be allocated in such a way as to create the greatest possible increase in population health status, even if this means that particular individuals do not benefit at all. Another aspect of utilitarianism which is relatively common is the belief that it is the results of actions which have moral value, not the intentions which lie behind them. Thus, for example, the claim that there is a moral difference between an act and an omission, where both the intention and the actual outcome is the same (which was crucial in the *ratio* of the *Bland* case), would be regarded as hypocrisy. (see author's footnote)

[Author's footnote. The *ratio* = the legal principles on which the case is decided.]

Rights-based approach. A very different approach would be a rights-based approach, according to which human beings, by their very nature as human beings, possess certain rights, such as the right to receive what treatment they need, to have their autonomy respected, or (perhaps the most basic right of all) the right not to be killed. The widespread nature of this approach is demonstrated by the existence of international organisations and treaties upholding human rights, such as the *European Convention on Human Rights*.

Two problems which tend to arise in connection with rights-based theories are *firstly* the fact that there is no clear consensus on what exactly constitutes a "right" or who may claim entitlement to one, and *secondly* the difficulty with dealing with situations where rights appear to conflict. While, in the latter case, it may often be possible to argue that some rights come higher in a pecking order than others and will take priority in any conflict, again there is no necessary consensus over this pecking order. The debate over the morality of abortion, for example, is often phrased in terms of a woman's "right" to determine what happens in her own body versus the "right" of an unborn child not to be killed. The opposing sides on that argument may not even agree over the very existence of the "right" claimed by the other, and will certainly be in conflict about which should take precedence. Nevertheless, despite the theoretical arguments about how rights can be "proved" or how conflicts between different rights can be dealt with, most "rights" do reflect widespread and fundamental beliefs about the nature of human beings and how they ought to behave towards each other.

A duty-based approach. A third approach to ethics, and one which underpins the approach of most **religions**, is a **"deontological"** (duty-based) one. Deontological ethics start from the premise that human beings have duties and obligations; in "revealed religions" such as Christianity, Judaism and Islam, these duties and obligations may be made manifest through prophets , through sacred texts, and, in Christianity, through the incarnation of God as a human being. The ten commandments and the sermon on the mount are famous examples of deontological codes by which Christians are urged to live their lives. Another, rather less well known, example of a deontological code is the "categorical imperative" of Immanuel Kant (according to which we should only undertake an action if we could will it to become a universal law- in other words if we would think it right for anybody else to take exactly the same action). Unlike rights-based theories, which do not tell us *how* to behave, except by respecting the rights of other, deontological theories tend to include moral absolutes: certain actions are regarded as *intrinsically* immoral, even if one could argue that no-one is harmed by them, or even that in a particular case people will benefit.

One of the ethical arguments surrounding the withdrawal of medical treatment falls very clearly into the deontological and religious category: the principle of respecting the *"sanctity of life"*. This principle is obviously of crucial importance, although it is interpreted very differently by various groups, with quite different meanings attached to both "sanctity" and "life". Thus in one interpretation, the principle of the sanctity of life is taken to mean that human life must always be preserved if the means to do so exist, if necessary against the will of the individual whose life it is. Life in this definition might be seen as a gift from God which we are not at liberty to refuse. Under another interpretation, the principle is taken to refer to the intrinsic value of human life: the belief that human life is valuable by its very nature, even if the person involved does not value it, or is not aware of it (for example because of severe learning difficulties or unconsciousness). However, this interpretation need not make the same clear absolute claim as the first, that life must always be preserved if humanly possible. It could be argued, for example, that bare existence, with no possibility of future consciousness, should not be included in "life": that the life we are holding to be sacred must include at least some of the aspects which, taken together, appear to make human life distinctly different from that of other species, such as the ability to relate to other human beings, to experience joy and sadness, to reason, to have aesthetic responses and so on. Moreover, stating that life is intrinsically valuable does not automatically "trump" any competing factors, such as the individual's own wish not to be treated (whether expressed contemporaneously or previously through an advance statement). The first interpretation of "sanctity of life", on the other hand, does not admit of any "balancing" of this principle against another.

The principle that is most often set against the sanctity of life principle by those who argue that it can, in certain circumstances, be permissible to cease life-prolonging medical treatment, is the *"respect for autonomy"*, or the more limited "right to bodily integrity". These principles state that human beings have the right to determine what happens to their own bodies, and ultimately to determine when they no longer desire medical assistance in prolonging their life. The legal principle that it would be a battery to treat a competent patient against their will, or an incompetent patient where they have made an advance statement refusing treatment in these circumstances, appears to depend heavily on the ethical principle of respect for autonomy.

As discussed above, in the context of rights-based theories of ethics, there is no simple resolution between those who uphold the more "absolutist" definition of the sanctity of life and those who would give primacy to autonomy: the two principles derive from separate value systems which, in the case of life-sustaining treatment refused by the patient, are simply incompatible (although they may produce the same answer in many other cases). An adherent of the primacy of autonomy might argue that the two principles are *not* in conflict: that the ability to exercise autonomous decision-making is a basic part of one's human nature and that to be denied it by others is to be denied what makes life "sacred" in the first place. However such an argument would be quite unconvincing to those holding the belief that it is "life" itself that is sacred, not what particular individuals choose to define as the most important aspects of that life.

Bishops' views. The Church of England House of Bishops and the Roman Catholic Bishops Conference of England and Wales addressed the potential conflict between the sanctity of life and autonomy as follows, in a joint submission to the House of Lords Committee on Medical Ethics in 1993 on the subject of euthanasia.

The sanctity of life and the right to personal autonomy

7. Attention is often drawn to the apparent conflict between the importance placed by Christians on the special character of human life as God-given and thus deserving of special protection, and the insistence by some on their right to determine when their lives should end.

8. This contrast can be falsely presented. Neither of our Churches insists that a dying or seriously ill person should be kept alive by all possible means for as long as possible. On the other hand we do not believe that the right to personal autonomy is absolute. It is valid only when it recognises other moral values, especially the respect due to human life as such, whether someone else's or one's own.

9. We do not accept that the right to personal autonomy requires any change in the law in order to allow euthanasia.

10. The exercise of personal autonomy necessarily has to be limited in order that human beings may live together in reasonable harmony. Such limitation may have to be defined by law. While at present people may exercise their right to refuse treatment (although this may be overridden in special but strictly limited circumstances), the law forbids a right to die at a time of their own choosing. The consequences which could flow from a change in the law on voluntary euthanasia would outweigh the benefits to be gained from more rigid adherence to the notion of personal autonomy. But in any case we believe that respect for the life of a vulnerable person is the overriding principle.

    Reproduced on the Church of England's website: http://www.cofe.Anglican. org/view/medical.html

Moreover, those who challenge a "balancing" between autonomy and the sanctity of life could argue that there are serious *practical* dangers involved in an approach which allows one to pick and choose what aspects of life are to be held as sacred.

In the case of advance refusals of treatment, for example, individuals might guess quite wrongly how they might react in the future if faced with very serious illness or disability, or how they might value that life when it was the only life open to them. Similarly, it could be argued that there is no way of knowing if people have changed their minds since refusing particular treatments in an advance statement, or whether a refusal reflects a temporary depression rather than a deeply-held view.

The relative weights to be given to respect for autonomy and respect for the sanctity of life, and indeed how respect for the sanctity of life is to be defined, become crucial when considering some of the central terms used in debates over the withdrawal of life-prolonging treatment such as "best interests", "burdensome" and "futile". This is especially the case where the patient in question is not competent to accept or refuse treatment, for reasons such as severe learning disability or stroke.

Defining terms: "best interests", "burdensome", "futility", "justice"

Best interests: As discussed in earlier parts of this Paper, the legal position is that such patients may be treated in their "best interests", with the current case law leaving the determination of "best interests" very much to doctors. An approach that placed great emphasis on autonomy might query why such a decision should be a matter for doctors at all: while medical assistance is certainly needed either to continue or withdraw treatment, and for diagnosis and prognosis, it could be argued that the actual issue of whether life should continue is one that only the person involved (or, in default of the patient being able to express a view, those who know them best) can take.

If, on the other hand, it is believed that sanctity of life must ultimately "trump" autonomy, then it could be argued that a person's "best interests" must always lie in remaining alive, or in remaining alive unless their pain is unendurable and uncontrollable, and hence there would be no real decision for either doctors or others to take. The doctors' role under either of these latter approaches would be limited to determining the most appropriate treatment (for example active treatment to prolong life, or palliative care where the patient is in such pain that active treatment is believed to be too burdensome) to achieve these aims. Recent attempts to define how best interests should be determined (for example by the Law Commission and the British Medical Association...) have tended to give greater weight to the autonomous approach.

Burdensome: Similarly, the term "burdensome" is used in a variety of ways. An approach emphasising the role of individual autonomy might describe treatment as "burdensome" if, for that particular patient, the pain or discomfort inherent in the treatment was not outweighed by the benefits the treatment brought (for example if the quality of continued life made possible by the treatment was not valued by the patient). On this understanding of "burdensome", treatment which some patients might regard as burdensome, might be accepted with gratitude by others in an identical position. Alternatively, "burdensome" could be understood to have a more objective meaning of causing an unacceptable degree of pain or distress to the patient.

Futility: One of the most contentious terms of all is perhaps "futility". Medical treatment could be deemed to be "futile" if it was not achieving its aim: but this begs the much bigger question as to what *is* the aim of medicine in cases such as these. Again, the range of answers would depend on one's views on the meaning and importance of the sanctity of life and the importance to be given to autonomy. If life in *any* form, including permanent unconsciousness, is sacred, then treatment cannot be futile as long as it is still assisting the patient to live. If sanctity of life is understood as the principle of accepting life as a "gift" which one cannot refuse, but which one is not required to prolong at all costs, then treatment may not be futile unless the patient is actually dying, or the treatment is causing unacceptable pain or distress. If, on the other hand, what is believed to be sacred about life is more than physical existence, then treatment might be regarded as futile if it cannot help return the patient to a state in which they can enjoy what *they* would regard as an acceptable quality of life.

Justice: Finally it may be helpful to raise the issue of the principle of justice. As with many other principles, there is no consensus on how it should be defined: definitions offered by philosophers include making decisions on people's *needs,* on their *entitlements* or their *deserts.* Other approaches would be to argue justice requires us to give equal consideration to people's interests or to satisfy claims in proportion to their relative strengths. Given that the NHS will always have a finite budget, the way justice is interpreted could have a major impact on decisions on the withholding or withdrawing of treatment.

An approach based on "need" or equal consideration of interests might suggest that treatment to preserve life should always take priority over treatment to improve the quality of life, on the basis that the need in the former case will always be greater. Alternatively, it could be argued that patients in pvs are not aware of any benefit from the treatment they are receiving, and hence could not be said to "need" it.

An argument based on "entitlement" might be developed in quite different directions: either that everyone is entitled to the same amount of healthcare resource (and hence spending large amounts treating very incapacitated patients could not be justified if this would reduce the amount left over for everyone else), or that life itself is such a basic "entitlement" that it should always be given priority.

An emphasis on "desert" might bring in factors such as whether patients have themselves contributed to their own state of ill health. Finally, an approach which emphasised satisfying claims in proportion to their strength would lead to a greater proportion of healthcare resources being devoted to those with greatest need for treatment, but would always have to give *some* consideration to weaker claims.

Extracted from "Medical Treatment (Prevention of Euthanasia) Bill". House of Commons Library Research Paper No 00/8, Jan 24th 2000 with permission. © House of Commons Library 2000.

The Patients' Protection Bill

In 2003 Baroness Knight of Collingtree introduced The Patients' Protection Bill [HL] to Parliament in the House of Lords. The aim of the Bill was to "Prohibit the withdrawal or withholding of sustenance with the intention of causing the death of a patient." The Bill received its second reading on March 12th 2003. The debate was thoughtful and wide-ranging and was fully recorded in Hansard.[1]

Baroness Knight sought to protect countless vulnerable people whose lives have been put at risk by lax interpretation of the judgment in the Bland case. Their Lordships appreciated the gravity of the situation but failed to come up with the solution. The debate touched on extremely complex issues that could not be covered in the time available.

Baroness Finlay of Llandaff who is a Professor of Palliative Care raised concerns about the legislation on behalf of her colleagues in palliative care, who feared that their freedom to withhold or withdraw hydration or nutrition would be restricted.

Baroness Andrews also opposed the Bill and presented the Government view.

Earl Howe seemed to be in favour of the Bill at first but then expressed concern. He thought that the kindest approach to patients in PVS was not to strive to keep them alive. Speaking about the Bland case judgment he said:

"Whether the Law Lords were right or wrong to decide that nutrition and hydration constitute medical treatment is, in a sense, neither here nor there: debating that issue is like dancing on a pin. The issue for us is whether food and water should be regarded as separate and distinct from conventional medical treatment and whether the right for every patient, however ill, to receive food and water should be safeguarded in law." (Hansard [1] col 1426)

Lord Alton supported the Bill and said:

"...By calling nutrition and hydration medical treatments the courts, the Government, the BMA and the GMC have over-medicalised sustenance and have opened the way to the killing of vulnerable, particularly elderly patients in our hospitals. Regardless of whether nutrition and hydration is given by a spoon, by PEG or by nasogastric tube, it does not alter the substance itself. To talk of artificial hydration and nutrition is a complete misnomer..." He then quoted the views of Lord Hoffman in his judgment in the Bland case. (Hansard[1] col.1415).

Lord Brennan, a lawyer with a distinguished medical negligence practice, stressed that:

"less extreme cases than Bland should be approached with extreme caution...Parliament must have a role, this is not a medical question alone. Yet as a society we have accepted in large part that it is for the BMA and the GMC to determine the manner in which these decisions should be made by doctors. Do doctors have the moral or social capacity to do that? What role do families have in these decisions? What role do resources have in these decisions? Those are basic questions which we would expect this House and another place, to consider."

"In our society, the ultimate surety for the value of human life is Parliament, speaking for the moral will of the people. It is not, if I may respectfully suggest, government; it is not, if the noble Baroness will accept, necessarily in the Bill that she has presented; and it is certainly not in the Bill which the noble Lord, Lord Joffe, intends to present. We must be very clear that the issue of euthanasia, and that which might be thought to be euthanasia, will not go away. It is central in our social and moral debate in this country. If a resolution is not reached in this debate, there will be others in which we will have to grapple with it. I hope that in today's debate and later, that sentiment is borne in mind. We should be deciding questions which profoundly affect the way in which our society accepts and deals with the value of human life." (Hansard [1] col 1420)

Lord Carlile of Berriew, also a distinguished lawyer supported the Bill. He said: "The Bill seeks to declare unlawful a purpose which plainly is and should be unlawful- on moral, religious, utilitarian and legal grounds." He welcomed the fact that the Bill gave Parliament an opportunity to consider the moral, social and legal issues raised by the Bland case. As the son of a doctor he had been a lay member of the General Medical Council for 10 years. He knew that "Doctors need to know where they stand" but felt that the guidance given by the GMC in August 2002 was "not as clear as it could be".

"If the GMC is unable to tell them exactly where they stand, then the general law- and that means Parliament- has to tell them...Doctors have to make critical judgements on critical issues, at critical times. But they should be left to make their judgement with a clear understanding of where they stand if they cross the line and deliberately cause death- that is what is achieved by this Bill. What cannot be acceptable is the deliberate withdrawal of the very basis of human life-food and water, nutrition and hydration. The withdrawal of food and water cannot have a therapeutic purpose. On its own it can only lead to death...This Bill provides, at the very least, a basis for greater clarity in the law." (Hansard [1] col 1422.)

Lord Toombs felt that the proposition was a very simple one: "... doctors owe a duty of care to their patients. Any weakening of that long-recognised principle would have profoundly undesirable effects, leading to a breakdown in trust in the long-standing belief that doctors act in the best interests of their patients..." He was critical of the BMA guidance, and felt that the Bill "would uphold the respect for life that underpins our society and would provide a clear reminder of the purpose of medicine in that society."

"The courts in the Bland case called for parliamentary examinations of the overall position, which has not been forthcoming. The Government and their predecessors can take no satisfaction from their failure to do so. But the practices that have resulted from that inactivity, coupled with misreading of the Bland judgment, have produced a quite unacceptable position. The Bill provides a restatement of the present law in clear and unambiguous terms and, in doing so, reaffirms our society's respect for life and provides support for patients and their relatives. I believe that it is a modest and necessary measure that demands our support." (Hansard [1] col 1409-1410)

During the Committee stage the Bill was amended with several new clauses. The amendments were debated again in the House of Lords on May 20th 2003 [2]. Once more Earl Howe, Baroness Finlay and Baroness Andrews were prominent with expressions of concern. After an hour of discussion, time ran out. Nothing more has been heard of the Bill since.

In conclusion

The issue, as Earl Howe rightly said is 1) whether food and water should be regarded as separate and distinct from conventional medical treatment, and 2) whether the right of every patient, however ill, to receive food and water, should be protected in law.

Many people believe that the answer to the first question should be a resounding YES. Food and water should be regarded as separate and distinct from conventional medical treatment. The answer to the second question should be a qualified YES. In principle all people however ill should have the right to receive food and water and this right should be protected in law.

Given the disastrous effect that the Bland ruling has had on medical ethics Parliament must find a way to protect vulnerable patients. One possible solution might be to permit the withdrawal of ANH from patients who are undoubtedly in a permanent vegetative state with the prior approval of a judge, providing that their relatives do not disagree with such a decision, and providing that high technology brain scans show no evidence of significant brain activity such as a response to human speech. A very firm line should then be drawn to ensure that people in a "near PVS" state, or a "minimally conscious state" are protected [3].

Since the right of patients *to refuse* treatment including food and water is well established, the right of patients *to receive* food and water, howsoever given, should also be recognised and protected in law. However clinical factors will make it unwise or impossible to provide ANH under all circumstances.

References

1. Patients' Protection Bill [HL] Official Report; *Hansard,* March 12th 2003, cols 1402-1436 *HMSO.* © Parliamentary Copyright House of Lords 2003.
2. Patients' Protection Bill [HL] Official Report; *Hansard,* May 20th 2003, cols 768-784.
3. "The minimally conscious state. Definition and diagnostic criteria." A special article endorsed by the American Academy of Neurology and others. *Neurology.* **58**: 349-353.

Acknowledgement

Parliamentary copyright material from *Hansard* is reproduced with the permission of the Controller of Her Majesty's Stationary Office on behalf of Parliament.

The Mental Capacity Act (2005)

The Mental Capacity Act [2005] is an immensely complex and controversial piece of legislation. It has proved controversial for a number of reasons, but chiefly because of concerns that it will promote euthanasia by omission through the withdrawal of medical treatment including ANH. A Government Minister Mr David Lammy, speaking in the House of Commons in December 2004 promised that: "We want to ensure, however, that under the Bill it is not possible for someone by omission to act to assist suicide or euthanasia" [1]. The Lord Chancellor made a similar pledge in the House of Lords.[2] Many people hope there will be a genuine attempt to amend the Act in accordance with the promises made.

The Act makes advance refusals of treatment legally binding, but advance requests for treatment will not be enforceable. The Act will enable third parties to take life or death healthcare decisions on behalf of adults with mental incapacity. People while still compos mentis, will be able to appoint a relative or friend to take such decisions for them should they become mentally incapacitated.

Lord Rix speaking in the House of Lords in January 2005 thought that the Bill was: "…fundamentally about empowering people to make as many decisions as they can, or to be as big a part of the decision-making process as possible…" He stressed three crucial issues: *Firstly* the need to strike the right balance between autonomy and protection; *Secondly* the issue of End-of-Life decisions; and *Thirdly* the need for independent advocacy. [3]

Lord Brennan spoke at length and expressed concern during the Bill's Second Reading in the House of Lords in January 2005. He described three examples of incapacity. *Firstly* there are those who are born brain damaged and will never have capacity or cognitive function, yet can love and be loved. *Secondly* there are those who once had capacity, who by illness or accident have lost it, and *thirdly* there are the physically disabled, who suffer a head injury and are awkward or difficult to deal with, yet have capacity. Lord Brennan said:

> "Those three examples – of permanent incapacity, the onset of incapacity and the challenge of capacity – illustrate the enormously complex range of matters we are discussing. On the one hand those who are against the Bill should not find succour in the strident, either in the tone or content of their contributions. On the other hand those in favour should not find succour in the belief that the Bill has a good purpose and that all problems can be solved in the end by a good code of practice. That is not good enough for effective legislation in a complex area.

> *"What are the complexities? First, the matter is complex.* The code of practice, covering seven categories of people, runs to 136 pages. My noble friends Lady Pitkeathley and Lady Royall confirmed the importance of educating those who might be involved in those problems about everything related to the matter. On palliative care, a decision made about incapacity and what someone wants to be done about his life, taken when poorly informed, is not a fair, just or proper basis for ultimately terminating that

life. People must appreciate that palliative care has changed the horizon of death and created dignity for the dying, to a far greater extent than it ever did in the past.

"*The second point of complexity is the question of mental capacity*. It can vary from somebody who is teetering on the brink to somebody who is totally incapable in terms of mental function. Who is to judge? Should it be the local GP, if it is a difficult case- and how? Should it be a nurse or carer- and how? Who is to decide when the stage of incapacity has been reached and when a court, attorney or deputy can act as the proxy? These are serious issues, and the code of practice must include an effective way to determine capacity.

"*The third area of complexity relates to "best interests"*. Clause 4 deals with a process of acquiring evidence, but it does not give us criteria for what are the best interests, personal or financial, that will dictate a decision, yeah or nay, in favour of particular medical decisions. No criteria are given. Subsections (5) and (10) are on the periphery of criteria but do not give them. If the Bill does not tell us what best interests are- whether they depend on the opinions of the family, the quality of life, intolerability, which are nebulous concepts- who is to determine them and how? That is a serious question.

"*I turn next to the effect of advance direction*. That they should be in writing seems obvious, otherwise the person who is subject to incapacity might become the victim of his own capricious comment, which may have been oft-repeated. It should be in writing; but what of the state of affairs when, as time goes by, Clause 25(4) does not operate, and the doctor, whatever the terms of the advance direction, decides that he is medically satisfied that it is not in the patient's best interests to terminate treatment? What is then to happen? Is the doctor to go to court as the Bill envisages? Is the advance decision to become mandatory, even in circumstances in which pursuing the notion of autonomy actually damages the patient's best interests? How would one resolve the conflict between the doctor and the patients if the doctor genuinely believes that treatment should continue? If it is to be a decision of a court, I return to the question of "best interests." What are they? [4]

"*Finally, there is the question of the withdrawal of artificial nutrition and hydration*. The fear expressed by many is not that the Bill is intended to introduce euthanasia by omission- that is patently absurd- but that by its terms it might create the risk of that event. Therefore, they are saying, we must get the terms right. Clause 58 rehearses the existing criminal law: murder or manslaughter or assisted suicide involving acts of commission, not omission. The query then arises of how the Bill deals with the problem of termination of treatment which by omission- stopping the treatment- causes a death.

"Perhaps I may remind the House of what Bland was about: someone in a permanent vegetative state. The Official Solicitor's position was that to withdraw treatment was murder. The House of Lords decided that it was not murder because to withdraw treatment was an omission and did not come within the definition of murder. But the patient was in a permanent vegetative state, had no prospect of recovery and was completely insensate. In the House of Lords' finding for the doctor and the decision to withdraw treatment 2 of the 5 (Judges) said, "This is not for us to decide. This is an issue for Parliament to decide on behalf of the country."

"What the House of Lords had in mind surely was not the Bland case but where the patient is sensate to some degree. There may or may not be a question of recovery; prognosis as well as diagnosis may be exceptionally difficult. Are you then to withdraw treatment and rely on Bland or some notion of best interests that appears to be reasonable in the circumstances of the particular case? That seems to many to be extremely dangerous because it raises the prospect that somebody who is not in a permanent vegetative state and who is not dying can have treatment withdrawn, which will end his life. I know of no other way to describe that than euthanasia. If there is a risk, let the Bill clear away that risk by proper amendment...

"It does not really matter what we think the Bill means, what we hope it means or what we intend it to mean; a Bill like this means what it says. If it says that euthanasia by omission is acceptable by inference, I have counted seven or eight public statements- not just by pro-euthanasia lobbyists, but by health economists- saying that living wills should be given to every patient coming into hospital because it will save a lot of money as well as help those who favour euthanasia.

"These are genuine concerns. This House of ours is not a crystalline ethical world in which we are all capable of taking perfectly rational and enlightened decisions. That is not the real world. This Bill will be tested many times as to its scope and effect. It is our obligation to get it right..." [4]

The Mental Capacity Bill was passed in March 2005 amid scenes of chaos and confusion in the House of Commons. The legislation was so controversial that last minute negotiations went on behind the scenes, between the Lord Chancellor and a senior representative from the Roman Catholic Church as the Bill was being debated. At a late stage of the debate, copies of a letter fluttered down over the Labour Party benches. The letter appeared to promise amendments that appeased dissident Members of Parliament. Consequently many MPs who had planned to oppose the legislation, in defiance of Labour Party policy, voted in favour, and the Government narrowly escaped defeat. Many people will be watching very carefully to see whether the promised amendments materialise. The Mental Capacity Act is due to come into force in April 2007.

In summary

The Mental Capacity Act [2005] will enable people, when compos mentis, to indicate in advance, their preferences on matters such as life-sustaining treatment or the provision of ANH. It will also enable them to appoint a trusted friend or relative to act as their attorney or proxy to take life and death decisions on their behalf should the need arise, when they cannot communicate, or decide for themselves by virtue of mental incapacity. A doctor will be obliged to comply with an advance refusal of treatment including ANH or risk imprisonment. However those who refuse life-sustaining treatment in advance may live to regret their decision. If they are still able to tell people that they have changed their mind, all will be well. But if they can no longer communicate their wishes, they risk dying of some eminently treatable illness.

A Consultant Physician once told a cautionary tale about a patient who had been admitted after a severe stroke. The doctors worked very hard on him and pulled him through, only to discover that he had signed an advance directive prohibiting treatment under such circumstances. The doctor apologised to the patient and said that if it happened again they would let him go. "Oh, that's alright doctor,"- said the patient, "Please keep on treating me"!"

Life-sustaining treatment covers a wide range of interventions as listed in chapter 1 of this book, so a person chosen to give or withhold consent on behalf of a mentally incapacitated individual will have the power of life and death. Note that no one can demand any form of treatment, not even tube feeding. The offer of life-sustaining treatment must come from the doctor, to be accepted or rejected in accordance with an advance directive or on the decision of the patient's attorney.

According to an article in the *Daily Mail* of January 30th 2006, the Department of Constitutional Affairs has issued a 'lasting power of attorney' form that is out for consultation. When the final form of words is agreed the ten-page-long form will be available through GP surgeries, hospitals and solicitors. Under the heading "Life-sustaining treatment" the draft form invites people to tick a box to answer "Yes" or "No" to the statement *"I wish to give my attorney(s) authority to give or refuse consent to life-sustaining treatment on my behalf."* Once that statement has been ticked and the attorney chosen the form will be registered with the Office of the Public Guardian, and the information will be available to your doctor. [5]

So the worst fears of those who opposed this dangerous legislation will be realised. The Mental Capacity Act will indeed increase the risk of euthanasia by omission. In our brave new world you will be able to sign away your life with a tick in a box! Beware and think very carefully before you do so.

References

1. Lammy D. Hansard. Official Report, House of Commons, December 14th 2004. Col 1580. *HMSO*. © Parliamentary Copyright House of Commons.
2. See comments by Lord Alton. Hansard. Official Report, House of Lords, Vol.668. No 18, January 10th 2005 col 80. *HMSO*. © Parliamentary Copyright House of Lords 2005.
3. Lord Rix. Hansard. As reference 2 above, cols 49-50.
4. Lord Brennan. Hansard. As reference 2 above, at cols 84-87.
5. Doughty S. Tick here to end your life. *Daily Mail*, January 30th 2006, pages 1 and 8.

Acknowledgement

Parliamentary copyright material from *Hansard* is reproduced with the permission of the Controller of Her Majesty's Stationary Office on behalf of Parliament.

Further reading

❑ Craig GM. Who decides? The law and mentally incapacitated patients. *Catholic Medical Quarterly* 2004; Vol. **LIV No 3**: 5-17.
❑ Craig GM. No man is an island: some thoughts on advance directives. *Catholic Medical Quarterly* 1999; **Vol. XLIV** No 3: 7-14.
❑ Draft Mental Incapacity Bill. Report of House of Lords, House of Commons Joint Committee, Session 2002-03. Volume 1: Report together with formal minutes. Volume II: Oral and written evidence. HMSO November 28th 2003.
❑ The Government Response to the Scrutiny Committee's Report on the draft Mental Incapacity Bill. *HMSO* February 2004.
❑ **Note**. A person can declare an interest in being kept alive, fed, hydrated and treated appropriately to sustain life and restore health where possible. While such a directive is not legally binding it may be a helpful guide to those responsible for making difficult decisions for the mentally incompetent. For further information see www. donoharm.org.uk/alert

Chapter 6

Further Guidance on Giving and Withholding Life-prolonging Treatment

Introduction

This chapter, compiled by Dr Gillian Craig, covers a number of sources of guidance on the thorny issue of giving, withholding and withdrawing life-prolonging medical treatment, including hydration and nutrition that is provided by means such as tube feeding. Some of the guidelines that are considered preceded the BMA guidelines others came into being in their wake. No guidance is perfect for the subject is exceedingly complex and controversial. Guidance on the ethical use of artificial hydration in terminally ill cancer patients is not included for that subject was covered in Challenging Medical Ethics Volume One. The European Palliative Care Guidelines of 1996 provide a useful basis for clinical decision-making on the provision of hydration and nutrition in terminally ill cancer patients, and could also prove helpful in other clinical situations, for example in stroke patients who cannot swallow. The chapter shows how carefully these matters have been considered by the medical profession and by respected judges, yet a nagging doubt remains as to the legality of some of the guidance on offer. Guidance that permits the withholding of artificial nutrition and hydration from sentient patients may yet be shown to contravene the European Convention on Human Rights.

1. The Views of the Medical Ethics Alliance

The Medical Ethics Alliance (MEA) came into being in 1999 in protest against the publication of the BMA's guidance document *Withholding and Withdrawing Life-prolonging Medical Treatment*. The MEA is an association of World Faith organisations and individuals, who share a common ethos, as stated in the Hippocratic Oath or Code of Practice and the Declaration of Geneva of 1948. The MEA is respectful of life. It is sure of the dignity of all persons. It places sound ethics at the centre of good practice. It seeks to promote open and informed debate within the profession and elsewhere. Since its formation in 1999 the MEA has organised several conferences and joined in professional, public and parliamentary debates on medical and ethical matters.

The Medical Ethics Alliance affirms the unique value of all human life, its God given dignity and consequent right to protection in law. We are certain that all persons are of inestimable worth, irrespective of illness or disability. The pursuit and practice of medical excellence is dependent upon sound ethical principles. The alliance looks to the Declaration of Geneva for inspiration.

The Medical Code of Ethics Declaration of Geneva 1948

NB. The Declaration of Geneva is the Hippocratic Oath reformulated.

"At the time of being admitted as a Member of the medical profession I solemnly pledge myself to consecrate my life to the service of humanity. I will give to my teachers the respect and gratitude which is their due. I will practice my profession with conscience and with dignity. The health of my patients will be my first consideration. I will respect the secrets which are confided in me. I will maintain by all means in my power, the honour and noble traditions of the medical profession. My colleagues will be my brothers. I will not permit considerations of religion, nationality, race, party politics or social standing to intervene between my duty and my patient. I will maintain the utmost respect for human life, from the time of its conception, even under threat. I will not use my medical knowledge contrary to the laws of humanity. I make these promises solemnly, freely and upon my honour…"

Note. The Declaration of Geneva was a post-war response to the atrocities committed by doctors in Nazi Germany. The Medical Code of Ethics was formulated at the Second General Assembly of the World Medical Association in 1948. It remains relevant and necessary. The Declaration of Geneva is fully supported by members of the Medical Ethics Alliance, by the World Federation of Doctors Who Respect Human Life (WFD), and by First Do No Harm- (a British offshoot of the WFD.)

Doctors who say "no" to death

Writing in *The Catholic Herald* of 20th August 1999 Dr Anthony Cole the chairman of the MEA expressed concerns about the BMA guidance and indicated, with reference to events in the Netherlands, the dangers of the direction in which events in the UK are moving. He noted that in 1994 the House of Lords' Select Committee on Medical Ethics concluded that there were no sufficient arguments to weaken society's prohibition of intentional killing, since the prohibition was the corner stone of law and social relationships. Their Lordship's report was accepted by Parliament but the Rubicon had already been crossed. Dr Cole explained the situation as follows:

"…The Rubicon had already been crossed in the case of Airedale Trust v Anthony Bland. This Hillsborough victim in the so-called persistent vegetative state (PVS) was believed to be unaware and to have no interest in remaining alive. It was ruled that water given by tube constituted part of his medical care. As such it was optional and dependent on clinical judgement. With the proviso that all such cases must be brought into court an appeal was eventually upheld in the House of Lords and the homicide law was effectively changed. The intentional causing of death by removing one of life's necessities, namely water, was allowed.

This thinking was to trickle down to the next stratum: that of demented and severely brain-damaged patients. This took a significant step forward with the publication of the BMA's guidance…(which) was explicitly meant to apply to patients with weeks, months, and years to live. Severe stroke patients and the senile demented were particularly mentioned.

"The guidance is cold and legalistic throughout. It is almost totally bereft of ethical argument or moral reasoning. Under its terms the stroke patient who has difficulty in swallowing, a not uncommon eventuality, would depend for survival on the opinion of two doctors or the willingness of their relatives to fight for them in court. Even here the cards would be stacked against them as the courts would be expected to be influenced by the guidelines- the work of seven people and never endorsed by the BMA membership.

"Despite the timing of the release of the document so as to forestall debate at the annual representatives meeting 13 days later, doctors in faith groups, others as individuals and members of avowedly Hippocratic medical associations rapidly came together to mount a challenge to the death ethic. The Medical Ethics Alliance came into being following the strong action of Cardinal Thomas Winning, joined by the British Council of Muslim Health Committees and the Office of the Chief Rabbi. When before has such a group been so quickly united?

"The debate is also becoming more public as individuals question what happened to their relations, mainly elderly parents, some of whom were apparently neglected, sedated and dehydrated sometimes to death. Nurses have made complaints leading to investigations by the police, files have been forwarded to the Crown Prosecution Service and at least one private prosecution is pending. The extreme reluctance of judges to think ill of doctors is coming up against increasing calls from members of the public who want explanations of what is happening to their loved ones.

"It used to be obvious that if a patient needed water and would suffer from lack of it, it was part of basic care to relieve their thirst. A cup of water for the dying was the absolutely irreducible Christian and human act of solidarity.

"The words from the Cross "I thirst" carry the sting of reproach to this day."

© Dr Anthony Cole 1999. Extract reprinted with permission.

Medical Ethics Alliance Guidance

This guidance is based on submissions made in 1999 to the BMA's consultation on withholding and withdrawing medical treatment. It is both critical and complimentary to the document 'Withholding and Withdrawing life-prolonging treatments; a guidance on decision making' published by the BMA in June 1999. It is intended as a contribution towards an ongoing discussion within the profession.[1]

The decision to withdraw or withhold treatments is usually based on clinical considerations but certain ethical principles are involved. These principles will be discussed below. Many are also enshrined in laws and international treaties. They include a respect for life, sometimes referred to as the sanctity of life, arising from the concept that life itself is God-given. This right is central to the United Nations Universal Declaration of Human Rights and is also foremost in the European Convention of Human Rights. It has long been established in national law as the law of homicide.

The concept of justice is fundamental and the first consideration is to whom is justice owed? The United Nations Universal Declaration of Human Rights makes this clear. It is owed to all members of the human family. No distinctions based on illness are made- justice is owed to all persons.

Within medicine there is also a strong tradition of ethics concerning obligations towards patients. This is what one must do, as well as what one may not do. It is at the heart of the doctor/patient relationship. Justice also recognises the fundamental equality, value and dignity of persons. These are not diminished by illness or disability. No person should be subject to arbitrary discrimination. In the medical context a judgement about a person's essential worth should not be made on the basis of some quality that they may have, such as the ability to communicate or enter into a relationship with others. Lack of these qualities do not in themselves provide a reason for aiming to end their lives.

Who should receive assisted food and fluid?

Any decision is likely to be clinically based and made on the basis of limited information. It may need to be adjusted as new evidence emerges. Two general principles may be taken into consideration, however. First is the patient in need of food and water given this way? Secondly would they suffer if it was not given?

Very occasionally the risk to the patient or evident burdensomeness of the method of giving the food and fluid may make it contraindicated.

The discontinuation of assisted food and fluid does involve more than the emotional problems referred to in the BMA guidance and there are differences in law and medicine between a decision *ab initio* from one made after review.

Leaving aside the legal requirements which vary between Scotland and England and Wales, when may food and fluid itself dependent on a medical procedure, be withdrawn?

The report of the Select Committee on Medical Ethics, House of Lords 1994 which followed the Bland Judgment, is helpful. Its conclusions were accepted by Parliament (but strangely are not mentioned in the BMA's guidance). In its conclusion the report stated:

' …development and ultimate acceptance of the notion that some treatment
is inappropriate, should make it unnecessary to consider the withdrawal
of nutrition and hydration except…where its administration is in itself
evidently burdensome to the patient.' [2]

We think this represents helpful and authoritative guidance. It also seems to be in conformity with the overwhelming practice of clinicians caring for permanent vegetative state patients.

Euthanasia

It has been defined as an'easy death' or as 'mercy killing'. Here we will suggest the definition- the intentional killing by act or omission of a person where life is felt to be not worth living.[3]

To have as the intention, aim and object the taking of life is contrary to justice and the doctor/patient relationship and is furthermore unnecessary because compassion does not require us to kill the patient to kill the symptoms. A respect for people is also to recognise that they are mortal. Ultimately death must be accepted and inappropriate treatment withdrawn.

Curing and Caring

The objects of medicine have been traditionally threefold. The restoration of health, even when this may only be partial, but which serves the patient's well-being. The prolongation of life, but not by any or all means. A proportionality should be sought and a balance struck between the benefits to the patient and burdens of treatment. When death itself approaches the role of medicine changes to palliative care. This is a holistic concept of relieving symptoms and offering spiritual and psychological support. Here the aim of treatment is to enable the patient to continue human flourishing through interaction with friends and family. When this is not possible the duty of care remains. There is never a duty to kill.[4]

Which doctor?

Patient care is now usually delivered by medical teams. These comprise senior and junior doctors, nurse and paramedics and the carers themselves. When decisions have to be made, especially major management ones, they are best made by the senior doctor with the agreement of the rest of the team. It should not be forgotten that the nurses and carers are closest to the patient. It is important that all are comfortable with decisions. Members of the team with a conscientious objection to a course of action should not be overridden, least of all eliminated from that area of medicine or considered as acting anomalously. Where grave issues are concerned and there is no agreement say between the medical team and the relatives or carers, the Family Division of the High Court is available to help. It should not be left to relatives to get their own legal advisers. Trusts should come to their immediate assistance with appropriate advice as to where and how help can be obtained.

Conscientious Decisions

All patients have a general right to a second opinion if they are not in agreement with decisions regarding their treatment. They may, themselves, or through their relatives request this. It is not part of a doctor's responsibility though to find another doctor to do something which he himself considers to be medically or ethically wrong.

Doctors or nurses on a team may conscientiously withdraw if they are not in agreement with decisions taken. They should not be put under an obligation to prove that their objection is on conscientious grounds.

There is a large and settled body of medical opinion for administering food and water by such techniques as inserting a feeding tube or a percutaneous endoscopic gastrostomy (PEG). Since the Bland Judgment in 1993 only a tiny number of PVS patients have had withdrawal decisions made in court. This may reflect difficulties in diagnosis or prognosis but in particular the views of doctors, nurses and relatives. It remains very uncommon to intentionally cause death by dehydration even in PVS.[5] In effect this reflects a strong view which is at variance with that implicit in the BMA guidance document.

Best Interests

The duty of care requires doctors to treat patients in their best interests. This should normally be concerned with their restoration to health, prevention of death or disability and relief of symptoms.

Treatment choices depend upon free and informed consent. There is no obligation to treat in a disproportionate or burdensome way and indeed, futile treatments should be withheld or withdrawn bearing in mind that clinical situations change. 'The art of medicine involves making decisions on limited amounts of information and expecting to adjust or correct them as new evidence emerges.'[2]

Advance Decision Making

This may be of a general nature and could be verbal or written. It becomes an advance directive seeking to bind when it takes the form of an advance refusal of treatment. Contrary to the impression in the BMA guidance, there is at present no case law on written advance refusals.

It seems likely that the patient would have had to have at least the competence to make a valid will. That is to say not acting under undue influence and in health decisions, also possessing sufficient information to make a valid decision. The circumstances arising, in fact, must be those that were foreseen and where there is uncertainty, the treatment given should be that which is in the patient's best interests. In practice doctors confronted with a document should treat the patient rather than a piece of paper. It is also the case that it is far more likely that if the patient suffers permanent harm that claims for damages will follow. When in doubt about the applicability or otherwise of an advance directive, it would be wise to seek legal assistance. Where the patient is unconscious the patient should be treated with the general presumption of preserving life.[6]

What about the dying?

For the dying patient, fluids should be offered by mouth and in such amounts as the patient wishes. Other forms of administration may be required but in accordance with the needs of patient comfort rather than to maintain organic systems per se. [7]

Conclusion

The Hippocratic moral tradition and the insights of the Major World Faiths reinforce one another. The ethical framework of medicine crosses frontiers and contains ageless concepts. The conscientious doctor will seek to act with integrity and within an ethical frame. Law is not a substitute for ethics but through the law society protects the vulnerable and the common good.

© 2000. Medical Ethics Alliance. Reprinted with permission.

References

1. Medical Ethics Alliance, PO Box 11582, Edgbaston, Birmingham B16 9XE, United Kingdom.
    e-mail: ethicsalliance@aol.com   www.medethics-alliance.org
2. Report of the Select Committee on Medical Ethics. House of Lords. *HMSO* 1994. Para. 257.
3. *Christian Medical Fellowship Bulletin* No. 7, 1999.
4. Consultation - *The Linacre Centre* London.
5. Christian Medical Fellowship submission to the BMA 1999.
6. *Catholic Medical Quarterly* Vol XLIX. No. 280. 1998.
7. Note. This was the view of the MEA in 1999. For further discussion please see Challenging Medical Ethics Volume 1. "No Water-No Life: Hydration in the Dying". Ed Craig GM, *Fairway Folio*. 2005.

2. European Palliative Care Association Guidelines of 1996

Bozzetti F (coordinator) Guidelines on artificial nutrition versus hydration in terminal cancer patients. Nutrition. 1996, Vol. 12, No.3: pp 169-172. © 1996 by Elsevier Science Inc.
All copyright material is used with permission from Elsevier.

Some helpful guidelines were published in 1996. They were prepared in 1995 by a Committee convened under the auspices of the European Association for Palliative Care. The issue of "whether a terminally ill cancer patient should be actively fed or simply hydrated through subcutaneous or intravenous infusion …(was) a matter of ongoing controversy at the time." The aim of the Committee was "to prepare guidelines to help clinicians make a reasonable decision on what type of nutritional support should be provided on a case-by-case basis to terminally ill cancer patients".

The Committee of seventeen experts was co-ordinated by Federico Bozzetti of Milan. The Committee had members from North America (Eduardo Bruera of Canada, and Mark Mantell from the USA) and members from Australia, France, Belgium and Switzerland but none from the UK. Committee members included physicians, a nurse expert in the provision of home parenteral nutrition (HPN), a relative of a cancer patient treated with HPN and a young patient who was on HPN.

The aim of the Committee was to determine whether artificial nutrition or simple hydration should be recommended for the terminal phase of the disease in cancer patients. Since the Committee had difficulty reaching agreement they decided to present "the pivotal elements involved in making such decisions, avoiding rigid treatment guidelines." The end result of their deliberations was a useful three step, clinically orientated process that could be applied not only in terminally ill cancer patients, but also in a wide range of other conditions where the provision of hydration and nutrition is problematical.

The Bozzetti Three Step Process for decisions on the provision of assisted nutrition versus hydration in terminal care

Step 1   Assess patient according to eight key clinical criteria.
        1. Clinical condition.
        2. Symptoms
        3. Expected length of survival.
        4. Hydration and nutritional status.
        5. Spontaneous or voluntary nutrient intake.
        6. Psychological attitude
        7. Gut function and route of administration.
        8. Need for special services based on type of nutritional support prescribed.

Step 2   Make the decision about provision of food and or fluids.

Step 3   Reassess patient and therapy at specified intervals.

Each element in the decision-making process is discussed in detail in the paper in *Nutrition*. Symptoms that may arise from dehydration and protein-calorie malnutrition are listed, as are symptoms that may interfere with food ingestion, and symptoms that are independent of nutritional status. The Committee make the point that: "Identification of symptoms and their relevance makes it easier for the clinician to provide a treatment regimen tailored to the expectations of the individual patient…"

Although devised for terminal cancer patients, the Bozzetti Three Step Process could prove useful in the management of other patients whose life expectancy and response to nutritional support is uncertain. Such patients might include patients with swallowing difficulties due to strokes or other neurological disorders. The European approach of 1996 offers a constructive alternative to the death-orientated end-of-life guidance that dominates current thinking in the UK and the USA.

Some symptoms and consequences of dehydration and starvation, according to Bozzetti and others, are shown in Tables 1 and 2 below.

Table 1   Some symptoms and consequences of dehydration

Thirst * dry mouth and impaired speech
Confusion and restlessness *
Increased risk of bedsores*
Circulatory failure.
Kidney failure* with low urine output
Cardiac arrest.
DEATH
                    [* After Fainsinger et al 1994.]

Table 2   Some symptoms and consequences of starvation.

Weakness, fatigue, anorexia, and nausea
Irritability, loss of concentration, poor judgment
Apathy, dementia-like state, psychosis / depression
Tingling and painful sensations in the limbs,
Hypersensitivity to noise and light,
Swollen legs and weakened heart muscle.
Low body temperature
Diarrhoea, abdominal cramps and vomiting
DEATH.
                    [After Bozzetti 1996 and others.]

---

3. The Views of The Royal College of Paediatrics and Child Health

The Royal College of Paediatrics and Child Health (RCPCH) issued a framework of practice in 1997 after years of discussion and research, prompted by the 1994 House of Lords' Select Committee Report on Medical Ethics. Their Lordships noted evidence from the British Paediatric Association- (later to become the RCPCH)- that the practice of withdrawal of treatment "might not be rare." The Ethics Advisory Committee of the RCPCH felt that the matter should be formally explored and undertook some research. They took advice from people of different beliefs from within the UK and involved parent and patient groups and many other people. Their report of 1997 was entitled "Withholding and Withdrawing Life-Saving Treatment in Children. A framework of practice."

The Ethics Committee of the RCPCH issued a second edition of their report in May 2004. This differed from the first in certain respects, but the basic framework was the same. The publication was entitled "Withholding and Withdrawing Life-Sustaining Treatment in Children: a framework for Practice." In the account that follows all quotes are taken from the May 2004 document unless otherwise stated.

The RCPCH identified five situations where the withholding or withdrawal of curative medical treatment might be considered.[1] These were:
1. The 'Brain Dead' Child.
2. The 'Permanent Vegetative State'
3. The 'No Chance' Situation.
4. The 'No Purpose' Situation and
5. The 'Unbearable' Situation.

These situations were summarised as follows:

1. *The "Brain Dead" Child* [2]. In the older child [3] where criteria of brain death are agreed by practitioners in the usual way [4] it may still be technically feasible to provide basic cardio-pulmonary support by means of ventilation and intensive care. It is agreed within the profession that treatment in such circumstances is futile and the withdrawal of treatment is appropriate.

2. *The "Permanent Vegetative" State* [5,6]. The child who develops a permanent vegetative state following insults, such as trauma or hypoxia, is reliant on others for care and does not react or relate with the outside world. It may be appropriate both to withdraw current therapy and to withhold further curative treatment.

3. *The "No Chance" Situation.* The child has such severe disease that life-sustaining treatment simply delays death without significant alleviation of suffering. Treatment to sustain life is inappropriate.

4. *The "No Purpose" Situation.* Although the patient may survive with treatment, the degree of physical or mental impairment will be so great that it is unreasonable to expect them to bear it.

5. *The "Unbearable" Situation.* The child and/or family feel that in the face of progressive and irreversible illness further treatment is more than can be borne. They wish to have a particular treatment withdrawn or to refuse further treatment irrespective of the medical opinion on its potential benefit.

"In situations that do not fit into these five categories, or where there is uncertainty about the degree of future impairment or disagreement, the child's life should always be safeguarded by all in the Health Care Team until these issues are resolved.

"Decisions must never be rushed and must always be made by the team with all evidence available. In emergencies it is often doctors in training who are called to resuscitate. Rigid rules, even for conditions that seem hopeless, should be avoided and life-sustaining treatment should be administered and continued until a senior or more experienced doctor arrives.

"The decision to withhold or withdraw life-sustaining therapy should always be associated with consideration of the child's overall palliative or terminal care needs. These include symptom alleviation and care, which maintains human dignity and comfort."

On Palliative Care in Children
In 1997 the RCPCH Ethics Advisory Committee said:

"Where treatment aimed at alleviation or cure of a condition has been withdrawn, the clinical team has a duty always to offer palliative care. Palliative care should consider the child's physical needs including the relief of pain and other symptoms and also address the emotional and social and spiritual aspects of care. The child should be nursed in a pleasant, child-centred environment with staff they can trust. The child's dignity should be respected. They should be kept clean, and food and fluid should be offered (but not forced) on a regular basis. The role of assisted feeding for infant or child (by naso-gastric tube or gastrostomy) should be considered very carefully and discussed fully with the family. It may be entirely appropriate, for example, in a child with a swallowing disorder due to progressive neurodegenerative disease, but would rarely be introduced for a child with a rapidly progressive, disseminated malignant disease." (Report at paragraph 3.1.4)

By 2004 the wording had been modified and read as follows:

"The clinical team has a duty always to offer palliative care to children with life-threatening and life-limiting illnesses. It may begin whenever it becomes apparent that the illness may result in premature death. It can be provided alongside treatment aimed to cure or significantly prolong life and should continue as the main focus of care when these treatments are withdrawn or withheld [7]. Palliative care should respect the child's dignity and consider their physical needs including the relief of pain and other symptoms, and also address the emotional, social and spiritual needs of both the child and their family. All these aspects of palliative care can be provided wherever a child and family are cared for- whether in hospital, at home, or in a children's hospice. Careful planning and communication is needed to ensure continuity of care for the child, particularly when they are moving between hospital and home. A key worker (often the paediatric community care nurse) is essential to co-ordinate this, especially where it is anticipated that palliative care may be needed for an extended period of time and involve a number of health care professionals. If the illness is prolonged respite care should be available. (Report at paragraph 3.2.3)

How do you define a severe/intolerable handicap or disability?
The RCPCH Ethics Advisory Committees of 1997 and 2004 agreed that:

"A severe/intolerable disability is indefinable; there are ways of making a disability more tolerable, and an individual sufferer, even with extreme disability, may still attach some value to existence. Judgements of disability are bound up in people's fears and attitudes to disability and can be altered by a change in the environment. Note:
❏ Intolerable may mean "that which cannot be borne" or "that which people should not be asked to bear".
❏ An individual may believe that he/she is an intolerable burden.
❏ An impossibly poor existence may not be recognised by an individual, depending on that person's cognition.
"It is possible to envisage a level of disability that doctors believe to be intolerable, i.e no reasonable person would want to live with it, and yet an individual sufferer may attach value to their existence." (Report of 2004 at para 2.7.3.)

On dissent and conflict
The RCPCH Ethics Committee of 1997 said that where a second opinion is sought:

"It is of course easy for a doctor to secure a second opinion which supports his own. This should be recognised and guarded against...If parental dissent continues, but the Health Care Team agrees on withdrawal of treatment, it would be advisable to consider seeking the involvement of the courts...If time and condition permit, the parents should be at liberty to...move to another consultant if they so wish...The Official Solicitor's Office can be telephoned for advice... Legal support for medical matters would usually be sought from a judge in a High Court..."
(Extract from RCPCH Report of 1997 paras. 3.4.1, 3.4.2, and 3.4.3.)

The report of 2004 contains much helpful advice about how to discuss and communicate decisions to withhold or withdraw treatment, but it does not appear to contain a warning of the need to guard against a second opinion that simply supports the first.

In para 3.4 'Resolution of different opinions', the report of 2004 states:

> "...Unanimity on the part of the Health Care Team is not essential... **Resolving a difference of opinion between the team and the family is** essential and may occasionally require additional input. Under these circumstances the family should still be supported by the team."

In para 3.4.1 'Medical Input' it is suggested that if the problem is one of uncertainty, a second medical opinion could come from a senior clinician "from within the team", but if the disagreement between the health care team and the family is more fundamental "an expert opinion from a senior clinician opinion from outside the unit/ hospital may be preferred... "

The RCPCH Ethics Advisory Committee identified three fundamental ethical principles:
1. Duty of Care and Partnership of Care.
2. The Legal Duty and
3. Respect for Children's Rights.

1. *Duty of Care and Partnership of Care*
The report of 1997 states that:

> "The Healthcare Team has a *Duty of Care* with the primary intention of sustaining life and restoring their patients to health. They and the parents will enter a *Partnership of Care* whose function is to serve the best interests of the child."

By 2004 the wording is more emphatic and reads at paragraph 2.3.1.1:

> "Granted the compelling presumption in favour of life, the Health Care Team has a duty of care with the primary intention of sustaining life and restoring their patients to health. Whether or not the child can be restored to health, there is an absolute duty to comfort and cherish the child and to prevent pain and suffering.
>
> "In fulfilling the obligations imposed by the duty of care, the Health Care Team and parents will enter a partnership of care, whose function is to serve the best interests of the child. This duty of care involves respecting the ascertainable wishes and views of children in the light of their knowledge, understanding and experience. Children should be informed and listened to so that they can participate as fully as possible in decision making."

2. The Legal Duty

Box 1. "All health care professionals are bound to fulfil their duty of care within the framework of the law. The law governing issues of withdrawal or withholding treatment is complex and arguably inconsistent, but it is clear that any practice or treatment given with the primary intention of causing death is unlawful..." (RCPCH reports of 1997 and 2004: para 2.3.1.2)

The RCPCH Ethics Advisory Committee report of 2004 contained additional material on legal matters. Professor Jonathan Montgomery considered the Human Rights Act and the United Nations Convention on the Rights of the Child (1989). The following comments are taken from the RCPCH report of 2004.

2.4. *The Legal Framework*

"The courts have accepted that it is lawful to withdraw life-prolonging treatment when the quality of life the child would have to endure if given the treatment would be so afflicted as to be intolerable to that child.[8] Although there has not yet been a case involving a child, the implementation of the Human Rights Act 1998 has not altered the court's view that withdrawing such treatment in appropriate cases is consistent with patient's human rights.

"Although it is necessary and fundamental to practice within the framework of the law, the Ethics Advisory Committee of the RCPCH believe it is important to define best practice in relation to the interests of the family and the child, rather than presenting the minimal legal requirement. We must look at what is legally permitted and required, but also at what is ethically appropriate, which may exceed the minimal standards set by the law.

"If a doctor wishes to continue treatment of a very ill child, but there is room for reasonable doubt about the benefit, the doctor may be in a difficult position if he continues when the parents have withheld or withdrawn consent. A court might say that the doctor did not act in the child's best interests. In cases of dispute it is good practice to consult the court*. In the meantime, the treatment should be given in the expectation that the court will support the action." (2004 report para.2.4)

*Box 2. "Matters regarding health would normally be considered in the High Court. Court "orders" can only prohibit an intervention or authorise one if medically expedient and in the person's best interests. They cannot oblige doctors to any specific intervention. In Scotland a doctor must take responsibility for treatment decisions and the courts have little or no authority to give sanction to such decisions in advance." (Footnote RCPCH report of 2004, para. 2.4)

3. Respect for Children's Rights

"The United Nations Convention on the Rights of the Child (1989) which has been ratified by the British Government, sets out fundamental principles which govern how children should be treated." (For further information see the RCPCH report of 2004, at paragraph 2.3.1.3).

The case of baby J.

Summarised by Dr Craig.

Legal precedent on the subject of withholding life-prolonging treatment in a child with a seemingly intolerable disability was established in 1990 in the case of a baby known only as J. This case is referred to in the RCPCH Framework and may well have influenced much of the discussion. For the benefit of readers a brief summary of the case may be illuminating.

According to official court records baby J was born on May 28th 1990, some 12 weeks premature. He suffered severe and permanent brain damage at birth and required ventilation and intensive care. Attempts to wean him off the ventilator proved difficult. A brief attempt to send him home in September failed: he was readmitted within days and subsequently collapsed but was resuscitated. By October 1990 the most optimistic medical evidence available was that he was epileptic, and likely to have a spastic paraplegia- that is paralysis of all four limbs. He would also be blind, deaf and severely intellectually disabled. It was thought that he would feel pain to the same extent as a normal child. He had by that time been ventilated twice for long periods when his breathing stopped, this treatment being described as long and painful.

The question arose as to whether doctors should reventilate him if his breathing stopped again. Since baby J was a ward of court, it fell to a High Court Judge, Mr Justice Scott Baker, to make the decision early in October 1990. He made an order that baby J should be treated with antibiotics if he developed a chest infection but should not be reventilated if his breathing stopped unless the doctors caring for him deemed it appropriate.

The Official Solicitor promptly appealed against the order, contending that "except where a child was terminally ill the court could never be justified in approving the withholding of life-saving treatment from a ward of court whatever the quality of the life preserved, or, alternatively, that it ought to do so only if it was certain that the child's life was going to be so intolerable that such drastic action was justified, but that had not been shown to be the case of J."

The Court of Appeal considered the matter on October 15th 1990, the judges being Lord Donaldson, sitting with Mr Justice Balcombe and Mr Justice Taylor. Lord Donaldson spent some time on the general issues raised by the case and the role of the court in decision-making. He did not consider that words such as "demonstrably so awful" or "intolerable" should be used as "a quasi-statutory yardstick" in such cases for "severely handicapped people find a quality of life rewarding which to the unhandicapped may seem manifestly intolerable..." All three judges agreed that the appeal should be dismissed.

Reference. Re J [1990] 3 All ER.

On Impairment and Disability

The RCPCH framework of 1997 contained some wise comments about living with handicap, and tried to define what might be considered an intolerable handicap. The term handicap does not appear in the report of 2004 being replaced by the words "Impairment or Disability." There are other significant changes to note as well.

Both reports state that:

"In 1991 the Court of Appeal accepted that it is unlawful to withdraw life-prolonging treatment when the quality of life the child would have to endure, if given the treatment, would be so afflicted as to be intolerable to that child. The court recognised that a quality of life which could be considered intolerable to an able-bodied person, would not necessarily be unacceptable to a child who has been born disabled. The Ethics Advisory Committee of the RCPCH believes that this means when there is little or no prospect of meaningful interaction with others or the environment. In this situation no reasonable person would want to lead such a life, nor impose on a doctor a duty actively to strive to bring it about." (para.2.7).

Thereafter there were some changes in the wording of paragraph 2.7.1, between 1997 and 2004. Although the wording was similar in most respects one important sentence was omitted in 2004. The relevant text is printed below. The report of 1997 contained the following sentences:

"Many people with severe handicap describe a life of high quality. *The Ethics Advisory Committee of the RCPCH do not support the withdrawal of life sustaining treatment from individuals whose prognosis is such that they may well experience an enjoyable life of high quality; neither does it support the withdrawal of life-sustaining treatment from those who are likely to be able to make judgements about their own future.* Impairment is not incompatible with a life of quality…"

Italics have been added to indicate the sentence that was omitted from the framework of 2004. This suggests that there may have been a major change in attitude to the withdrawal of life-sustaining treatment at the RCPCH between 1997 and 2004. Both reports emphasise the importance of care, but that is not the same as treatment.

The report of 2004 said:

"Many people with severe impairment describe a life of high quality and say they are happy to be living it. Impairment is not incompatible with a life of high quality. Children and adults may not view their disability as negatively as some able-bodied people do, provided adequate support is available. It is important that society does not devalue disabled people or those living with severe impairment. **The Ethics Advisory Committee of the RCPCH strongly believes that the provision of care to those with disability should not be reduced and there must always be a commitment to the provision of high quality care for those with disability.** Sadly there are indications that such children are being discriminated against when they compete for surgery.[9]

"There is a degree of impairment which includes a loss of awareness and an inability to interact. Perhaps this is intolerable disability. Spastic quadriplegia with very severe cognitive and sensory deficits might be one such condition. The burden is not only for the child but also for the parents or their surrogates, and society must also determine how best to share it." (para 2.7.1)

On the subject of Ethics Committees

The RCPCH committee of 1997 felt that:

"An ethics committee is likely to be too remote from the individual case to understand all aspects…usually the medical team has more to contribute to the decision-making process….If ethics committees are to be created they will have to be easily convened and their role would have to be not only supportive but educational [10]…Whichever kind of committee is created the legal and professional responsibility would still lie with the consultant in charge of the case. Any committee created in the UK should be independent of trusts. Both NHS trusts and fund holding GPs may be considered to have financial interest in some management decision. If there is an appeal against a decision to withdraw treatment, the appeal should be considered by medical staff in a trust or practice unassociated with the case."

(Report of 1997, extract from para 3.4.4.)

The report of 2004 said:

"Any UK Clinical Ethics Committee needs to retain its independence so as to secure its moral integrity. It is not clear how this is to be protected in the current Hospital and Primary Care Trust since both may be considered to have some financial interest in the decisions made. It is not clear how these tensions will develop in the future, or what means may be used to reduce them. Whichever model of Clinical Ethics Committee is created, it remains the case that the legal and professional responsibility for decision making still rests with the consultant in charge of the case.

"It is possible that Clinical Ethics Committees may have a role if there is an appeal against a decision to withdraw or withhold treatment made in another Trust and an independent analysis of the case is required."

(Report of 2004 at para 3.4.3).

Acknowledgement. For further information please read the current (2004) RCPCH Framework in full. Copies can be obtained through a good reference library or can be purchased from Direct Books (e mail: elt@bebc.co.uk). Extracts, quoted with permission, are © Royal College of Paediatrics and Child Health. London.

References and notes on the RCPCH Framework

References 1-10 listed below, are as cited in the RCPCH publication of 2004.

1. Withdrawal of curative medical treatment should signal the initiation of palliative care if this has not already been introduced...see section 3.2.4.

2. Definition- Brain death occurs when a child has sustained either (1) irreversible cessation of circulatory and respiratory functions or (2) irreversible cessation of all functions of the entire brain including the brain stem. A determination of death must be made in accordance with accepted medical standards.

3. Original definitions of brain death were not applied to neonates as criteria were thought to be affected by brain immaturity.

4. Task force for the determination of brain death in children: Guidelines for the determination of brain death in children. *Annals of Neurology*, 1987; **21**:616-617. *Pediatrics*, 1987; **80**:298-299.

5. The vegetative state-guidance on diagnosis and management. A Report of a working party of the Royal College of Clinical Medicine (2003) **3**:249-254. Defines the vegetative state and uses the terms "persistent" to mean a vegetative state that has persisted for weeks or more and "permanent" when the vegetative state is deemed to be permanent and it is predicted that awareness will never recover. (See note 11 below)

6. " The persistent vegetative state." Conference of Medical Royal Colleges and their Faculties of the United Kingdom. *Journal of the Royal College of Physicians of London*. 1996; **30**:119-121. (See note 11 below.)

7. Palliative Care for Young People. Report of the Joint Working Party of ACT (The Association for Children with Life-Threatening or Terminal Conditions and their families), the National Council for Hospice and Specialist Palliative care Services and the Scottish Partnership Agency for Palliative care and Cancer Care. 2001.

8. Re J [1991] Fam 33 and Re C (1998) 1FLR 384.]

9. Smith GF et al. The rights of infants with Down's Syndrome. Journal of the American Medical Association. 1984; 251:229. Bull C et al. Should management of complete atrioventricular canal defect be influenced by coexistent Down's syndrome. *Lancet* 1985; ii:1147-1149. A heart for Jo. *The Guardian Weekend*. 10.8.96. Controversy over disabled girls' death in casualty unit. *The Sunday Telegraph*. 29.12.96.

10. Larcher VF, Lask B, McCarthy J. Paediatrics at the cutting edge: do we need clinical ethics committees? *Journal of Medical Ethics* 1997; **23**:245-249.

11. *Note added by Dr Craig.* The RCPCH Framework of 1997 referred to a permanent vegetative state as being- "A state of unawareness of self and environment in which the patient breathes spontaneously, has a stable circulation and shows cycles of eye closure and eye opening which simulates sleep and waking, for a period of twelve months following a head injury, or six months following other causes of brain damage." This is a helpful description.

4. General Medical Council Guidance

The General Medical Council (GMC) issued guidance on "Withholding and withdrawing life-prolonging treatments: good practice in decision-making" in August 2002.[1] The guidance was intended to clarify decision-making at the end of life, and to set a framework for practice that would be ethically and legally permissible when patients are mentally incapacitated and unable to contribute to decision-making. Artificial nutrition and hydration are given special attention in paragraphs 78 to 83.

Paragraph 38 states:

Always consult a clinician with relevant experience (who may be from another discipline such as nursing) in cases where:

❑ You and the health care team have limited experience of the condition.

❑ You are in doubt about the range of options, or the benefits, burdens and risks of a particular option for the individual patient.

❑ You are considering withholding or withdrawing artificial nutrition or hydration from a patient who is not imminently dying, although in a very serious condition, and whose views cannot be determined (see paragraph 81 below).

❑ You and other members of the health care team have a serious difference of opinion about the appropriate options for a patient's care.

Paragraph 81 states:

Where patients have capacity to decide for themselves, they may consent to, or refuse, any proposed intervention of this kind. In cases where patients lack capacity to decide for themselves and their wishes cannot be determined, you should take account of the following considerations:

❑ Where there is a reasonable degree of uncertainty about the likely benefits or burdens for the patient of providing either artificial nutrition or hydration, it may be appropriate to provide these for a trial period with a pre-arranged review to allow a clearer assessment to be made.

❑ Where death is imminent, in judging the benefits, burdens or risks, it usually would not be appropriate to start either artificial hydration or nutrition, although artificial hydration provided by less invasive measures may be appropriate where it is considered that this would be likely to provide symptom relief.

❑ Where death is imminent, and artificial hydration and/or nutrition are already in use, it may be appropriate to withdraw them if it is considered that the burdens outweigh the possible benefits to the patient.

❑ Where death is not imminent, it usually will be appropriate to provide artificial nutrition or hydration. However circumstances may arise where you judge that a patient's condition is so severe, and the prognosis so poor that providing artificial nutrition or hydration may cause suffering or be too burdensome in relation to the possible benefits. In these circumstances, as well as consulting the health care team and those close to the patient, you must seek a second or expert opinion from a senior clinician (who might be from another discipline such as nursing) who has experience of the patient's condition and who is not already involved in the patient's care. This will ensure that, in a decision of such sensitivity, the patient's interests have been thoroughly considered, and will provide necessary reassurance to those close to the patient and to the wider public.

❑ It can be extremely difficult to estimate how long a patient will live[2] especially for patients with multiple underlying conditions. Expert help in this should be sought where you, or the health care team, are uncertain about a particular patient.

Paragraph 82 states:

Where significant conflicts arise about whether artificial nutrition or hydration should be provided, either between you and other members of the health care team or between the team and those close to the patient, and the disagreement cannot be resolved after informal or independent review, you should seek legal advice on whether it is necessary to apply to the court for a ruling.

Paragraph 83 states:

Where you are considering withdrawing artificial nutrition and hydration from a patient with a permanent vegetative state (PVS), or a condition closely resembling PVS, the courts in England, Wales and Northern Ireland currently require you to approach them for a ruling. The courts in Scotland have not specified such a requirement, but you should seek legal advice on whether a court declaration may be necessary in an individual case.

© General Medical Council 2002. Reprinted with permission.

Is the GMC Guidance lawful?

The case of Lesley Burke
Reviewed by Gillian Craig

The GMC Guidance was subjected to severe legal scrutiny in 2004 and 2005 when a patient by the name of Oliver Leslie Burke challenged the legality of the guidance and forced a judicial inquiry in the High Court. Mr Burke had a progressive brain disorder that would, in the course of time prevent him from expressing himself. It would also make normal eating and drinking so difficult that he would require tube feeding to prevent death from dehydration or starvation. He sought reassurance that his wish to receive food and water- by means of tube feeding (ANH) if need be- would be respected.

The case brought many important issues to the surface and revealed chasms of disagreement between the judges concerned. Although a detailed discussion of the legal arguments is beyond the scope of this book, some key points will be considered briefly.

Mr Justice Munby presided over the judicial enquiry in the High Court 2004 and considered the issues carefully. In July 2004 he ruled that several paragraphs of the GMC Guidance were unlawful.[3]

The General Medical Council appealed against the ruling "primarily because it seemed to make important changes in the law. First, it made competent patients' requests for life-prolonging treatment 'in principle determinative' of the treatment they should be given. Second, it redefined the best interests test-used where a patient is incapacitated- so that the 'touchstone' for deciding best interests would be the 'intolerability' of providing or not providing the treatment. Third, it made it a legal requirement in a range of situations, to seek the court's view before withdrawing a life-prolonging treatment." [4]

The Government supported the GMC in their appeal. It was revealed in the *Daily Mail* of February 5th 2005 that John Reid, then Secretary of State for Health, had written to the Appeal Court Judges to express concern about the cost implications of keeping patients alive [5]. John Reid's leaked submission mentioned concern about expenditure of 'scarce resources, regardless of whether those resources might be more effectively deployed elsewhere.' Within days there were questions in Parliament, but the Government spokesman shrugged them off. Within a week John Reid and the Prime Minister were seen on television promising more money for the National Health Service in Kettering- a Midland town in a marginal Labour constituency. When votes are needed and an election looms, money is available!

The legal arguments put forward by Mr Justice Munby were wide-ranging and thorough, his judgment detailed and long. The Appeal Court Judges, Lord Phillips, sitting with Lords Waller and Wall chose to take a more restricted view of the case. They refrained from speculation, declined to give Mr Burke the advance declaration that he sought, and overturned all Mr Justice Munby's Declarations.

All the judges were critical of the wording in paragraph 81. Mr Justice Munby ruled it unlawful, but the Appeal Court Judges would go no further than to say that part of the drafting was "inadequate". There was a difference of opinion about the interpretation of paragraphs 38 and 82. When taken in isolation, each paragraph was judged to be unlawful by Mr Justice Munby. When taken together by the Appeal Court Judges both of these paragraphs were ruled to be lawful.

The end result of the legal scrutiny was that the GMC Guidance emerged shaken but essentially unchanged. However that is not necessarily the end of the story for the case may yet go to the European Court of Human Rights in Strasbourg.

The High Court Judgment

At the outset, in the second paragraph of his judgment Mr Justice Munby said:
"The case plainly raises issues of great importance. Central to these issues are fundamentally important questions of medical law and ethics. In particular the extent to which we should respect the patients autonomy: the personal autonomy which our law has now come to recognise demands that the choice of medical treatment- the choice of how we are to live and how we are to die- should be left to the individual....To the claimant these are

quite literally matters of life and death. They are issues which potentially affect us all. For all of us must die, and any of us may at some tine need ANH."

The Judge expressed concern that "the emphasis throughout the Guidance is on the right of the competent patient to refuse treatment, rather than on his right to request treatment." (paragraph 219)

He examined the issues in the light of *English Common Law*, and declared that several paragraphs of the GMC guidance including paragraphs 38, 81 and 82 were unlawful. He also considered various hypothetical scenarios that might arise during the course of Mr Burke's illness in the light of the *European Convention on Human Rights*, and said:

> **214:e** "…I find it hard to envisage any circumstances (other, perhaps, than those envisaged by Professor Higginson) in which a withdrawal of ANH in such circumstances- that is from a sentient person, whether competent or incompetent-could be compatible with the Convention."
>
> **214:f** " But the position will be different once the claimant has entered into the final stage of his illness and has finally lapsed into a coma. Assuming that the patient is otherwise being treated with dignity, and in a manner which is in all other respects compatible with his rights under Articles 3 and Article 8, there will not be any breach either of Article 3 or of Article 8 or of Article 2 if ANH is withdrawn in circumstances where it is serving absolutely no purpose other than the very short prolongation of the life of a dying patient who has slipped into his final coma and lacks all awareness of what is happening. For it can then properly be said that the continuation of ANH would be bereft of any benefit at all to the patient and that it would indeed be futile."

Some general points made by Mr Justice Munby

❑ Paragraph 81 was ruled unlawful because it "(a) it fails to recognise that the decision of a competent patients that ANH should be provided is determinative of the best interests of the patient and (b) it fails to acknowledge the heavy presumption in favour of life-prolonging treatment and that such treatment will be in the best interests of the patient unless the life of the patient, viewed from the patient's perspective, would be intolerable. And (c) provides that it is sufficient to withdraw ANH from a patient who is not dying because it may cause suffering or be too burdensome in relation to the possible benefits." (Judgment Declaration 4)

❑ Paragraphs 38 and 82 were unlawful because "…they fail to reflect the legal requirement that in certain circumstances ANH may not be withdrawn without prior judicial authorisation but provide that it is sufficient to consult a clinician with relevant experience or take legal advice." (Judgment Declaration 6)

- When considering whether to withhold or withdraw ANH from an incompetent patient the assessment of best interests has to be made from the point of view or perspective of the particular patient, and the touchstone of best interests in this context is intolerability. (Judgment paragraph 111)
- ANH can legitimately be withheld or withdrawn from an incompetent patient where it would not in fact prolong life, or would in fact provide *no* benefit at all for the patient. (Judgment paragraph 112.)
- If ANH is providing *some* benefit, then it should be provided unless the patient's life, if thus prolonged, would from the patient's point of view be intolerable. Alternatively if the test is to be framed in other terms then it must be set at a threshold which is no lower than intolerability…" (Judgment paragraph 113.)
- Decisions should be referred to court if there is a dispute between any of the medical professionals and relatives or carers as to whether artificial feeding should be withdrawn or withheld (See Judgment paragraph 214:g and Table 1 below).
- "There is a very strong presumption in favour of taking all steps which will prolong life, save in exceptional circumstances, or where the patient is dying, the best interests of the patient will normally require such steps to be taken. In case of doubt, that doubt falls to be resolved in favour of the preservation of life. But the obligation is not absolute. Important as the sanctity of life is, it may have to take second place to human dignity. In the context of life-prolonging treatment the touchstone of best interests is intolerability. So if life-prolonging treatment is providing *some* benefit it should be provided unless the patient's life, if thus prolonged, would be from the patient's point of view intolerable." (Judgment paragraph 116).

Mr Justice Munby listed a number of situations where, in his opinion, doctors should seek court approval as a matter of law, before withholding or withdrawing ANH. These are shown in Table 1. Had his advice been accepted it would have extended court supervision quite considerably. However when the matter came to the Appeal Court, his views were rejected. Nevertheless all the situations listed in Table 1 indicate the need for further discussion, if not by the High Court, then by other people who are competent to adjudicate in such matters. It is noteworthy that in June 2005 the Royal College of Physicians of London issued a report on "Ethics in Practice" in which they made a series of recommendations on how ethics advice in the NHS might be improved. They argued that the role of ethics committees should be strengthened and their role clarified, and that the provision of ethics support should be central to the mission of the modern NHS.

Table 1 Circumstances where prior judicial authorization is required as a matter of law before withholding or withdrawing ANH according to Mr Justice Munby.

   i.   where there is any doubt or disagreement as to the capacity (or competence) of the patient, or,

   ii.   where there is a lack of unanimity amongst attending medical professionals as to either (1) the patient's condition or prognosis or (2) the patient's best interests or (3) the likely outcome of ANH being withheld or withdrawn; or (4) otherwise as to whether ANH should be withheld or withdrawn; or

   iii.   where there is evidence that the patient when competent would have wanted ANH to continue in the relevant circumstances: or

   iv.   where there is evidence that the patient (even if a child or incompetent) resists or disputes the proposed withdrawal of ANH; or

   v.   where persons having a reasonable claim to have their views or evidence taken into account (such as parents or close relatives, partners, close friends, long-term carers) assert that withdrawal of ANH is contrary to the patient's wishes or not in the patient's best interests.

The Appeal Court Judgment.[6]

In July 2005 Appeal Court Judges, Lord Phillips, Lord Waller and Lord Wall overturned all Judge Munby's declarations. They did not find paragraph 81 unlawful but considered the drafting inadequate. They found that paragraphs 38 and 82 were "proper and lawful" and felt that their net effect was to direct doctors to consult a clinician *and* take legal advice before withholding ANH in certain situations. Having made that reasonably clear they went on to distinguish between a directive to take legal advice and a legal duty to obtain court approval. In paragraph 70 of their judgment they stated " …we do not consider that the judge is right to postulate that there is a legal duty to obtain court approval to the withdrawal of ANH in the circumstances that he identifies." It would seem from paragraph 71 of the their judgment that even in cases of PVS "it is a matter of good practice" and not a legal duty to seek the court's approval before withdrawing ANH. The Judges were clearly swayed by concerns that the courts would be swamped with work if Mr Justice Munby's criteria were applied.

Court supervision of disputed end-of-life decisions.

As mentioned above Mr Justice Munby attempted to increase court supervision of difficult end-of-life decisions involving non-provision of ANH, but his views were over-ruled by Appeal Court Judges. The trend now is for judges to leave crucial end-of-life decisions involving mentally incompetent adults in the hands of the medical profession. This leaves doctors and patients in a precarious situation. In cases of serious disagreement legal advice should be obtained as to the need for a court directive.

If the patient is mentally incompetent the advice of the Official Solicitor should be sought. He may deflect the decision back to solicitors acting for the NHS Hospital Trust, or try to persuade dissenting relatives to accept medical advice. Undue deference to NHS Trust solicitors carries a risk of conflict of interests. Relatives should seek their own advice.

When the Mental Capacity Act [2005] comes into force in England and Wales in 2007, court supervision will be reduced for mentally incompetent patients who have made a valid advance directive, or appointed a proxy healthcare decision maker. If senior judges and doctors have difficulty reaching agreement, it is surely unwise to expect members of the public to take such decisions without first consulting well-informed and independent professionals.

Most judges have no first hand experience of what goes on at ward level. Yet the Appeal Court Judges in the Burke case had some inkling of the situation because the Medical Ethics Alliance (MEA), acting as interveners, brought some cases to their attention. The case reports were thumbnail sketches that had been presented as evidence to the House of Lords and House of Commons Joint Committee on the draft Mental Capacity Bill in 2002, and were published in the Committee Report in 2003.[7]

The Appeal Court Judges found the MEA case reports "disturbing" and referred to them in paragraphs 60, 61 and 63 of their judgment. They said:

"These were cases where patients who were terminally ill appear to have been denied water and nutrition in circumstances where this was contrary to the demands of palliative care…These reports do not constitute admissible evidence, but underline the importance of clear law and guidance in this area...the disturbing cases referred to….if correctly reported, were cases where the doctors appear to have failed to observe the Guidance. They are not illustrative of any illegality in the Guidance. The (GMC) Guidance expressly warns against treating the life of a disabled patient as being of less value than the life of a patient without disability, and rightly does so."[8]

If judges distance themselves from involvement and do not take their part in enforcing the law, matters will not improve on the wards. Many worried relatives whose elderly relations have died in hospitals in the UK have the utmost difficulty in being heard by a Coroner, let alone by a High Court Judge. It is regrettable that despite the best efforts of those who intervened in the Burke case, the Appeal Court Judges did very little to improve the situation of patients at risk. However clear the law and professional guidance if it is not enforced it is useless. History may well see this as a missed opportunity.

Some key points and paragraphs from the Appeal Court Judgment

❑ **Paragraph 66**. " …We do not consider that the terms of paragraph 81 are unlawful. We do, however, feel that the wording of that part of the paragraph that deals with the position where death is not imminent could be better drafted. We believe it is attempting to set out the circumstances in which it may be lawful to withdraw ANH in a case such as Re J. The statement that the provision of ANH "may cause suffering or be too burdensome in relation to the possible benefits" is not a clear or helpful description of the circumstances in which life is so burdensome that there is no duty to prolong it. This inadequacy of drafting does not, however, justify the Judge's declaration."

- **Paragraph 31**. "The proposition that the patient has a paramount right to refuse treatment (has been) amply demonstrated. The corollary does not, however, follow…Autonomy and the right to self determination do not entitle the patient to insist on receiving a particular medical treatment regardless of the nature of the treatment. Insofar as a doctor has a legal obligation to provide treatment this cannot be founded simply upon the fact that a patient demands it. The source of the duty lies elsewhere.

- **Paragraph 32**. So far as ANH is concerned, there is no need to look for the duty to provide this. Once a patient is accepted into a hospital, the medical staff come under a positive duty at common law to care for the patient.…A fundamental aspect of this positive duty of care is a duty to take such steps as a reasonable to keep the patient alive. Where ANH is necessary to keep the patient alive, the duty of care will normally require the doctor to supply ANH. This duty will not, however, override the competent patient's wish not to receive ANH.…

- **Paragraph 33**. "Insofar as the law has recognised that the duty to keep a patient alive by administering ANH or other life prolonging treatment is not absolute, the exceptions have been restricted to the following situations: (1) where the competent patient refuses to receive ANH and (2) where the patient is not competent and it is not considered to be in the best interests of the patient to be artificially kept alive. It is with the second exception that the law has had most difficulty. The courts have accepted that where life involves an extreme degree of pain, discomfort or indignity to a patient, who is sentient but not competent and who has manifested no wish to be kept alive, these circumstances may absolve the doctors of the positive duty to keep the patient alive. Equally the courts have recognised that there may be no duty to keep alive a patient who is in a persistent vegetative state ('PVS'). In each of these examples the facts of the individual case may make it difficult to decide whether the duty to keep a patient alive persists."

- **Paragraph 34**. "No such difficulty arises, however, in the situation that has caused Mr Burke concern, that of the competent patient who, regardless of the pain, suffering or indignity of his condition, makes it plain that he wishes to be kept alive. No authority lends the slightest countenance to the suggestion that the duty on the doctors to take reasonable steps to keep the patient alive in such circumstances may not persist. Indeed it seems to us that for a doctor deliberately to interrupt life-prolonging treatment in the face of a competent patient's expressed wish to be kept alive, with the intention of thereby terminating the patient's life, would leave the doctor with no answer to a charge of murder."

The intolerability test

Mr Justice Munby's suggestion that, in the context of life-prolonging treatment, the touchstone of best interests was the intolerability of life, gave rise to concern. In paragraph 63 of their judgment the Appeal Court Judges said: "…We do not think that it is possible to attempt to define what is in the best interest of a patient by a single test, applicable in all circumstances…"

Mr Justice Balcombe took a similar approach in Re J, for he said: "…I would deprecate any attempt by this court to lay down such an all-embracing test since the circumstances of these tragic cases are so infinitely various." [9]

On suffering, burdens and benefits

The phrases in paragraph 81 of the GMC Guidance that were criticised by both Mr Justice Munby and the Appeal Court Judges contained advice of a vague but broadly helpful nature. The concept of balancing burdens and benefits has proved useful in clinical practice, and is widely accepted. The basic principles, as set out by the House of Lords' Select Committee on Medical Ethics at the time of the Bland case in 1993/94 can be found on page 3 of this book. Their Lordships rightly said that "such matters cannot be defined or legislated for and consensus must be developed on a case- by- case basis, inching forwards as best we can." They considered that "progressive development and ultimate acceptance of the notion that some treatment is inappropriate, should make it unnecessary to consider the withdrawal of nutrition and hydration, except in circumstances where its administration is evidently burdensome to the patient."

Unfortunately despite a decade of experience, there is no consensus about how to approach these difficult problems. Attempts to force the pace of change for reasons that are primarily political and financial should be discouraged. These matters must be decided with the utmost wisdom and sensitivity, taking into consideration all the problems, medical, psychological, social and spiritual that affect a particular patient. Doctors must concentrate on medical matters, since that is their area of expertise, but good doctors, like good judges, also consider the broader aspects of the case.

Comments from the Disability Rights Commission (DRC)

❑ The DRC issued a press release on July 28th 2005, and noted that the High Court ruling had created a Catch-22 situation for Mr Burke by upholding his right to life-saving treatment if he requested it, but allowing doctors to make the decision to remove the treatment, once he had lost the ability to express his wishes, or lacked mental capacity.

❑ The DRC said that the Court of Appeal ruling underlined a competent patient's right to autonomy and self-determination. Such a patient can refuse treatment, but cannot demand treatments that have no clinical benefits. The DRC drew attention to the wording of paragraph 34 of the judgement but …were very concerned that the Court of Appeal failed to take the opportunity to provide equal protection for patients who lack capacity.

❑ They noted that the definition of lack of capacity as defined in the Mental Capacity Act is as follows: "A person lacks capacity in relation to a matter if at the material time he is unable to make a decision for himself in relation to the matter because of an impairment of, or a disturbance in the functioning of, the mind or brain."

❑　As the ruling stands Mr Burke's lawyers would be forced back to court to request ANH if he loses capacity. Mr Burke and the DRC are seeking leave to appeal to the House of Lords.

❑　When a patient lacks capacity it will be up to the doctors to decide what is in the patient's 'best interests'. The DRC is extremely concerned that 'best interests' could be based on a doctor's discriminatory attitude or negative stereotypical assumptions of a disabled person's quality of life. The GMC guidance also fails to set out clear tests and considerations for doctors to arrive at what is best for the patient. The GMC guidelines use a variety of undefined terms such as; benefits and burdens; net benefit; burden and risk; benefits and disbenefits; clinically indicated; clinically appropriate; and futile.

❑　The Appeal Court emphasised that disabled people should be "treated properly and in accordance with good practice, and that they will not be ignored or patronised because of their disability." (para 83). The DRC believes that without clear tests and considerations for doctors on the circumstances to give or withhold life-prolonging treatment, that those laudable sentiments will remain just that- laudable sentiments!

In conclusion

Since the General Medical Council has a statutory duty to deal with cases of serious misconduct and criminal offences involving doctors, it was a source of concern and embarrassment to the profession when the legality of the GMC Guidance was called into question. It remains to be seen whether the GMC will attempt to redraft paragraph 81 to the satisfaction of all concerned.

Perhaps the time has come for high-level collaboration between the medical profession and the judiciary to evolve professional guidelines that are acceptable to all concerned. However care should be taken to ensure that the interests of patients are given priority over the self-interest of doctors or judges.

Lord Hailsham established in 1987/88 that *issues of public policy cannot prevail over the interests of a ward of court* [10]. The same should apply to the interests of mentally incapacitated adults. Resource and financial considerations, such as concerns about the cost of tube feeding, should not be allowed to influence judicial decisions. All attempts to interfere with such decisions should be resisted. If doctors have a duty to provide ANH as necessary in the best interests of their patients, the State has a duty to provide the NHS with the necessary resources.

Under the present circumstances doctors in the UK would be well advised to tread cautiously, rely on their good judgment, take into account the Appeal Court Judges views *and* current GMC guidance *and* take legal advice- before withholding or withdrawing ANH from patients who are not imminently dying.

Decisions to withhold hydration and/or nutrition will inevitably prove fatal unless the patient dies of their primary disease before dehydration or starvation reaches a critical level. The provision of hydration and nutrition will give the patient the best possible chance to survive, and perhaps improve. When patients with chronic or progressive disease want to survive they should receive all reasonable help to do so. Provision of ANH can help to prevent many unpleasant symptoms that are caused by dehydration and starvation.

A doctor must use his skill to do what is best for the patient under all circumstances. We should respect the age-old guidance "Thou shalt not kill" and offer food and water, by ANH if need be, to all who may benefit from its provision. If the patient refuses the offer- so be it.

References on GMC Guidance

1. Withholding and Withdrawing Life-prolonging Treatments: Good Practice in Decision-making. *General Medical Council* London, August 2002.
2. For example see 'Accuracy of prognosis estimates by four palliative care teams: a prospective cohort study.' Higginson IJ, Constantini M. *BMC Palliative Care* 2002; 1:1.
3. R (Burke) v General Medical Council. [2004] EWHC 1879 (Admin) In the High Court of Justice. Before: The Honourable Mr Justice Munby.
4. (Anon.) The appeal court ruling on our end-of-life guidance. *GMCtoday*, 2005; 04:15.
5. Doughty S. Too costly to be kept alive. *Daily Mail* Feb 5th 2005, pages 1 and 6.
6. R [Burke] v General Medical Council. [2005] EWCA 1003. In the Supreme Court of Judicature Court of Appeal (Civil Division) on Appeal from the High Court.
7. Report of Joint Committee on the draft Mental Incapacity Bill. Session 2002-3, Volume 2: Oral and written evidence. Ev 163.HMSO 2003.
8. See reference 6 above, paragraphs 60-63.
9. Mr Justice Balcombe in Re J [1990] 3 All ER. At 942 g–h.
10. Lord Hailsham quoted by Mr Justice Balcombe in Re J.[1990] 3 All ER. At 941 e and f, and 942 c.

Summary

Key features of some guidelines on the provision or non-provision of ANH in patients who are not imminently dying.

❑ **European Association for Palliative Care Guidance of 1996**. "Guidelines on artificial nutrition versus hydration in terminal cancer patients." A useful three-step process devised for terminally ill cancer patients, but of wider potential relevance. [Bozzetti F. *Nutrition* 1996; 12: 163-167. © 1996 by Elsevier Science. Inc.]

❑ **RCPCH framework of 1997 (updated in 2004)**. The Ethics Advisory Committee of the RCPCH identify five situations where withholding/withdrawing curative medical treatment might be considered in children. Emphasise duty to offer palliative care; find it impossible to define intolerability; somewhat wary of ethics committees and second opinions. Consider it good practice to consult the court in cases of dispute.

❑ **National Council For Hospice and Specialist Palliative Care Services Guidance of 1997**. "Ethical decision making in palliative care. Artificial hydration for people who are terminally ill." Basic guidance published by the National Council in London. For the background to these guidelines see Challenging Medical Ethics Volume 1. "No Water-No Life: Hydration in the Dying." (Ed. Craig GM). Fairway Folio 2005 [ISBN 0 9545445 3 6.]

❑ **BMA guidelines of 1999 and 2000**. Permit withdrawal/non-provision of ANH if patients lack self-awareness. Require a formal second opinion in all cases. Obtain legal advice in patients with PVS as a Court Declaration is required. Seek legal advice in cases resembling PVS.

❑ **Medical Ethics Alliance Guidance of 1999**. Multifaith consensus. Guidance based on the Hippocratic Oath and Declaration of Geneva 1948, and in keeping with advice of House of Lords' Select Committee on Medical Ethics of 1993/4.

❑ **British Association for Parenteral and Enteral Nutrition (BAPEN) 1999**. "Ethical and legal aspects of clinical hydration and nutritional support." A report by J.R. Lennard-Jones. This report (ISBN 1 899467 25 4) gives advice about tube feeding in stroke patients.

❑ **BAPEN**. "Standards and Guidelines for Nutritional Support of Patients in Hospitals." (Ed. Sizer) [Basic assessment of nutrition and maintenance of satisfactory nutritional levels.]

❑ **General Medical Council Guidance of 2002**. Permits cautious withdrawal/ non-provision of ANH if patients are mentally incapacitated. Where death is not imminent, the prognosis is poor and treatment is burdensome, seek a second opinion before withholding ANH. Seek legal advice in cases of unresolved disagreement. Legal advice obligatory in cases of PVS.

❑ **See also**: 'Assessment of nutritional status and fluid deficits in advanced cancer.' Sarhill N, Mahmoud FA, Christie R, Tahir A. *Journal of Terminal Oncology*, 2003, 2:1, 29-37.

Chronological Sequence of Events in the UK

1993 Bland case decision. ANH defined as medical treatment.
Tony Bland, a patient in PVS has ANH withdrawn and dies.

1994 Report of House of Lords' Select Committee on Medical Ethics.

1997 RCPCH Framework for treatment withdrawal in children.

1999 January. *The Times* warns of 'backdoor euthanasia'.
June. BMA issues guidelines on treatment withdrawal.

2000 The debate reaches Parliament.

Medical Treatment (Prevention of Euthanasia) Bill fails.

European Convention on Human Rights becomes operative throughout UK.

2002 General Medical Council issues guidelines on withholding and withdrawing life-prolonging treatment.

2003 The Patients' Protection Bill [HL] fails.

The Patient (Assisted Dying) Bill [HL] fails.

2004 The Assisted Dying for the Terminally Ill Bill [HL] fails, but the House of Lords' appoints a Select Committee to consider the issues.

Lesley Burke challenges GMC Guidance in the High Court and wins.

2005 Appeal Court overturns High Court ruling in the Burke case.

Mental Capacity Act passed. Advance refusals of treatment and proxy decision makers to be introduced in 2007.

Report of Select Committee on Assisted Dying for the Ill Bill debated.

Lord Joffe reintroduces Assisted Dying for the Terminally Ill Bill [HL]

99

Part 2

The American Experience

Introduction

The American experience as portrayed by American authors in case reports and papers, shows only too clearly the road that we in the UK are about to follow, unless we pause for thought and handle matters differently.

Since there is no national health service providing free health care for all citizens in the USA, the cost of health care falls on individuals or on their insurance companies. Not surprisingly therefore questions of cost loom large in the minds of American economists and bioethicists. Some years ago they hit on the idea of withholding basic sustenance to hasten death. Daniel Callahan, then director of the Hastings Centre, wrote in 1983:

> "…a denial of nutrition may, in the long run, become the only effective way to make certain that a large number of biologically tenacious patients actually die…Given the increasingly large pool of superannuated, chronically ill, physically marginal elderly, it could well become the non-treatment of choice." [1]

Thus we come face to face with the stark reality that death by dehydration and starvation has been advocated for over two decades by mainstream bioethicists in the USA. In line with this thinking in 1986 and 1989 the American Medical Association declared that treatment, including artificial nutrition and hydration may be withdrawn from patients who are in a permanent vegetative state. The limitations specified were not heeded, and it is alleged that conscious as well as comatose patients have been dehydrated or starved to death in the USA.

Wolfensberger sounded the alarm in 1987. Writing from a North American perspective he said:

> "We are facing a conservative estimate of 200,000 deaths a year of handicapped and other devalued people whose lives have been taken either directly or indirectly, and at the very least by readily preventable abbreviations of life, motivated by social devaluation or outright death wishes. Canadian figures can be assumed to be about one tenth of that i.e. 20,000. Thus the term 'genocide' seems warranted, and in order to give such genocide its proper historical context and recognition, it may deserve a special name, such as 'Holocaust 2'" [2].

In 1994 the American Medical Association revised its guidelines and, (to quote Wesley J. Smith) 'expanded the list of those eligible for withholding of "artificial nutrition" to include the conscious but mentally incompetent who cannot make medical decisions for themselves.' Thus the rules were relaxed to take account of prevailing practice.

Writing in the San Francisco Chronicle in December 1995, Wesley J Smith, an author and advocate based in California warned:

' All over the country, in hospitals, nursing homes and other facilities, conscious but cognitively disabled and aged people are being denied adequate care and/or are being starved and dehydrated to death in the name of patient autonomy, "quality of life" and "best interests of the patient" determinations. But what is really going on is the creation of a disposable caste of people, whom we, the healthy, find too emotionally painful, too expensive, or too inconvenient to care for, and whose intentional killing we increasingly find all too easy to rationalise'[3].

This state of affairs is the outcome of widespread use of advance directives, and the application of 'futile care policies' that permit the withdrawal of treatment and the provision of 'comfort care only' for countless people with terminal illness or severe chronic disabilities. Advance directives or 'living wills' are discussed in some detail elsewhere [4]. Suffice it to say at this stage that they have their uses, but can be extremely dangerous. Take for example the case of the late Mrs Marjorie Nighbert of Florida. As Wesley J. Smith explained:

' Her brother decided to cut off her tube feeding, allegedly because of the terms contained in her advance directive. Marjorie was not unconscious. During starvation she specifically asked nurses for food. This was so upsetting to one nurse that she blew the whistle. Enter the court, where, after a hurried investigation, it was determined that Marjorie was not medically competent to retract her advance directive (in other words to ask for "treatment" of food.) Thus even though she asked to be fed, the starvation was allowed to continue. Mrs Nighbert died on April 5th 1995'[3].

Live and let die

Comments from an article by Richard John Neuhaus. First published in the National Review on April 4th 1994. © by National Review, Inc., 215 Lexington Avenue, New York, NY 10016. Reprinted by permission. Father Neuhaus is the Editor-in-Chief of FIRST THINGS.

'...In its current phase the "right to die" debate goes back more than twenty years. Most states have now enacted "living will" and "health care proxy" laws. The living will specifies what kinds of life support are to be withdrawn or withheld in the event of mental incompetency; health care proxy allows patients to appoint someone else to make decisions for them.

'The first living-will law, enacted by California in 1976, authorised only the refusal of extraordinary measures in cases of advanced terminal illness. Laws have now been greatly expanded to allow the withdrawal of basic forms of care such as food and fluids from patients who are not "terminal" in the traditional sense. The federal Patient Self-Determination Act of 1990 requires hospitals to inform patients of their rights under state laws. Today the "right to die" movement advocates "automatic proxy" statutes that would give a designated person broad powers to make life and death decisions for the incompetent patient who never appointed a proxy or signed a living will.

'The courts have also been in expansive mode. In the Karen Quinlan case, the New Jersey Supreme Court in 1976 based the right to refuse a respirator on broad constitutional grounds, including the "right to privacy" that was key to *Roe v. Wade.*[4] In that and other cases, courts have, somewhat ironically, cited individual freedom and "privacy" to justify making decisions for incompetent patients who never indicated their own wishes. In addition, the right to refuse life support has been exercised by others, usually by family members, employing substituted decision-making to include the withdrawal of food and fluids.

'Courts in New York and Missouri have been more cautious, requiring "clear and convincing evidence" of the patient's own past wishes before feeding tubes are withdrawn. From Missouri the *Cruzan* case went to the U.S. Supreme Court, which in 1990 ruled that, even if patients have a right to refuse life support, the state is not required to give family members such a right when there is no clear evidence of the patient's own wishes. Yet Nancy Cruzan was allowed to die of dehydration after new witnesses came forward to claim that she had told them she wished to die in the event of permanent disability. In 1993 Missouri allowed Pete Busalacchi to arrange for the death of his daughter Christine, although there was no evidence regarding her own wishes.

'There is also a move to deny life support even when patients or their families clearly do want such support. A "reasonable person" standard is used to limit treatment. Thus a seriously ill person may be denied treatment on the grounds that he is making an irrational claim on scarce resources. Moreover, in May 1993, the *Journal of the American Medical Association* editorialised in favor of a "futile care" standard for withdrawing life support. The Clinton Administration has granted a Medicaid waver to Oregon for a rationing plan that denies some forms of life-sustaining care to seriously ill indigent patients. Rationing life-sustaining treatment-turning the legal "right to die" into an economic "duty to die"- could become a major controversy in the debate over health care reform.

'Then there is active euthanasia and physician-assisted suicide. In the late 1980s, initiatives to legalise such practices failed to qualify for state ballots in Oregon and California. They did make it to the ballot in Washington in 1991 and in California in 1992, but were turned down by margins of 54 to 46 %. A more artfully worded initiative was prepared for vote in Oregon…[and was enacted following a state-wide referendum in November 1994. Ed.]…Euthanasia bills have been considered by several other state legislators, but none has been enacted. In fact, Michigan and other states have enacted new laws making it clear that assisted suicide is illegal.

'Having failed so far in the democratic process, euthanasia backers are going to court. Two Michigan judges have found that state's new law unconstitutional, but their decisions are being appealed. In Washington State a suit has been brought in federal court claiming that laws against assisted suicide violate the "equal protection" clause of the U.S. Constitution. The argument is that competent patients can exercise their "right to die" while incompetent patients cannot. Critics and supporters alike have suggested that one of these cases may become "the *Roe v. Wade* of euthanasia."

'Sobered by the mushrooming of involuntary euthanasia in the Netherlands and mindful of the mandate "always to care, never to kill," medical associations in this country are opposing physician-assisted suicide. Despite polls indicating high public support for this practice, when confronted with the choice voters have so far had second thoughts. But then, as always, there are the judges, and they may discover that "the living constitution" comes down on the side of death.' [5]

Richard John Neuhaus

The U.S.Supreme Court ruling on physician-assisted suicide

In January 1997, according to Willke, the U.S. Supreme Court ruled that assisted suicide was not a fundamental Constitutional right. The Supreme Court stated that "Anglo-American common law has punished or otherwise disapproved of assisted suicide for over 700 years." States however remained free to make their own decisions [6].

In November 1997 the State of Oregon legalised physician-assisted suicide by a referendum. Doctors in Oregon are allowed to write a prescription for a lethal drug that can be taken by the patient. They are forbidden to give lethal injections. The patient must be terminally ill and have less than six months to live. They must be capable of making a rational decision. If depressed they must be referred to a psychiatrist and there is a 15 day waiting period before the drug can be dispensed by a pharmacist. Shortly after the law was passed the Drug Enforcement Administration stated that if a physician prescribed a lethal dose of medicine for the purpose of assisting a patient to die, that physician's licence would be automatically revoked. Eventually in November 2001 the American Attorney General, John Ashcroft, ruled that it was not permissible to use federal drugs to kill people. This should have nullified Oregon's law according to Willke,[6] but doctors in Oregon continued to dispense lethal potions under the terms of their State legislation.

Following the Ashcroft Directive the Oregon Attorney General took prompt action in the federal district court to protect Oregon's physician-assisted suicide law. Judge Robert Jones of the U.S. District Court then issued a restraining order barring the Drug Enforcement Agency from taking action against Oregon doctors who prescribed lethal barbiturates, or any federal controlled substance, for the purpose of assisting suicide. Having heard the case Judge Jones ruled, in 2002, that it was for individual states to determine what constitutes a legitimate medical practice of purpose in that state.

Thereafter the case of *Oregon v. Ashcroft* became a battle between the State of Oregon and the U.S. Department of Justice. In 2004 a Court of Appeal in San Francisco upheld Judge Jones' ruling and took the view that the U.S. Attorney General had overstepped his authority. When Alberto Gonzales took over as U.S. Attorney General, the Justice Department petitioned the U.S. Supreme Court to rehear the case, which was thereafter called *Oregon v. Gonzales*. Eventually, in January 2006, the U.S. Supreme Court ruled in favour of Oregon. So ended a long battle to block physician-assisted suicide in Oregon.[7]

Under Oregon's "Death with Dignity" Act of 1997 the Oregon Health Division (OHD), now called the Oregon Department of Human Services (DHS) is required to collect information, review a sample of cases and publish a yearly statistical report. Opponents of the law say that due to major flaws in the law and the state's reporting system, there is no way of knowing for sure how many patients have died from assisted suicide in Oregon, or under what circumstances. The only physicians interviewed for official reports are those who admit to prescribing lethal drugs for patients. The law contains no penalties for doctors who do not report their actions. The OHD is not authorised to investigate how physicians determine the diagnosis or life expectancy of their patients. Thus regulation of assisted suicide in Oregon is unsatisfactory and official reports do not tell the whole story. [7]

On the right to refuse life-saving hydration

In the case of Washington v Glucksberg, as quoted by Willke, the U.S.Supreme Court said that "The constitutionally protected right to refuse lifesaving hydration and nutrition that was discussed in Cruzan... was not simply deduced from abstract concepts of personal autonomy, but was instead grounded in the Nation's history and traditions, given the common-law ruling that forced medication was a battery, and the long legal tradition protecting the decision to refuse unwanted treatment."[6]

Further, (in Vacco v Quill) the U.S. Supreme Court said: "Everyone, regardless of physical condition, is entitled, if competent, to refuse unwanted lifesaving medical treatment; no one is permitted to assist a suicide....The distinction between letting a patient die and making that patient die is important, logical, rational, and well established: it comports with fundamental legal principles of causation...and intent... The line between the two acts may not always be clear, but certainty is not required, even were it possible." [6]

Several high profile cases of death after withdrawal of tube feeding and hydration have gone through the courts in the USA, the most recent and controversial being that of the late Terri Schiavo of Florida. The U.S. Supreme Court refused to intervene in her case and she died amid storms of protest in 2005.

Thus in the USA, as in the UK, a rational person's refusal of life-saving treatment, including hydration, must be respected. Both countries permit treatment to be withheld from permanently unconscious patients under some circumstances. In both countries there is evidence that conscious patients are also denied life-prolonging treatment at times. Regrettably Judges have been slow to recognise that such omissions may, on occasions, seem tantamount to murder.

Chronological sequence of events in North America

1976 First advance directive enacted in California.

1976 Karen Quinlan case- New Jersey Supreme Court approved end of life support.

1986 American Medical Association (AMA) Guidelines approve withdrawal of food and fluids from terminally ill people, and those who are without doubt permanently unconscious.

1987 Wolfensberger warns of 'Holocaust 2'.

1990 U.S.Supreme Court ruling in the Nancy Cruzan case.

1994 AMA guidelines revised to include the conscious but mentally incompetent who cannot make decisions for themselves.

1994 Editorial in New England Journal of Medicine proposes that doctors treating the profoundly disabled should be allowed to refuse treatment they consider futile or inappropriate. Proposal to redefine "death" discussed.

1996 U.S. Supreme Court upholds right to refuse life-saving nutrition and hydration. Cases of Washington v. Glucksberg and Quill v.Vacco.

1997 U.S. Supreme Court ruled physician assisted suicide unconstitutional. States make decisions for themselves.

1997 Oregon legalises physician-assisted suicide by lethal medication.

1999 AMA publish report on "Medical Futility in End-of-Life Care."

2003 Governor of Florida intervenes to save Terri Schiavo.

2005 Terri Schiavo dies. U.S. Supreme Court refuses to intervene.

2006 U.S. Supreme Court confirms Oregon's right to allow physician-assisted suicide.

References

1. Callahan D. On feeding the dying. *Hastings Centre Report*, October 1983, page 35.
2. Wolfensberger W. The new genocide of Handicapped and Afflicted People. Syracuse University Division of Special Education and Rehabilitation 1987. Quoted by Sinason V. See Mental Handicap and the Human Condition, p. 317. *Free Association Books Ltd.* London 1992.
3. Wesley J.Smith. Creating a disposable caste. *San Francisco Chronicle.* December 8th 1995.
4. Roe v Wade [1973] was a landmark case that undermined restrictive laws on abortion.
5. Neuhaus R.J. Live and Let Die. *National Review*, April 4th 1994, page 40.
6. Willke. J.C. Assisted Suicide and Euthanasia. Chapters IX and X, p118-129. *Hayes Publishing Company* Ohio 1998.
7. Attorneys in *Gonzales v. Oregon* take battle to U.S. Supreme Court. International Task Force Update-Volume 20, Number 1. January 2006. http://www.internationaltaskforce.org/iou35.htm
8. Six years of assisted suicide in Oregon. Report by the International Task Force on Euthanasia and Assisted Suicide. http//www.internationaltaskforce.org/orrpt6.htm

Chapter 7

The Role of the American Medical Association

Is the Code of Ethics of the American Medical Association ethical?

Comments by Richard C. Eyer. D. Min., Assistant Professor of Philosophy at Concordia University, Wisconsin, USA.

'The American Medical Association (AMA) was founded in 1847 under the original name of the National Medical Association. In part, harbouring less than noble reasons for its creation, it appears to be founded to a large degree on self interest, *'for the protection of their interests, for the maintenance of their honour and respectability, for the advancement of their knowledge, and the extension of their usefulness'.*[1] The specific intent was aimed at the exclusion of quacks which were understood to be homeopathic doctors and apothecaries. An article in the Journal of the American Medical Association (JAMA) recounts:

The introductory remarks constantly emphasized quackery and the duty of physicians to stamp it out. 'Physicians, as conservators of the public health are bound to bear emphatic testimony against quackery in all its forms', even when masked as philanthropy or religion... *Ministers of the gospel often 'give their countenance, and at times, direct patronage, to medical empirics'.* And Apothecaries, through sale of 'quack medicines and nostrums', often seemed allied to 'empirics of every grade and degree of pretension'. The fight against quackery was an important part of medical ethics.[2]

The Code of Ethics of the American Medical Association is an outgrowth of the attempt to maintain control of the practice of medicine. The Code claims to be in the tradition of the Hippocratic Oath, but it has gone much further than that and is in constant flux. The Code of Ethics has undergone many revisions since the founding of the AMA, changing already in 1993 and more recently in 1996. An editorial for August 5, 1996 in JAMA reports, 'The AMA's Code of Ethics today is a constantly evolving document that serves as a contract between physicians and their patients. Responding to current trends, the code is developing new boundaries for the business of medicine.' This editorial comment in JAMA, although intended as a compliment, raises some red flags regarding the purpose of a code of ethics.

First, that the standard of moral behaviour with reference to the Code of Ethics should change according to 'current trends' makes one wonder whether doctors are expected to abide by the Code or whether the Code is to be adapted to the practices of doctors. If the Code is a standard to live by it seems a strange matter to revise the Code to conform to the behaviour that is obviously beyond the limits set by the Code. The same editorial elaborates, 'the ethics which govern it (AMA) must keep pace with (that) progress'. How interesting that moral behaviour in medicine *should* change and that such change is necessarily seen as 'progress'.

Second, it will not come as any surprise to most that the word 'business' has replaced the word 'profession' in reference to medicine. What is a surprise is that the medical profession should boldly acknowledge the word. It would seem that the same self interest that founded the AMA in 1847 is alive and well in the 1990s. Lester King MD, writing in JAMA in 1982, reports that physicians at the founding considered themselves a 'superior class' with a 'definite obligation to maintain the honor and dignity, a sort of noblesse oblige that rested on status'. Perhaps it is for this reason that membership in the AMA is declining among young doctors who feel differently about the status of their profession. In spite of this decline in membership and the fact that the AMA represents only half the doctors in America, the Courts continue to recognise the AMA as representative of physicians in America in making judgements on ethical questions in medicine.

In many ways the issue of control seems to have guided the founding and the continuance of the American Medical Association and its Code of Ethics rather than a genuine concern for the moral behaviour of its physicians. The criteria for physician acceptance into the AMA in the early days at times came to rest on his *belief* more than his *educational* level.'…the AMA code, ignoring the educational deficiency of many of its members, stressed orthodoxy in medical beliefs'. The political nature of the AMA is inherent in its foundations. It would appear to be a highly politically motivated organization even today as evidenced in its boast that it is the final appeal in the courts in matters of ethical/legal decision-making. If this is true, then the need for 'keeping pace with trends' seems all the more expedient lest the AMA lose status and control for its own political aggrandizement.

Arthur Caplan, writing in JAMA in 1995, says, 'Up until 1995 the AMA Code had far more to do with matters of etiquette and professional comportment than with substantive matters of morality.' He claims that it was in 1980 that the first significant revision of the Code appeared identifying the new Principles of Medical Ethics that exceeded the norms that ought to be followed by physicians in private practice 'into the much more murky ethical waters'. Caplan concludes, 'The AMA has grown feisty, ornery, and even courageous.' One's appreciation for the courage of the AMA must depend on one's appreciation of the ethical directions in our culture today. I, for one, do not believe our culture, much less medicine, is headed in a direction that makes ethics anything more than expediency glorified.

In March of 1997 the American Medical Association met in Philadelphia to 'celebrate American medicine' by celebrating the 'common bond that has linked physicians over the year- our professional code of ethics'. The object of celebration was the latest revision of the Council on Ethical and Judicial Affairs (1996-1997 edition), *Code of Medical Ethics: Current Opinions with Annotations*. The 'annotations' are legal judgements establishing the practice. There are no moral judgements throughout the Code. Although the Introduction to the Code contains a disclaimer that ethical and legal may not be equivalent, it is clear that *ethics* for the AMA has, for all practical purposes, become a synonym for *legal*. The Code bears little resemblance to Aristotle's meaning of the word *ethics* as moral character development. In the remainder of this paper I propose to run through some of the more controversial aspects of the Code of Ethics.

The principles of medical ethics identified in the prologue of the Code of Ethics is a general appeal to the physician to provide *competence, honesty, responsibility, respect for patient's rights, continued study, provision of appropriate care, and participation in the AMA.* Although laudable these Principles are also vague. Most significant is the highlighting of ' patient's rights' as an indicator of the value placed on autonomy. The best illustration of this is found in the first ethical issue taken up in the Code, abortion. It is boldly stated, against Hippocratic tradition, that 'The Principles of Medical Ethics of the AMA do not prohibit a physician from performing an abortion...' The ethical justification is cited as the Supreme Court Ruling in 1973.

The issue of patient autonomy spreads quickly to the other end of life's spectrum when, five pages later, the issue of end of life decision-making is addressed. Under 'Futile Care' there is an attempt to place limits on patients autonomy when it infringes on the physician's interests. The physician is not obligated to meet all patient demands when, in his judgement, such demands are futile. Denial of treatment on the basis of futility is to be based, not on clearly defined meaning of futility however, but on the general Principles of the Code. In former times of moral conviction this might have worked, but in today's world of economic interests and moral relativity the Code's Principles are an empty guideline....

Euthanasia and Assisted Suicide

The issue of euthanasia is addressed in the Code as unacceptable. However, it is defined narrowly enough to enable us to think of euthanasia only as 'the administration of a lethal agent....for the purpose of relieving the patient's intolerable and incurable suffering'. The subject of euthanasia is dispensed with in 18 lines, one of which reads, '...to engage in euthanasia would ultimately cause more harm than good'. Does this imply that it might cause some good in the penultimate sense? Is the implication here that it is not so much a moral issue as it is a practical one? The practical issue, it is pointed out, is that it might confuse the role of the doctor as healer with the role of doctor as killer. Whereas this is a legitimate concern, one wonders whether keeping up with the pace of change in medicine as mentioned earlier in this paper, might not cause change in the acceptance of euthanasia if it becomes expedient, or is politically correct to do so.

Conclusions

The Code of Ethics of the American Medical Association follows the trends of society and has all but abandoned the Hippocratic Tradition. Although there may, on the part of some, be a well-intentioned attempt to define right and wrong and to set limits for physicians to follow, such ethics are built on a distortion of the Kantian notion of autonomy, the perversion of a Kierkegaardian existentialism, and the Machiavellian doctrine of expediency. More importantly, there is a growing credibility gap between what the AMA now stands for and the Christian physicians who reject a purely utilitarian ethic which justifies itself in the name of 'progress'...

*Acknowledgement. These comments are taken from an article that was first published in Ethics and Medicine, 2000;Volume **16:2**: 47-50. They are reprinted with permission. References and full bibliography cited by Eyer are listed at the end of this chapter.*

Medical Futility Guidelines in the USA

Introduction

Attempts have been made to develop guidelines for treatment ablation in the USA for a number of years. The main driving force behind this undertaking has been a desire to reduce the cost of medical intervention in elderly patients transferred from nursing homes to hospitals. Elderly economically unproductive people, especially those who have lost their faculties, can become social outcasts and are at risk of death-hastening activity. There is also concern that technology can be used inappropriately to keep hopelessly ill people alive too long- a fate that some view as being worse than death. Americans are not alone in their fear of becoming 'prisoners of technology', so it is not unreasonable to try to develop guidelines for treatment ablation. The problem lies in deciding where to draw the line between legitimate and predominantly therapeutic medical decisions, and euthanasia by neglect or omission. Inevitably concerns about a doctor's intent can cause much dispute and grief, hence the need for guidelines.[1,2]

Various projects to develop guidelines in the USA have been reviewed by Johnson and Potter, in a book on Medical Futility published by Cambridge University Press in 1997.[3] They describe projects in Santa Monica and Sacramento California, in Minnesota, in Denver Colorado, in Houston Texas, in Ohio, and at Appleton in Wisconsin. The prime purpose of guidelines in Minnesota was said to be to protect patients from harmful or useless treatment, and secondarily to protect doctors if they were sued for refusing to give treatment they regarded as futile. A city task force in Houston Texas recognised the need for dialogue between the physician and the patient, or surrogate decision maker. A conference at Appleton Wisconsin tried to develop guidelines for the responsible use of intensive care, recognising the need for public education and involvement of an informed public. They realised that guidelines should not become legal mandates, and considered it vital to strike a balance between autonomy and paternalism. Public meetings were planned to discuss draft guidelines, and the educational aspects of the programme were carefully coordinated. The pattern of activity in Appleton was similar to that adopted in Denver Colorado, where churches, synagogues and community groups were contacted.[3]

Wesley J. Smith, author and attorney for the Anti-Euthanasia Task Force based in California, is a close observer of the American scene. Writing in 1998 he warned:

"Pay close attention to this ongoing dialogue in the medical world today, and it becomes vividly clear that Futile Care Theorists seek to create public policies that promote death as the answer to the problems of old age, debilitating and terminal illnesses, and dependency caused by cognitive disability."

In 1999 the American Medical Association devised a step-by-step process for dealing with disputes about medical futility.[4] The process devised received approving comments in the British Medical Journal [5] and may influence conflict resolution procedures in the UK. Our procedures are embryonic in comparison with experience gained in the USA, so advice offered by colleagues in the USA must be studied carefully. Dissenting relatives in the UK, and no doubt in the USA, have to be determined, vocal and well informed to be heard, for the kindest of doctors can become difficult when their professional judgement is questioned. Members of the public may find themselves in a weak bargaining position. An account of the American approach to conflict resolution follows.

Medical Futility in End of Life Care

Report of the Council on Ethical and Judicial Affairs of the American Medical Association (AMA) March 1999.

Reviewed and summarised by Gillian Craig

The following account is based on the AMA report as published in the Journal of the American Medical Association in March 1999.[4] The full text can be obtained through a good medical library. Extracts are quoted with permission. The report limits discussion to "the use of interventions in patients with life-threatening illnesses." The Council recognise that "What constitutes futile intervention remains a point of controversy in the medical literature and in medical practice..." Consensus is unlikely to be achieved since "definitions of futile care are value laden... A full objective and concrete definition of futility is unattainable." Nevertheless, the AMA take the view that "a workable understanding of futility is necessary. Some interventions must eventually be stopped." Therefore they have devised a complex step-by-step approach to decision making for use when there is serious disagreement about the care of patients with life threatening illness.

Situations in which conflict may arise

1. A discrepancy between the values or goals of individuals. For example one party may wish to prolong life, while another thinks this simply prolongs the dying process. Alternatively one party may feel that the other is "inappropriately pursuing life-prolongation when death is inevitable."
2. Doubt about who has decision-making authority. In cases that have reached the courts in the USA some judgements have upheld the right of the patient or designated health care proxy to decide, while others have "upheld the prerogative of the profession to decline medical intervention that is considered to be futile."
3. The issue of resource allocation. The AMA note that "There is a danger that judgements about futility mask a covert motive to conserve resources." The AMA stress that "whether or not futility standards might realize cost savings, they should not be used as covert rationing mechanisms."
4. Avoidance of discussion. The AMA stress that "Futility claims should not be used to avoid difficult discussions with patients and families."

Attempts to define futility

Given that a fully objective and concrete definition of futility is unattainable, attempts to define it will inevitably be flawed. The AMA discuss various approaches and attempts to define futility, namely:

- *A quantitative approach.* According to the AMA the best known proposal in this category is that of Schneiderman et al who are reported to assert "that if an intervention does not work in more than 1% of attempts, it should be considered futile." [6] They are said to define whether the intervention has worked in a particular case according to physiological outcome. This is problematic argues the AMA, "for individuals do not judge the worth of an intervention by physiological outcomes alone." For example preserving normal kidney function in a person who has no capacity for interpersonal reaction, (or in BMA terms one who lacks self-awareness) may not be regarded as worthwhile. There is however the problem that "one person's assessment of sufficient mental function may not be the same as another's…" [4] Quality of life factors enter the equation. There is also the problem of who should decide what is an acceptable level of mental function, and on what grounds?
- *Intervention that is intended to prolong dying.* This is not necessarily futile according to the AMA, because firstly, "some intentions to prolong dying are justifiable…" and secondly " the occasions when futility disputes arise usually involve disputes about intervention and intent."
- *The use of community standards to determine intervention* is controversial and exceedingly difficult, given the range of different opinions within a community, the problem of defining the relevant community, allowing for exceptions and so on.
- *The use of institutional standards.* It has been suggested that these could be used "to define proactively, what interventions are considered futile for defined circumstances." [4] However the AMA argue that institutional standards would be subject to the some of the same problems as community standards. This is certainly true. I find myself thinking of the problems that may arise when fit and successful professional men and women on institutional committees make pronouncements about the value of the life of another individual. The spectre of ageism, racism, intolerance of disability, marginalisation of the poor and disabled could, only too easily, rear its ugly head! The medical profession is not immune to prejudice.

The AMA conclude that "Since none of these previous attempts at defining futility is truly adequate, the challenge now is to find a suitable approach that allows for quality decision making when there is a possibility of futility."

The AMA proposal for a fair process in futility cases

The AMA consider that:
- ❑ "In medicine and for futility policies, fair process approaches would likely be adopted at the institutional level for use in individual cases, but could be adopted for larger communities of, say, religious institutions or even states. The emphasis of the approach is on fair process between parties rather than having

a definition that is externally imposed on the parties. Professional standards including those of clinical outcome measures, patient rights, intent standards, and family or community involvement usually should be accommodated in the process of deliberation. For this reason Council favours the fair process approach.

❑ "The fair process approach for declaring futility in a particular case would be defined within the parameters set by a regulatory body of the institution or the community…"

At this point their report becomes fearfully bureaucratic and beset with management jargon! For example there is a statement to the effect that:

"The regulatory body would itself have an appropriate legitimising composition and mechanisms to establish its authority. The body would, for instance, likely have a composition or structure to allow patient/public representation as well as professional and expert guidance. To foster ownership by those who must adhere to it, the fashion of its development, as well as the fair process adopted, should be openly published and accessible to members of the community and enrolled patients."

Phew! The heart sinks, but the aim is to create arbitration "in a setting that is usually more convenient, more knowledgeable in medicine, more rapidly responsive, and less expensive in financial and emotional terms than court action." [4]

Features of the fair process

The AMA state: "Ideally, a fair process approach to futility would include at least four distinguishable steps aimed at deliberation and resolution, two steps aimed at securing alternatives in case of irresolvable differences, and a final step aimed at closure when all alternatives have been exhausted."

The fair process in outline is as follows:

1. The AMA give precedence to the wishes of the patient if he or she is able to give an opinion. If the patient is unable to take part in discussions the wishes of their proxy decision maker will be heeded.
2. The AMA recommend that decisions about care should be made before the patient reaches the terminal stage.
3. Outcome data, giving the likely consequences of intervention should be used in discussions. There is however the problem that good data may not exist.
4. Consultants should take part in the discussions to help the parties reach agreement. However the term Consultant in this context may not mean a medical Consultant in the English sense.
5. There should be an ethics committee, to give the patient or his/her proxy a full voice, either in person or through a lay representative on the committee, or both. The patient or proxy should be able to call for ethics committee involvement.
6. If a dispute cannot be resolved despite going through all these stages, the doctor and patient/proxy should consider transferring the patient to another doctor in the same institution, or transferring the patient to a different institution where a different approach to treatment may be acceptable to the staff. [4]

Having expounded the fair process scheme in some detail the AMA Council Report states:

"Finally if transfer is not possible because no physician and no institution can be found to follow the patient's and/or proxy's wishes it may be because the request is considered offensive to medical ethics and professional standards in the eyes of the majority of the health care profession. In such a case, by ethics standards, the intervention in question need not be provided, although the legal ramifications of this course of action are uncertain."

"This fair process approach insists on full and fair deference to the patient's wishes, placing limits on this patient-centred approach only when the harm to the patient is so unseemly that, even after reasonable attempts to find another institution, a willing provider of the service was not found. The approach has the further advantage of being open, allowing for a sense of fairness and accountability for all parties in an era when cost containment and other driving forces compromise trust."

"If a patient enters an institution's care, perhaps on an emergency basis, but disagrees with the futility policy, cases may arise of irresolvable disagreement without options for a full, fair process and transfer. Some institutions may allow patients and/or proxies to opt out of the policy, but other institutions may insist on the eventual option to cease unseemly intervention even if it leads to court action to arbitrate."

In the final paragraph of recommendations the AMA return to the question of prolonging the dying process, a subject that is at the heart of grave ethical concerns about withholding and withdrawing life-prolonging medical treatment including the provision of hydration and nutrition by means such as tube feeding. Note the death-orientated terminology used- with the emphasis on prolonging dying rather than prolonging life! The AMA Council state:

"...When the physicians primary purpose of the treatment seems to be to prolong the dying process without much benefit to the patient or others with legitimate interest, this will be taken into account among fairly heard perspectives, and may become determinative but only if all institutions share this perspective. The fair process approach also provides a system for addressing the ethical dilemmas regarding end-of-life care without need to recourse to the court system. The Council therefore recommends that health care institutions, whether large or small, adopt a policy of medical futility, and that policies on medical futility follow a fair process approach such as that presented above." [4]

The AMA must be commended for they have tried very hard to create a reasonable process for resolving disputes at the end of life, but clearly there are serious flaws in their proposals. The AMA Council admit that "futility" is value-laden and cannot be defined objectively. They note that community and institutional approaches to the problem are "exceedingly difficult". Nevertheless since they insist that "some interventions must eventually be stopped" all these objections are put aside, and they opt for the institutional approach, controlled largely by the medical profession.

Who, one may well ask, are those others "with legitimate interests" who do not want to prolong life, or prolong dying? Are they economists perhaps, or relatives due to inherit, or insurance companies who are paying the bills, or transplant surgeons seeking spare parts? Or are they simply honest and compassionate people who realise that life, for the patient, has lost its purpose and it is time to let them go? How can all these conflicting factors be weighed in the balance to decide what is truly in the patient's best interest? How can we ensure that distraught and grieving people are treated kindly and have their concerns addressed? These issues must be at the heart of the fair process for it must be humane as well as fair. Only time will tell whether the fair process is indeed fair. Sadly some disputes will still need to be resolved in a court of law.

The current situation in the USA

In the wake of high profile cases of ANH withdrawal the American public have started to question long-held medical policies on the use of ANH.[7] Some States have made it more difficult to withdraw ANH than other life-sustaining measures.[8] Concerned that public opinion may turn against them, some doctors have taken defensive action in *The New England Journal of Medicine*. Their paper published in December 2005 examined "the ethical principles that have guided the appropriate use of ANH" in the USA for the past 20 years.[7] The authors recommend ways to overcome "obstacles to ethical decision making." Some of their recommendations are listed below. Attempts will be made to persuade legislators, regulatory agencies and those who pay the bills for nursing care to promote these recommendations. The prospects for those who wish to receive ANH in years to come are not good.

Overcoming obstacles to ethical decision-making on ANH
according to Casarett , Kapo and Caplan 2005[7]

❑ Train clinicians to negotiate with patients and their families.
❑ Pay physicians for the time spent discussing end-of-life decisions.
❑ Shield nursing homes from "financial and regulatory pressures"
❑ Reduce inducements that may promote ANH use in nursing homes.
❑ Do not report weight loss after decisions to forego ANH.
❑ Promote advance directives that include preferences about ANH
❑ Document patient preferences on ANH carefully.
❑ Defend right of choice on ANH against legal, financial and administrative challenges at the bedside.
❑ Treat symptoms due to ANH withdrawal.
❑ Offer palliative care, including hospice care.
❑ Improve care for all patients with serious illness.

Acknowledgement

Extracts from the AMA Council Report "Medical Futility in End-of-Life Care" published in the Journal of the American Medical Association of March 10th 1999, Volume 281 number 10, pages 937- 941, are reprinted with permission. "Copyrighted 1999, American Medical Association."

References on Medical Futility Guidelines in the USA

1. AMA Council on Ethical and Judicial Affairs. Withholding or withdrawing life-prolonging medical treatment. *JAMA* 1986; **236**:471
2. AMA Council on Scientific Affairs. Persistent vegetative state and the decision to withdraw or withhold life support. *JAMA* 1990; **263**:426-430
3. Johnson L. Potter RL. Professional and public community projects for developing medical futility guidelines. Chapter 14, pages 155-167 in "Medical Futility" Ed Zucker M and Zucker H.D. *Cambridge University Press* 1997.
4. AMA Council Report. Medical Futility in End-of-Life Care. *Journal of the American Medical Association.* 1999; **281**: 937-941.
5. Charaton F. AMA issues guidelines on end of life care. *British Medical Journal* 1999; **318**: 690.
6. Schneiderman L.J., Faber-Langendoen K, Jecker N.S.Beyond futility to an ethic of care. *American Journal of Medicine* 1994; **86**:110-114.
7. Casarett D, Kapo J, Caplan A. Appropriate use of artificial nutrition and hydration- fundamental principles and recommendations. *The New England Journal of Medicine*, 2005; **353**: 24, 2607-2612.© Massachusetts Medical Society. Quoted with permission.
8. Sieger CE, Arnold JF, Ahronheim JC. Refusing artificial nutrition and hydration: does statutory law send the wrong message? *Journal of the American Geriatric Society.* 2002; **50**: 544-50. Cited by Casarett in ref 7 above.

Bibliography cited by Eyer

❑ American Medical Association, Council on Ethical and Judicial Affairs, Code of Medical Ethics: Current Opinions with Annotations (1996-1997 Edition).
❑ *American Medical News*, editorial for August 5th 1996.
❑ Caplan, Arthur L. pH Book Reviews: Code of Medical Ethics: Current Opinions with Annotations, *Journal of the American Medical Association,* 1995: **272**, No 15,1232.
❑ Johnson, Daniel H. Jr.MD. American Medical Association, Opening remarks, 1997 AMA Ethics Conference, Philadelphia, March 14th, 1997.
❑ King, Lester S.MD. 'Medicine in the USA: historical vignettes, V, The "Old Code" of medical ethics and some problems it had to face.' *Journal of the American Medical Association*, November 1982: **248**, No 18, 2329-2333.
❑ Pellegrino, Edmund D. *Journal of the American Medical Association*, Contempo 1996.
❑ Veith, Gene Edward. Postmodern Times. *Wheaton: Crossway Books,* 1994.

Chapter 8

Futile Care Theory In Practice

Based on articles by Wesley J. Smith

Killing Grounds

Extracts from a paper by Wesley J Smith. First published in the National Review of March 6th 1995. © by National Review Inc., 215 Lexington Avenue, New York, NY 10016. Reprinted by permission.

Those we would kill we must first dehumanise. That truism has been demonstrated repeatedly throughout history. Today in the United States, disabled people with brain damage are being systematically dehumanised so that society will accept the "compassion" and utility of killing them. "He is an empty shell, a vegetable," a person may say of a relative in a coma. "He is no different than a corpse," another may agree, as if the disabled person were already dead.

Physicians and lawyers representing families who wish to end the lives of their disabled loved ones can be even more brutal. "They, as human beings have long since departed from the world," Dr Fred Plum of Cornell University Medical Centre recently told the *American Evening News*. "They're stealing from the mouths of others." Or consider the statement from Paul Armstrong, a lawyer who represented the parents of Nancy Ellen Jobes in the ultimately successful quest to withdraw food and fluids from their disabled daughter. People with profound brain damage, he said, are "nonmentatiative [sic] organ systems, artificially sustained like valued cell lines in cancer laboratories." The medical terminology for such patients, who are said to be in a "persistent vegetative state" (PVS), reflects this attitude.

Since the truly dead often get more respect than the disabled living, it's hardly surprising that the killing of PVS patients by starvation and dehydration has become routine. The American Medical Association has given its blessing to the practice since 1986, when it approved starving or dehydrating terminally ill people on the brink of death and those who are "without doubt permanently unconscious." Nutrition through a feeding tube is now deemed "medical treatment" (which may be withheld) rather than "humane care" (which must be supplied).

Despite the limitations supposedly imposed by the AMA guidelines, conscious as well as comatose patients have been dehydrated to death. Nurses who cared for Nancy Cruzan- perhaps the most famous dehydration victim, because her case went all the way to the U.S. Supreme Court- insist to this day that she was conscious when her parents decided to withdraw her nutritional support. Indeed she had been able to take food orally before a feeding tube was utilized to make her care easier. Likewise Christine Basalacchi, whose care givers swore she smiled at jokes and responded to music, died by dehydration at the request of her father. Then there were the cases of Ronald Comeau [1] and Michael Martin [2]. Both were indisputably conscious but judges nonetheless authorized their dehydration and starvation. Mr Comeau was saved only because a pro-life minister succeeded in finding his relatives, who intervened...Mr Martin was also saved after a lengthy court battle.[3]

These and many other cases fly in the face of the 1986 AMA guidelines, which require terminal illness or permanent unconsciousness. Not to worry. In 1994 the AMA revised its ethical rules to comport with the practices of physicians and the courts, expanding the list of those eligible for withholding of "artificial nutrition" to include the conscious but mentally incompetent, who cannot make medical decisions for themselves. "Even if the patient is not terminally ill or unconscious," the AMA now says," it is not unethical to discontinue all means of life-sustaining medical treatment in accordance with a proper substituted-judgement or best-interests analysis."

Furthermore, some who sanction the killing of the profoundly brain damaged would not limit it to those who make their wishes known in advance or whose families choose to have nutrition withdrawn. They are pushing the nation toward a medical ethic that would eliminate the right of these patients to live- even if the family wants medical care to continue. The charge is being led by the prestigious *New England Journal of Medicine*. In a May 26, 1994, editorial, the journal's executive director, Dr. Marcia Angell argues that doctors treating the profoundly disabled should be permitted to refuse treatment they consider futile or inappropriate. Dr. Angell describes three ways of accomplishing this.[4]

First, death could be redefined to include permanent unconsciousness. The current definition "brain death," was intended to permit organ harvesting. But after brain death, the body cannot be kept functioning more than a few days. By contrast, patients diagnosed as permanently unconscious can often survive without assistance, other than food and fluids, indefinitely. Dr. Angell sees a problem with redefining death to include those diagnosed as permanently unconscious: it would be unseemly to bury a breathing body. Thus the "corpse" of an unconscious person considered "dead" would have to be killed.

Second, states could prohibit medical care for the unconscious after a specified time. The beauty of this approach, according to Dr. Angell, is that the decision to let a person die would be made in advance by society without regard to any particular case. In other words, the family words, the family would know that the decision to let their disabled relative die was nothing personal.

Third, states could create a legal presumption that people with brain damage would not want treatment after a specified time. A family that held the "idiosyncratic view" that their loved one should not be starved to death would have to prove that he had expressed a specific desire to be treated under these circumstances.

When the Doctor is wrong

The equanimity with which much of society has accepted euthanasia by dehydration of these profoundly disabled people is disturbing to those who hold the old-fashioned view that all human life is sacred. But even those who have doubts about the moral status of comatose patients should recognize that people deemed by doctors to be permanently unconscious often aren't. In more than a few cases, such people have awakened. (If the definition of death is ever changed to include the supposedly unconscious, we could say they were resurrected.)

According to a growing body of medical literature, misdiagnosis of the permanent vegetative state is a real problem. A study published in the June 1991

Archives of Neurology found that, of 84 patients with a firm diagnosis of PVS, 58 per cent recovered consciousness within three years.[5] Moreover, researchers were unable to identify objective "predictors of recovery" to differentiate between those who would awaken and those who would not. So it is likely that many who would recover consciousness given sufficient time are being killed in the name of compassion, cost containment, or "quality of life."

Dr. Angell suggests that such mistakes can be prevented by allowing sufficient time to pass after the brain injury. But as the dehumanising of the profoundly brain damaged has progressed, the urge has grown to get them out of the way as soon as possible. "What we are seeing in too many cases is a completely improper rush to judgement that a patient is suffering PVS," says Pasadena neurologist Dr.Vincent Fortanasce. "It takes at least three to six months before a firm diagnosis of persistent vegetative state can be made. However many doctors make such diagnoses within a week or less, often without objective testing. Eighty to ninety per cent of the cases I see have been improperly diagnosed, often by doctors who are not qualified to make the diagnosis. Unfortunately, that's the real practice of medicine today."

To illustrate his point, Dr. Fortanasce describes a case in which he was involved. A sixty-year old patient who had collapsed received a PVS diagnosis from his internist, who strongly recommended against continuing life support. The family was reluctant to see their loved one die, so they demanded a second opinion from a neurologist. "I came in and diagnosed a severe brain seizure, not PVS," Dr. Fortanasce says. "I prescribed continued life support and medication. Within a week the patient walked out of the hospital in full possession of his faculties. If the family had listened to the internist that man would be dead today."

And there is another twist. The Japanese may have discovered a way to wake up some patients from PVS. An article in the September 24 *St. Louis Post-Dispatch* [6] reported that Japanese doctors have awakened seven of twenty patients diagnosed as permanently unconscious by stimulating their mid-brains with electrodes. This news comes at an awkward time. Just when society seems to have accepted brain-damaged people as disposable, it turns out that they may not be "dead" after all. Indeed, Dr. Christopher M. DeGeorgio, an assistant professor of neurology at the University of Southern California, reports that some PVS patients who have awakened report that they were aware of their surroundings while "unconscious." Such findings make it more difficult to starve brain-damaged patients to death and still get a good night's sleep. Perhaps that is why the Japanese study has received little attention from bioethicists, who increasingly focus on determining which vulnerable group will be the next to be deemed expendable. If that seems harsh, consider what the director of the Hastings Centre for Bioethics, Daniel Callahan, wrote in 1983: "Denial of nutrition may in the long run be the only effective way to make certain that a large number of biologically tenacious patients actually die. Given the increasingly large pool of the superannuated, chronically ill, physically marginal elderly, it could well become the non-treatment of choice." He said the practice could be kept under control "if there remains a deep-seated revulsion at the stopping of feeding even under legitimate circumstances." But given the current trend, that revulsion is fast becoming a thing of the past.

Futile Care Theory and Medical Fascism. The Duty To Die

Extracts from an article by Wesley J. Smith that was first published in March 1998 in 'Heterodoxy' 1998; 6: 9-11. Published by the Centre for the Study of Popular Culture of Los Angeles, USA. It is reprinted with the author's kind permission.

"My mother's doctor is refusing to give her antibiotics," the woman caller told me in an urgent voice. "Why is he refusing to prescribe antibiotics?" I asked. "He says that she's 92 and an infection will kill her sooner or later. So it might as well be this infection."

As disturbing as this call was, and as outrageous the doctor's behaviour, I wasn't particularly surprised. I have been receiving such calls with increasing frequency over the last several years. Not every day. Not every week. But with enough frequency to know that something frightening is happening to American medical ethics.

There was the case of the Indiana teenager whose doctor refused to treat the boy's 107 degree fever because he was severely brain damaged from an auto accident. Had the boy's father not been a powerful corporate executive capable of bringing great pressure to bear on the doctor, his son would have died. Today, the young man is conscious, back home, and slowly recovering.

Then there was the Oregon woman whose nursing home doctor placed a DNR (Do not resuscitate) order on her medical chart over her, and her family's objections. Even though the patient was competent to decide for herself, it took the lawyer's threat of litigation to get the DNR removed from her chart.

Lawyers were also required by the brother of a Colorado woman with brain cancer. When he insisted on continuing treatment after the disease went into remission- a decision with which his sister agreed- the health insurer sued to disqualify him as the surrogate decision-maker. Not only that, threats were made to charge the family with the entire cost of treatment. The case ended when the woman died after surgery to repair a severe bed sore.

These cases show that something is rotten in the state of our current medical system and getting more rotten every day. Patients are entitled to make their own health care decisions based on "informed consent," that is they may accept or reject medical treatment based on information supplied by the doctor as to its hoped-for benefits and potential risks. Instead they are being precipitately shunted toward the "exit" sign and being urged to take early checkout from life.

Back when a lot of money could be made in medicine keeping people alive on machines, some patients and families complained bitterly that their right to reject unwanted medical treatment was violated by doctors who refused to disconnect life support when it was no longer desired. This was seen, correctly, as an unwarranted interference by doctors with the personal autonomy of their patients. The problem was addressed by enacting laws protecting people's right to refuse unwanted medical treatment, even if the likely result was death. If anything we now err on the other side. The imperative for personal autonomy in medicine has now grown so strong that the feeding tubes of cognitively disabled people who are not terminally ill can (inappropriately in my view) be removed at the request of surrogate decision-makers, with the explicit intention of causing their death by dehydration.

If people can say no to life-saving medical treatment in the name of autonomy, consistency requires that they also be allowed to say yes. But that is not how things are working out. In the emerging brave new world of medicine, personal autonomy applies strictly only when the "correct" end-of-life health care decision is made. Patients or families who make treatment decisions disapproved of by doctors, government bureaucrats, and health insurance executives, in Dylan Thomas' famous words, to rage against the dying of the night- frequently discover to their dismay that personal autonomy has its limits.

Futile Care Theory

While society and the media have focused primarily on the importance of personal autonomy in the context of the "right to die," little attention has been paid to concurrent efforts to disregard autonomy when a dying or disabled patient wants care that bioethicists, moral philosophers, doctors, and managed-care health insurance executives deem "futile". Futile Care Theory goes something like this: When a patient reaches a certain predefined stage of age, illness or injury, any further treatment other than comfort care shall be deemed "futile" and shall therefore be withheld, regardless of the desires of the patient or family. The personal values and morals of the patient are no longer relevant. End of story, and often end of life.

If Futile Care Theory were an objective concept, this would not be cause for alarm. Using an extreme example to illustrate the point: in simple objective terms, a doctor would properly and ethically refuse a patient's request that a kidney be removed as treatment for an ear infection (even though this request was an act of personal autonomy) because the requested "treatment" would have no possible medical benefit to the patient. Indeed it would be unethical to remove the kidney since it would cause the patient very real harm.

But this objective approach is not what Futile Care Theory is all about. Rather, as preached by the medical intelligentsia, the notion of futility is based on the perceived subjective value- or better stated the lack thereof- of the patient's life. In this context, futilitarianism becomes an exercise in raw Darwinism in that it views some patient's lives as having so little quality, value or worth that the treatment they request is not worth the investment of resources or emotion it would cost to provide.

The first group of patients attacked by futile care theorists were the permanently unconscious. Unsatisfied with limiting the removal of feeding tubes to those circumstances where dehydration is specifically requested futilitarians have begun to promote ethical policies that *require* food and fluids to be withheld from such patients regardless of the desires of patient or family.

Advocacy of this position comes from the highest levels of the medical establishment. For example, in May 1994, Dr. Marcia Angell, executive editor of the *New England Journal of Medicine* wrote in the Journal that the legal presumption in favour of life as applied to patients diagnosed with permanent unconsciousness should be removed so that "demoralized" care givers won't be forced to provide care they believe is futile or which wastes "valuable resources." [4] How? One way suggested by Dr.Angell would be to change the definition of "death" to include the diagnosis of permanent unconsciousness .

People with severe brain damage are not the only ones futilitarians want to push out of the life boat. In 1993, Daniel Callahan, one of the world's foremost bioethicists, urged in *The Troubled Dream of Life* that health care be rationed on the basis of age.[7] He has since gone further, arguing that treatment should be deemed futile if "there is a likely, though not necessarily certain, downward course of an illness, making death a strong probability," or when "the available medical treatments for a potentially fatal condition entail a significant likelihood of extended pain or suffering," or when care would "significantly increase the likelihood of a bad death."

These definitions are so vague that almost any serious life-threatening medical condition potentially qualifies. Moreover, they beg the question: what if patients *want* to assume such risks of treatment in order to save their lives?

All of this sounds suspiciously like the creation of a duty to die. Indeed, the idea that people deemed done for by the medical intelligentsia have such a duty is under active discussion within bioethical circles. A peer reviewed article, "Is There a Duty to Die?" in the March-April 1997 *Hastings Centre Report*- one of the world's most respected bioethical journals- is a case in point. According to the author John Hardwig, an East Tennessee State University medical ethics professor, among those with a "duty to die" are the elderly above the age of 75 and people whose continued life will "impose significant burdens- emotional burdens, extensive care giving, destruction of life plans." Among others who are expendable are people whose loved ones "have already made great contributions- perhaps even sacrifices- to make their life a good one," and people whose illness or disability renders them "incapable of giving love." People who don't accept this duty, according to Hardwig, suffer from "a moral failing, the sign of a life out of touch with life's basic realities." [8]

It is important to realise that these advocacy articles are not the ranting of some fringe. They are being published in the most prestigious medical and ethical journals in the world and insinuating their way into a status of respectability. It is the beginning of the route to consensus which effectively excludes public input. The "experts" argue among themselves in professional publications and seminars about what a specific health care policy should be. Agreement is eventually reached and then it is on to the courts and legislatures to solidify these agreed upon policies into legal precedent and statutory law.

We have seen this routine before. Fifteen years ago, (in 1983) journals such as the *New England Journal of Medicine* and the *Hastings Centre Report* led the way in moulding an ethical consensus that tube-supplied food and fluids should be considered medical treatment, leading directly to current laws and court decisions permitting intentional dehydrating of people- both conscious and unconscious- suffering from severe cognitive disabilities. Ten years ago (in 1988) the discussion concerned living wills. Five years ago (and continuing), the hot topic was assisted suicide. In some sense, Jack Kevorkian is merely a battering ram for those who follow him but never have to deal with the outrage his activities occasion.

Pay close attention to this ongoing dialogue in the medical world today and it becomes vividly clear that Futile Care theorists seek to create public policies that promote death as the answer to the problems of old age, debilitating and terminal illnesses, and dependency caused by cognitive disability. Futile Care advocates view people who reach these stages of life as better off dead- for their own benefit, for that of their families, and for society. If "choice" achieves the death goal, thereby preserving the ideal of personal autonomy, all well and good. But if the claims of personal autonomy are a hindrance, then "choice" will be discarded as counterproductive and the decision will be made for the patient and family.

Futile Care Theory is not merely some ominous possibility lurking in the future. It is already being imposed on some patients. In Michigan, when the parents of the prematurely born infant, Baby Terry, refused doctors' advice to turn off their child's life support, they were brought up on charges of child abuse and stripped of their right to make decisions for their baby- solely because they insisted on continuing medical treatment. (The child died before the trial court's decision could be appealed.)

In Massachusetts, a 71 year old woman Catherine Gilgunn, explicitly instructed doctors and family that vigorous efforts be made to keep her alive. After she became unconscious from a stroke, rather than obeying her instructions as reiterated by Mrs Gilgunn's daughter, the doctor instead removed her from the respirator, resulting in death. The family sued for malpractice but lost the case when the judge instructed the jury that any treatment that did not promise a cure was futile.

In the state of Washington, another family was turned in for child abuse by a hospital administrator when they obtained a court injunction ordering kidney dialysis to continue for their prematurely born son, known as Baby Ryan. Next, the doctors and administrators vigorously fought the parents in court over who had the right to decide the level of Ryan's care. Doctors even signed sworn affidavits that the child had "no chance" of surviving, arguing that continued treatment thereby violated *their* ethics. Happily the doctors were dead wrong. Baby Ryan survived when his care was transferred to another medical team. Today, at age 5, Ryan struggles to overcome health problems associated with his premature birth, but he no longer needs kidney dialysis. Had the doctors' "values" prevailed over the autonomy of the parents, Ryan would be but a painful memory.

These legal cases are the first drops of a coming torrent. All over the country and to an ever increasing degree, policies permitting the refusal of desired care for the frail elderly, very prematurely born infants, those who are diagnosed as permanently unconscious, the severely disabled, and the terminally ill- the weakest and most vulnerable among us- are being formally implemented and put into clinical practice.

In February 1997, the Alexian Brothers Hospital in San Jose, California, instituted a formal Futile Care ("Non-Beneficial Treatment") policy. Its stated purpose: "to promote a positive atmosphere of comfort care for patients near the end of life" and to insist that "*the dying process must not be unnecessarily prolonged.*" Who decides what is unnecessary prolongation? The hospital, of course.

The Alexian Brothers policy presumes that requests for medical treatment or testing, including cardio-pulmonary resuscitation (CPR), is "inappropriate" for a person with any of the following conditions:

❑   Irreversible coma, persistent vegetative state, or anencephaly.
❑   Permanent dependence on intensive care to sustain life.

- Terminal illness with neurological, renal, oncological, or other devastating disease.
- Untreatable lethal congenital abnormality.
- Severe, irreversible dementia.

The only care such patients are entitled to is comfort care. This is devastating to such people who want treatment. Under the policy, healthy severely mentally retarded people could be denied CPR that their families want for them as well as other medical treatments such as antibiotics to fight infection and reduce fever. Dying people may be denied the extra weeks of months of life that desired CPR might provide them. People who are deemed permanently unconscious (a condition notoriously misdiagnosed) will have tube-supplied food and fluids withheld whether their families agree or not.

Worse yet, doctors who violate this policy must "provide written justification" for the treatment provided. Moreover, to ensure that doctors toe the line, snitching is encouraged by nurses and others against physicians who provide treatment or testing "such as antibiotics, dialysis, blood tests, or monitoring," that the hospital's policy has declared inappropriate. The punishment for deviation from the policy is unmentioned, but it can be presumed that a doctor who consistently refuses to follow the hospital's dictates would be in jeopardy of losing staffing privileges.

Patients and families are also subjected to pressures that are hard to withstand. If the patient or family "insists on continuing treatment after advisement that it is non-beneficial," the matter is sent to the bioethics committee, an anonymous group whose deliberations are held in private. "If the recommendations of the bioethics committee are not accepted by the patient (or surrogate), care should be transferred to another institution." And if, as is often the case, there is no other institution willing to take the patient? The policy is silent, but one presumes the care will be refused despite patient and family desires.

Towards Collective Medical Decision-Making

Futilitarians are working to replace the current medical system in which private health care decision-making between patient and doctor is sacrosanct with a legally enforceable collective standard of allowable- and disallowable- medical care. So admits Dr. Donald J. Murphy who heads up the Colorado Collective for Medical Decisions (CCMD), a futilitarian think tank that expects to distribute futile-care guidelines throughout the nation by 1999.

In an interview given during my research for *Forced Exit*,[9] Dr. Murphy described the future he and other futilitarians envision: Health will be a community concept as much as an individual one, and will include other community considerations such as the need for "recreation and transportation." Doctors' duty to their patients will be subsumed by their overarching responsibility to the collective. Consequently, the parameters of private health care decision-making will be limited to those choices considered appropriate by the community. (For example, according to Dr. Murphy, mammograms would be permitted for women who are middle aged but not for women who are elderly.) And when people reach certain predefined stages in life,

123

in the infamous words about the elderly by CCMD co-founder, former Governor Richard Lamm, they will have a "duty to die and get out of the way."

Futile Care Theory has already poisoned Oregon's Medicaid Program, the first in the nation to explicitly ration health care. The rationing program seeks to expand eligibility for Medicaid by cutting costs through limiting certain treatments. Here's how the program works: A list was created consisting of 745 medical treatments. The lower the number, the more beneficial the treatment is deemed. Every two years, a cut-off line is determined based on budget estimates. If the number of the treatment a poor person needs is below the cut-off line, it will not be funded- which of course, means that it will not be provided. In 1994, for instance, the cut-off number was 606. In 1998 it was 578.

The number each treatment received in the rationing hierarchy was established, in part, by the kind of futilitarian political determination advocated by CCMD. The effect was to pit some poor, sick people against other poor, sick people. Not surprisingly, those with political clout generally did well, while the relatively powerless found their treatment needs excluded from coverage. For example, as initially proposed, curative treatment for late stage AIDS would have been excluded from coverage based on the futilitarian concept that such treatment is "ineffective." When the gay community heard of the plan, it organized and successfully maintained coverage for AIDS treatment. At the same time, lacking an organized political constituency, some late-stage cancer patients were excluded from coverage.

Considering the philosophy behind Futile Care Theory, it should come as no surprise that the Oregon Department of Health recently declared assisted suicide to be a form of "comfort care," a covered treatment in Oregon's Medicaid rationing scheme. Thus does the ultimate death agenda which underlies futile care theory come full circle. Imagine the scenario: a poor Medicaid patient wants treatment not covered by the rationing plan Denied desired care by the new bureaucratic rules, in desperation she turns to assisted suicide. The woman's early death is seen by the powers-that-be as best for her, her family, and the budgetary needs of Oregon's Medicaid Program.

CCMD's Dr. Murphy sees the coming battle over Futile Care as the key to the future ethics of American medicine. He is right. The 92 year-old woman mentioned at the top of this story, who was initially denied antibiotics was eventually able to secure treatment that saved her life. But if Futile Care Theory is imposed on the American people through formally enacted guidelines and enforceable public policies, similar cases will not have equally happy endings. For if Futile Care Theory becomes the law of the land, health care decision-making will have little to do with personal autonomy- unless the choice is the politically correct one of choosing to die- but will become primarily a matter of "doctor knows best," with available choices limited by the dictates of the collective will. No problem for the young, healthy, and productive, but devastating for everyone else.

There is a term that aptly describes the health care system that futilitarians seek to impose on us: medical fascism. Its implementation may be closer than you think.

Acknowledgement. The author of these articles, Wesley J. Smith, is an attorney for the International Anti-Euthanasia Task Force and a senior fellow of the Discovery Institute in Seattle, USA. He has brought concerns about Futile Care Theory to the attention of the American public. His assistance in providing material for this book is greatly appreciated.

References

References were given in the text in the original articles. In the interests of uniformity these have been indicated by numerals in the text and are listed below.

1. Smith Wesley J. The right to die, the power to kill. *National Review*; p40-44, April 4th 1994.
2. Smith Wesley J. Better dead than fed. *National Review; p48-49,* June 27th 1994.
3. Legal case reference; Martin, 538 N.W.2d. 399 (Mich.1995). See account that follows later in this book. (Ed.)
4. Angell M. Editorial. *Archives of Neurology* June 1991.
5. *Archives of Neurology* June 1991
6. *St. Louis Despatch* September 24th. 1993.
7. Callaghan Daniel. Troubled Dream of Life. 1993.
8. Hardwig. J. Is there a duty to die? *Hastings Centre Report*. March-April 1997.
9. Wesley J. Smith, Forced Exit: The Slippery Slope from Assisted Suicide to Legalized Murder. *Spence Publishing*. 2nd Edition 2003.

Chapter 9

Some Cases That Reached The Courts In The USA

Based on published reports by Wesley J. Smith

Introduction

The cases described in this chapter illustrate the dilemmas that doctors, relatives, legal guardians and judges face when trying to decide whether life-sustaining assisted or artificial feeding and nutrition should be withdrawn. Families can be torn about by internal strife as court cases ebb and flow and verdicts are challenged or overthrown. It can be a nightmare for all concerned.

The American experience is that it is usually the families who involve the courts and demand that life support is ended. The first such case was that of Karen Quinlan whose respirator was turned off in 1976. Since then numerous American courts have allowed life-sustaining treatment to be withdrawn in patients with a permanent vegetative state (PVS). Observers in the USA find themselves on the proverbial slippery slope, for as the case of Ronald Comeau demonstrates, patients who are aware but mentally disabled are at risk of having their life-support ended.

The Ronald Comeau story. The right to die, the power to kill

The account that follows is an abridged version of a report that was first published in The National Review on April 4th 1994; p 40-48. It is used with the kind permission of author Wesley J. Smith.

'It was June 21, 1993. For thirty-year old drifter Ronald Comeau, the day seemed to mark the end of the road. Under arrest in the small community town of Bennington, Vermont, accused of robbing another homeless man, Ron was alone, seemingly with no one to turn to. It had been a long time since he had seen his father, and their relationship had never been good. His mother had no phone. He hadn't seen his brothers for nearly seven years. Even the police didn't care to watch him in the holding cell. Minutes after being locked up, police say, he was found hanging from a noose he had made out of the trim of a cheap jail blanket.'

So began Wesley J. Smith's article in 1994. He went on to explain that Ronald Comeau was cut down by the police, revived by paramedics and taken to the Southwestern Vermont Medical Centre where he had two shots of electricity to restart the heart. It worked. After about 15 minutes without a pulse Ron had a steady heart beat, but he was not expected to survive. The hospital located Ron's father in Maine within hours but he did not come to the bedside. It was decided that Ron needed a guardian to make decisions on his behalf, so one Joseph Schaff, known for his role in child-custody matters, was appointed as his guardian by Judge Buchanan in July.

By mid-August Ron had been diagnosed as being in an irreversible persistent vegetative state. He was awake and had reflexes, but there appeared to be no cognitive ability whatsoever. Therefore Mr Schaff instructed Stephen Saltonstall, an attorney, to seek permission in the Probate Court to remove the ventilator that aided Ron's breathing. This was expected to lead to death.

On August 17th a hearing was held before Judge Buchanan. Convinced it was in Ron's best interests she signed the order permitting the ventilator to be withdrawn. But Ron did not die. Not only that, he began to improve. By the middle of September he had emerged from his persistent vegetative state and was more aware. But this was not a cause for joy. Joe Schaff was said to be horrified by his condition saying " I saw a person who could register some feelings, but those feelings were pain, agony and fear. His hands were bent in towards his wrists. It appeared he was trying to remove his feeding tube. Whether it was a conscious act, I could not tell."…He decided to raise the question of withholding food and fluids. However a consultant neurologist Dr Edwards found it difficult to support this suggestion, so the medical ethics committee convened…

Wesley J. Smith continued 'Ron Comeau was neither terminally ill nor in an irreversible coma. He was awake and aware, if profoundly brain-damaged and disabled. But that did not seem to concern the ethics committee… They took the view that if being in jail made him so unhappy that he wanted to kill himself, then being in hospital partially paralysed would also make him unhappy. His emotions

usually looked like fear, anger, rage and sometimes sadness.' However a speech therapist saw things rather differently- she saw a man who could respond happily to human conversation. Other notes on file indicated that he took an intense interest in discussions about his future care. Nevertheless, noted Smith, the case for removing the feeding tube was presented to Judge Buchanan with information couched in terms of unbearable suffering. Two doctors testified in support of removing nutritional care, but Dr Edward's dissenting report was not mentioned to the judge. Accordingly the judge ruled that Ron would "beyond all reasonable doubt…ask that artificial hydration and nutrition be terminated." If all had gone to plan, observed Smith, Ronald Comeau would have been dead within a week.

To the rescue came Revd Mike McHugh, a controversial pro-life Christian minister and founder of the Vermont chapter of Operation Rescue. He saw it as his duty to seek to preserve life. Two days after Judge Buchanan's ruling McHugh got a phone call from a fellow believer who had heard a radio report that a young man was going to be legally starved to death. Was there anything McHugh could do? There was indeed! McHugh called Judge Buchanan at her home and told her he wanted to petition to be Ronald Comeau's guardian. She agreed to convene an immediate hearing. McHugh then went high profile, wrote Smith, issuing a press release announcing that he was going to fight to save Ronald Comeau's life.

At the court hearing on November 11th 1993, the judge ruled that McHugh had no standing in the case under Vermont law. This ruling was affirmed by another judge the next day, on appeal. So McHugh called a pro-life attorney who immediately prepared and presented an emergency motion to the Chief Justice of Vermont Supreme Court. A stay was granted pending a hearing on November 16th. The order was served on the hospital and Ron Comeau's food and fluids were restored as a temporary measure.

McHugh had one last card to play, wrote Smith- Ron's family. He drove down to Rhode Island in a fruitless search for Ron's mother, then back to Maine where he managed to trace Ron's father and uncle. The two men were persuaded to go to Vermont with McHugh to attend the hearing on November 16th, all expenses being paid by McHugh and his pro-life supporters. Ron's father and uncle visited him in hospital and came away convinced he should live. His father told the press "I said 'This is Dad'. When he heard that he had a smile on his face and started to move all over the place." His uncle added "If he's in a coma, it's the funniest coma I ever saw."

Meanwhile Ron's brother Renald Comeau in Massachusetts had heard a news report about the case and travelled to the bedside to be joined by other members of the family. It was the first family reunion there had been for a long time. Smith noted 'Ron delighted at being shown a shirt with the Harley Davidson logo on it. He and his brothers laughingly compared tattoos. The brothers came away quite upset at what had almost happened to Ron. "Imagine, they were going to kill this guy," said his half-brother later, "There's a lot of life there.""…Thereafter Joe Schaaf met with Renald Comeau, and it was agreed that Renald would take over as his brother's guardian. Any thought of starving Ron to death was abandoned.

In the month's since he was saved, Ron Comeau's condition slowly improved. Wesley J. Smith noted that according to Renald, Ron could recognize family, listen to music, sit up, roll over, use the television remote control, clumsily push himself in a wheelchair, and eat foods such as soup and pudding. He even flirted with pretty nurses, summoning them with his call button and blowing them kisses. He was later transferred to a rehabilitation facility in Massachusetts where he had good days and bad days. One very good day was when he was reunited with his mother, whom he had not seen for years.

It could happen anywhere

In the final section of his report Wesley J. Smith wrote 'What happened to Ron Comeau could happen anywhere. There are no villains here. Yet, the legal and medical systems almost permitted Ron to be killed, because a retired educator believed that the quality of his life was not worth living.

'One fundamental problem was the way the court decided to withdraw Ron's nutrition. The hearing took place in a kangaroo-court atmosphere with a predictable, almost predestined, conclusion. The only opinions Judge Buchanan heard were those favouring Ron's death. No one argued to maintain Ron's life, not even the guardian *ad litem,* appointed to represent Ron in the hearing. Moreover the judge knew, but apparently did not take into account, that Ron had improved since the August hearing…

'It is clear that those who advocated Ron's death did not do so out of malice but in the sincere belief that dying would be better than living a life so profoundly disabled. But, does anyone have the *moral right* to starve and dehydrate another human being to death? If this case teaches us anything, it is that once acts to *cause death* are allowed, so-called "protective guidelines" are easily broken and ignored.

'Rita Marker, director of the International Anti-Euthanasia Task Force, said: "Denying food and water to a person because we think he wouldn't want to live in his current condition doesn't change the fact that we're ending his life. Bluntly stated, we're killing him. Whether the motivation is benevolence, cost-containment, or ignorance, the bottom line is that we have become judge and jury in a process that ends with capital punishment for the 'crime' of being dependent."

'Ronald Comeau is alive and reunited with his family, not because the system worked, but because an unpopular, in-your-face pro-life radical threw a monkey wrench into its gears. And despite the widespread disdain for his zealotry and suspicion of his motives, *he* was the one who had it right: not the doctors, who said Ron would never improve; not the guardian, who essentially chose to kill his ward: not the medical ethics committee, which gave the guardian its blessing; and not the judge, who acted like a rubber stamp.

'Renald Comeau wonders, "How many more Ronnie Comeaus are there out there?" An important question, especially since the next Ron Comeau might not have a Mike McHugh.'

The case of Michael Martin

Compiled from information on the International Task Force for Euthanasia web site, attributed to Wesley J. Smith and Rita Marker. Used with permission. See also 'Better dead than fed?' by Wesley J. Smith. National Review June 7th 1994.

The case of Michael Martin is a sad example of a family at war, a wife who cannot see the person beneath the disability, and of legal indecision. Had Michael Martin put in writing his pre-accident views about life as a 'vegetable' he would now be dead. As it is his views after the accident were unequivocal- he wanted to live. Fortunately the courts found in his favour but it was touch and go.

Legal case reference. Re Martin, 538 N.W.2d 399 Mich.1995

Michael Martin, an American aged 41 was severely injured in a car-train accident in 1987. Experts said he was not in a persistent vegetative state (PVS). He had communicated through a computerised device that he wanted to live. Yet despite this wish, his wife Mary, who was also his legal guardian petitioned through the courts in Michigan to have his gastrostomy feeding tube removed and food and fluids withheld, claiming that Michael had made statements prior to the accident indicating that he would not want to live as a 'vegetable.' Michael's sister and mother fought for his right to live. The Probate Judge rejected the wife's request to have Michael starved and dehydrated to death, because his pre-accident statements were not in writing. Had Michael been terminally ill or unconscious the judge would have granted his request. The fact that Michael indicated that he wanted to live was ruled irrelevant because of his "impaired condition."

Yet we are told that Michael had been assessed as level five on the Los Amigos Ranchos scale, a scale used by rehabilitation doctors in the USA to assess a patient's improvement. A level of five means that the patient is interactive and ready for intensive rehabilitation. Court testimony also indicated that Michael had an I.Q, after the accident, ranging from 61-73, this being the range for someone who is *mildly* retarded. Thus, noted Smith and Marker, Judge Grieg's ruling raised serious questions regarding the autonomy of disabled patients, and just how 'impaired' a person has to be before he or she no longer has rights and interests.

The case was referred to the Michigan Court of Appeals who were critical of the Probate Court proceedings. They had failed to issue specific findings based on the evidence as to Michael's current decision-making capacity and his present level of physical, sensory, emotional and cognitive functioning. They had erred in denying the petition to Michael's mother and sister to have Mary Martin removed as legal guardian, without even holding a hearing concerning the "possible bias, prejudice, conflict of interest, or improper motive" on the part of Mary Martin. Finally they had erred in not granting his mother and sister legal standing.

The case was returned to the Probate Court and the Judge changed his original ruling and allowed the feeding tube to be removed. That ruling was then affirmed by the Court of Appeals, but a further appeal was lodged with a higher court, the Michigan Supreme Court.

This man was not in a permanent vegetative state. He was said to be alert, played cards, watched TV, loved country – western music, and appeared contented in the nursing home where he lived. While the Michigan Supreme Court was considering whether to grant an appeal, he spelt out "*Afraid*" on his alphabet board. When the speech therapist asked him "Are you afraid of somebody?" Michael shook his head *no*. "Are you afraid for somebody?" asked the therapist. Michael nodded *yes*. The therapist queried whether Michael was afraid for the nurses, aides, or his roommate. Michael indicated *no*. "Was he afraid that someone would remove him from the nursing home?" *Yes*. According to the chart notes, as reported by Smith and Marker, when Michael was assured that he would be at that facility for "quite a while," he produced a big smile. That nursing facility had refused to starve and dehydrate Michael to death. If his wife got her way Michael would have to be removed from his current home.

Writer and lawyer Wesley J. Smith who followed the case closely posed the question, "Why isn't the benefit of the doubt being given to the choice of life in these starvation cases?" Perhaps, he suggested, it is because we are becoming a society that increasingly believes that it is better to be dead than disabled.

In the end Mrs Mary Martin lost her case and her husband Michael Martin lived. Nevertheless the wife whose "possible bias and prejudice" was overlooked by one court, continued to advocate the removal of food and fluids from people who are disabled. Addressing a conference in Philadelphia in 1998 Mrs Martin said- "he (Michael) is not in PVS. He is conscious, awake..." Later, referring to the fact that her husband was injured in a car-train accident, she asked "Do you know why car insurance rates are so high? Because people like Mike are being forced to stay alive... He's in well enough health thanks to the feeding tube, he could outlive us all. And for what? Because his mother and sister aren't willing to let him go." She further stated it is alleged, "He does nothing but smile... Patients like this can smile and nod their head...They could be organ donors who are so desperately needed."

Seeking the death of Robert Wendland. A commentary by Wesley J Smith

This report was first published in the Sacramento Bee on November 14th 1997.[1] It is reprinted with the author's kind permission. Copyright Wesley J. Smith1997.

"Robert Wendland should die so that his family can 'be allowed to live their lives'," Dr. Ronald Cranford, a Minnesota neurologist and bioethicist, testified …in the Stockton, California courtroom of Superior Court Judge Bob McNatt (in 1997). The chosen method of death? Intentional dehydration and starvation.

What had Wendland, aged 45, done to deserve such a fate? He went into a coma in September 1993 from injuries sustained in an automobile accident. Sixteen months later, he awakened from the coma, paralysed on one side and unable to walk, talk or swallow enough to eat. He was physically and cognitively disabled and dependent on others for his care. He was not terminally ill. He was not hooked up to machines. He did require a feeding tube to sustain his life.

Those who sought to end Wendland's life downplayed his physical and cognitive abilities. That is because people who are diagnosed as permanently unconscious are being dehydrated in this country, all perfectly legal thanks to several court decisions. Now, "right to die" activists such as Cranford who has testified in support of dehydration in most of the nation's major dehydration cases of brain damaged patients' including that of Nancy Beth Cruzan want to stretch acceptable dehydration to disabled folk with brain damage who are awake and aware. This is the slippery slope in action.

A Wisconsin Supreme Court decision dealt a blow …to the right-to-die crowd's hopes when it ruled that it is not acceptable in Wisconsin to dehydrate conscious, brain-damaged patients (who would feel pain and agony) absent clear and convincing evidence probably through a written declaration executed by the patient before illness or injury, that dehydration is precisely and explicitly what the now-incapacitated patient wanted. In other words, general statements are not enough. The Michigan Supreme Court issued a similar ruling in 1995.

Cranford and others of his ideological persuasion were not amused by these decisions, seeing them as an impediment to the right to die. Wendland provided an opportunity to expand the law. Rose Wendland, Robert's wife, claimed that Robert would not want to live in his current condition. She based her claim primarily on her husband's statements made in the aftermath of her father's death, three months before Robert's injury, that he would not want to live if he could not "be a husband, father or a provider."

But is it right to kill someone because he might have said he would not want to live in a dependent state? Is it right to kill someone because he can't work and be productive? Is it right to kill someone because he is disabled? Robert Wendland's mother, Florence Wendland, and half-sister Rebekah Vinson, said no. They sued to prevent dehydration.

It is important to note that Wendland had slowly improved in the nearly two years since he awakened from his coma. For example, he had manoeuvred an electric wheelchair down hospital corridors and could manoeuvre a manual wheelchair with his unparalysed leg or arm. He had written the letter "R" of his first name when

131

asked, as well as some other letters of his name. He had used buttons to accurately answer yes and no questions some of the time. (Is your name Robert? Yes. Is your name Michael? No) In this regard, one of the doctors asked Wendland if he wanted to die. He didn't answer the question.

According to Cranford, these and other of Wendland's activities meant little. He also opined in his testimony that Wendland's therapists, who believed he had slowly improved, should be disregarded by McNatt because they were only "seeing what they want to see." Perhaps it is Cranford who is only seeing what he does not want to see!

It is disturbing that McNatt did not dismiss Rose Wendland's desire to end her husband's life out of hand when the case first came to his court in 1995. It is especially disturbing that a noted neurologist such as Cranford believes that one reason to dehydrate Wendland was to benefit his family, even though Rose Wendland has said she now only visits her husband once a month for about 30 minutes, and his children do not visit at all.

Dehydration begins when the feeding tube is removed, and death occurs usually within six to 30 days. Ironically to ensure that Wendland doesn't feel the pain of dehydration, Cranford testified it might be necessary to put him back into a coma with morphine.

It is said that a society is judged by the way in which it treats its weakest and most vulnerable members. Increasingly in the United States we kill them…[1]

Wesley J. Smith continued the story in the Weekly Standard in 1998 saying-

'The litigation has been bitter and prolonged. Robert's interests were supposed to be represented by a San Joaquin County public defender, Doran Berg. But in a nasty twist, Berg sided with the wife and argued even more vehemently and emotionally *for* Robert's dehydration than Rose did- perhaps the first time in the history of jurisprudence that a public defender has urged a judge to sentence a client to death. But Judge Bob McNatt reluctantly declined. Stating that he was making "the absolutely wrong decision for the right reasons," McNatt ruled wisely that such a momentous change in law and ethics should be decided in the legislature of the court of appeals, not by a trial judge…" [2]

On December 9th 1997 Judge McNatt ruled that Rose Wendland had failed to present clear and convincing evidence that starving and dehydrating Robert to death would be in his best interest. "If I have to choose life and death based on the evidence presented to me, I must err on the side of caution and choose life," the judge said. "I am not ready to start down that slippery slope without some form of guidance."[3]

'Judge McNatt's surprising ruling came after Rose and others had testified that, while Robert could do simple tasks, those functions were not sufficiently meaningful to justify letting Robert live. Robert was referred to as "minimally conscious." At least six doctors and ethicists testified that it would be ethically permissible to "let him die." But Janie Hickok Siess, the attorney for Robert's mother, Florence Wendland, argued that neither Rose's attorney nor the attorney appointed to the court to represent Robert had presented sufficient evidence to meet the "clear and convincing" burden of proof required under Californian law. Judge McNutt agreed…[3]

'McNatt's December 9th 1997 decision may have been only a reprieve for Robert Wendland' wrote Wesley J. Smith a year later. 'Berg quickly appealed and asked McNatt to authorise the use of San Joaquin County funds for a private attorney to argue for Robert's death in the appeal courts. McNatt agreed and permitted a maximum fee of $50,000. The power of the state of California and the money of its taxpayers are now being used to urge the death of one of its citizens, whose only "crime" is to be brain-damaged.'[2]

Three years later, as reported by Thomas Marzen in March 2000, the California Court of Appeal ruled that life-sustaining tube feeding and hydration may be withdrawn from a disabled person at the direction of the person's guardian, even if the patient is not unconscious, not terminally ill, and never said he or she would want food and fluids removed. [4] Thomas Marzen, J.D. general counsel of the National Legal Centre for the Medically Dependent and Disabled, found this decision "ominous" and "in conflict with the decisions laid down by the State Supreme Courts of Michigan and Wisconsin." In the view of the California Court of Appeal, "A guardian's withdrawal of life-sustaining treatment does not constitute a deprivation of life; rather it allows the disease to take its natural course." As Marzen explained, that ruling meant that all that a legal guardian in California was required to do was to say in good faith, and supported by medical evidence, that withdrawal of food and fluids was in the patient's "best interest." There was no requirement to prove that the patient, when competent, had expressed a desire to die, or to refuse the treatment offered. Thus in California, in the year 2000, a proxy decision-maker had a virtually free hand to make life and death decisions about medical treatment for a disabled person.[4]

However Florence Wendland battled on and took matters to the California Supreme Court, who (to quote Smith) 'overruled the Court of Appeal, and reinstated the trial judge's approach, noting *inter alia* that similarly fundamental decisions involving incompetent persons require very high standards of proof.'[5] Robert Wendland died of pneumonia shortly before this ruling was made.

The case of Hugh Finn with general comments about Futile-Care Theory

The following comments by Wesley J. Smith are taken from his article 'The deadly ethics of futile care theory' published in The Weekly Standard 1998; 4(12): 32-35. Extracts are used with the author's permission.

'Former news anchorman Hugh Finn was intentionally dehydrated to death last month, when doctors at a Manassas, Virginia, nursing home removed his feeding tube at the request of his wife. The act was legal. It had the explicit approval of federal and Virginia courts. It took eight days for Finn to die.

'Finn was not terminally ill. He was left severely brain damaged by a 1995 automobile accident. His doctors claimed he would always remain unconscious, in …a permanent vegetative state. But there was significant reason for doubt. His brother Ed claimed that Hugh was sometimes conscious and interactive, as did other members of the Finn family. A medical investigator had testified that Hugh Finn had said "Hi" to her upon first their first meeting, which if true proved Finn was conscious. Now Finn is dead and we will never know the truth.

'Finn's death made headlines because of the intervention of Virginia governor James Gilmore on the side of Finn's brothers and parents, who wanted feeding to continue. And many people around the country expressed shock at his fate. They shouldn't have. For years, the medical intelligentsia- philosophers, academics, and policy advisors known as bioethicists- have pushed lawmakers and judges to permit the death of patients like Hugh Finn who depend on feeding tubes for nutrition and water. In 1990, the Supreme Court gave its implied permission to the practice in the Nancy Cruzan case. Today, people diagnosed as being in a permanent vegetative state are deprived of food and water almost as a matter of medical routine. Moreover, *conscious* brain-damaged people meet the same end. Indeed, families of profoundly brain-damaged people are often pressured by doctors and social workers to cease "treatment" with food and fluids as a way of easing family burdens and ending lives deemed to have poor quality.

'It is only when families are divided, as they were in the Finn case, that such cases end up in court. But if the patient is in a vegetative state, it is almost impossible to stop a dehydration order by a spouse or other primary decision-maker, no matter how strongly other members of the family may object. If the patient is conscious, it remains a harder sell to obtain court permission for dehydration and starvation over family objections. But it is doubtful that the courts will resist much longer…

'Cases such as Hugh Finn's, Michael Martin's and Robert Wendland's are usually described in the media as promoting patient autonomy and private medical decision-making by families. But that is only partly true. Increasingly "choice" in medical cases involving profoundly disabled people is viewed by bioethicists and doctors as a one-way street. Should families choose death for their loved ones, their wishes are honoured and acted on with despatch. But if families insist that their loved ones continue to be nourished and cared for, these same experts proclaim instead that "autonomy has its limits."…

'Futile care decisions are already being implemented in many of the nation's hospitals. Little noticed by the mainstream media- but well documented in the medical literature- doctors and hospitals in Michigan, Massachusetts, Texas, Tennessee, and California have already refused to provide desired medical treatment to profoundly disabled and dying patients. This has led to a handful of court cases…

'Futile care theory is so new that the state of the law has not kept pace with clinical practice, leaving families, lawyers, and clinicians in doubt as to their respective rights and obligations. But many medical associations have now endorsed the doctrine, which means that desperately ill and disabled patients will increasingly be denied treatment against their families' and their wishes. Lawsuits are sure to follow…

'In New York, legislation has been introduced to clarify the rights and obligations of decision-makers and health-care providers when a patient is incompetent. Alarmingly, if passed in their current form, the bills would set futile care theory into legal concrete. The measures would permit hospitals to refuse desired treatment if based on a "formally adopted policy" predicted on "sincerely

134

held moral convictions." Physicians, too, could refuse to treat patients if doing so violated their moral beliefs. Disputes about treatment would be taken to committees that the legislation would require each hospital to create. If the person speaking for the patient disagreed with the decision of the ethics committee, he would have to move his loved one to a different hospital. Doctors and hospitals that acted in "good faith" pursuant to the law would be granted immunity to civil and criminal penalties. Opponents of the measures are hoping to require that care of the patient will continue until a doctor can be found willing to provide the desired treatment.

'Futile care policies are ostensibly designed to relieve the suffering of desperately ill and disabled people. But they are also underpinned, let's face it, by a cold-hearted, collectivist desire to save "scarce resources"... Futile care theorists could refuse desired end-of-life treatment to Grandma Jones in Florida, so that Little Suzie in Appalachia could have better access to medical care. Among bioethics professionals, for whom the restructuring of society is a deeply treasured goal, this is known as "distributive justice."...People on the medical margins are the first victims of the distributive-justice movement because they are widely viewed as having lives of little meaning or purpose. They can't or don't protest. And with remarkably few exceptions, no one else protests their fate either. As a result, futile-care theorists encounter surprisingly little opposition as they carve into the bedrock of American law the utilitarian principle that the lives of some people can be sacrificed for the benefit of others deemed more worthy of care.

'Futile-care policies, in and of themselves, won't save that much money. But once futile-care theory is legally entrenched, America's traditional medical system-organized round preserving the life and health of the individual patient and the Hippocratic obligation of the doctor to care for that patient- will be enfeebled beyond recognition.'

The case of Terri Schiavo

The following comments are based on information from Wesley J Smith and other sources.

Terri Schiavo collapsed at home in 1990 at the age of 26. She was admitted to hospital as an emergency with brain damage due to lack of oxygen. The precise cause of the collapse was somewhat uncertain, but the brain damage proved to be permanent. She required ANH to sustain her life for the next 15 years. The official diagnosis was a permanent vegetative state, but some observers doubted this, as videos seemed to indicate that she sometimes smiled and opened her eyes in response to her mother.[6,7] Wesley J Smith, speaking in Birmingham, England in 2005 said:

> "Vague statements became a death warrant for Terri. They were made when President Reagan was in office, when feeding tubes were not discussed. She was probably thinking about being hooked up to a respirator.[6]

> "In 1992 Terri's husband sued the hospital for malpractice, and said that he would take care of Terri for the rest of his life- she would have a normal life span. There was no mention of her desire to die at this stage. He won a

considerable amount of money for loss of companionship, and for her future care. He was not allowed to control the money as there was a conflict of interest, but when the money was safely in the bank he said that she would not want to live like this. Six months later he refused permission for her to have antibiotics for a urinary infection. Then her family started a bitter fight to save her… In 1996 the husband fell in love with someone else… In 1998 he started moves to get Terri's feeding tube stopped. Despite financial and emotional conflicts of interest he was allowed to pursue her death. Her property was more important than her life. This was an unbelievable paradox. The courts never strived for her life, and one has to ask "Why?"[6]

Eventually Judge Greer of Florida said that her feeding tube could be removed. This ruling was affirmed by the Florida Federal Court of Appeal and Terri's dehydration started in October 2003. But such was the public revulsion that there was a massive grass-roots political campaign to save her life. A petition was sent to Governor Jeb Bush of Florida, and the Florida legislature passed "Terri's Law" that enabled the Governor to intervene. He halted her dehydration on day 6 but the final outcome remained in doubt because there was a dispute about whether Terri's Law was constitutional.[7]

Terri's lawyers felt that her Catholic faith would be violated if her feeding tube was removed, but it was removed again in March 2005 following a court order. Her parents made a last-ditch appeal to the U.S Supreme Court to have the tube replaced, but the Supreme Court refused to intervene. Congress, supported by President Bush rushed through an emergency Bill giving federal courts the right to review her case- but the 11th Circuit Court of Appeals in Atlanta, Georgia refused to order the feeding tube to be replaced.[8,9] As her life ebbed away, passions ran high, and protesters gathered outside the hospice to plead for a last-minute intervention. But it was not to be and Terri Schiavo died.

Reactions to Terri Schiavo's death

The Bishop of Florida argued that the decision to remove the feeding tube was the right decision, and thought that the intrusion of politicians was "extremely inappropriate". He circulated a pastoral letter to this effect in the diocese of Southeast Florida. An edited excerpt from his letter was published in the Church Times.[10]

David Casarett who is an Assistant Professor of Geriatrics at the University of Pennsylvania School of Medicine and an investigator with the VA Centre for Health Equity Research and Promotion, said "That case was the ethical equivalent of an airplane crash- a highly visible tragedy that spurs investigation, analysis, and hopefully improvements and safeguards to prevent a recurrence." [11]

For Casarett the case was a tragedy because it challenged long-held "agreements" about ANH. He and his colleagues responded with a paper in the *New England Journal of Medicine* that set out various steps that could be taken to overcome "obstacles to ethical decision making" about ANH. (See page 115 of this book.)

The authors felt that the right of "patients and their families to make independent decisions about ANH and other medical treatment should be defended against legal, financial, and administrative challenges at the bedside." [12]

Sources

1. Smith Wesley J. Commentary. Seeking the death of Robert Wendland. First published in the *Sacramento Bee* on November 14th 1997. (In deference to the passage of time some verbs have been changed to the past tense. Ed.)
2. Smith Wesley J. *The Weekly Standard* Vol.4, No 12; p33: 1998.
3. Comments from the website of the International Anti Euthanasia Task Force, February 2000.
4. Marzen T. *National Right to Life News.* March 2000, page 10.
5. Smith Wesley J. The Wendland case and the treacherous road to nonpersonhood. In Ethical Issues in Modern Medicine. Eds. Steinbock B, Arras J D. London A J. 6th edition; p348-353 *McGrawHill.* 2002.
6. Wesley J Smith, speaking at a meeting of the Medical Ethics Alliance in Birmingham, England, May 13th 2005.
7. Wesley J Smith. Dehydration nation. *The Human Life Review.* Fall 2003; 69-79.
8. *Daily Mail*, March 25th, 2005. Judges doom right-to-life case woman.
9. Russell Alec. Passions run high as Schiavo vigil turns into 'death watch'. *The Daily Telegraph*, March 26th 2005, page 5, cols 1-5.
10. Leo Frade, Death's dominion. *The Church Times*, April 1st 2005.p16.
11. From a statement on http://www.med.upenn.edu/ December 15th 2005.
12. Casarett D, Kapo J, Caplan A. Appropriate use of artificial nutrition and hydration- fundamental principles and recommendations. *New England Journal of Medicine*, 2005, 353:24, 2607-2612. © 2005 Massachusetts Medical Society. All rights reserved. Quoted with permission.

Part 3

Children Matter

Introduction

People matter from the cradle to the grave. The articles that follow, based on experience in the United Kingdom, demonstrate the breadth and complexity of the ethical problems that may arise in the care of severely disabled children. With the advent of futile-care theory some children with severe disabilities and mental incapacity are at risk of having life-prolonging measures withheld or withdrawn with fatal results. The human being trapped within a disabled body can be overlooked only too easily, as happened in the case of David Glass. There is however a growing realisation that with skilled attention and a responsive environment, some meaningful interaction can be achieved to make the life of such children worthwhile.

A sensitive approach to decision-making in sick newborn infants, is described by Dr John Wyatt in a paper that was first published in Ethics and Medicine in 1998. This is reprinted with the author's kind permission. Dr Wyatt, a respected medical ethicist is Professor of Neonatal Paediatrics at University College Hospital London. In his paper, Wyatt states his view that within the traditional Hippocratic and Judaeo-Christian tradition of medical practice, there are basically two indications for withdrawal of treatment. Firstly, that the treatment is futile. Secondly, the patient is actively dying.

The following chapter consists of illustrative case reports in older children, compiled largely from reports in the media. "Remembering Susie" illustrates how a very handicapped child can be treasured as a person, and remembered with love long after her death. The management of her case gave no cause for concern and received no publicity. In contrast the notorious case of David Glass alerted the British public to the dangers that face very handicapped children these days. Sadly such children can no longer be guaranteed protection by the law. Moreover there are times when the wishes of the family regarding active intervention are overruled by doctors, as happened in the case of David Glass and that of child I. Such decisions are always difficult, and controversial.

There are times when the family would prefer to have no medical intervention, as happened in the case of conjoined twins Jodie and Mary from the Maltese island of Gozo. The doctors' plans to save Jodie would of necessity lead to the death of Mary, but the parents were devout Roman Catholics who found the decision in conflict with their religious belief. The case attracted great interest in the UK for the twins came to London for treatment. Permission for surgery was given by three judges in the Court of Appeal. Mary died, but happily Jodie survived and is now growing up at home on Gozo, with every prospect of living a normal life.

This section of the book ends on a note of hope, for in the UK severely disabled children with special needs have the best possible attention. Trained staff who work in this challenging field endeavour to create responsive environments which offer such children an opportunity to take part in positive, meaningful interactions.

Chapter 10

Non-treatment Decisions in the Care of the Newborn Infant

Author John Wyatt
*First published in Ethics and Medicine 1998; **14.2:** 45-49.*
Reprinted with permission.

In this article I am considering the specialist care of newborn infants and the sort of questions that arise from different forms of treatment. I will seek above all to provide some background to the decisions which we have to face. These concern, first, the explosive advances in neonatal care and, secondly, the ethical and philosophical debate which undergirds these issues. I would also like to talk about my own personal practice as a paediatrician at a major tertiary centre and the way forward for resolving, at least, some of the desperately difficult and painful issues in this area of medicine.

The very low birth-weight baby accounts for approximately 1% of all births. This means several thousand births in England and Wales- and across the world a far greater number. Over the last thirty years there has been a quite dramatic explosion in the use of technology. Although, as Dr Nicholson rightly says, medical technology as a whole has not had a dramatic impact on survival in this particular group of infants, the introduction of technology has undoubtedly had a dramatic effect.[1] The chances of survival of a very low birth-weight baby thirty years ago would have been approximately 20%. Now at major centres such as University College Hospital, London, the chances of survival are more like 80-85%. That change is mainly as a result of improvements in technology after birth, although not exclusively. There have been improvements in ante-natal obstetric care as well.

But the question is: is it appropriate to provide intensive neonatal care in the case of all low birth-weight babies? In particular, the spectre of brain injury is a major concern. The statistics vary, but approximately 10-15% of all extremely low birth-weight babies will suffer permanent brain injury. The commonest cause for this is hypoxic-ischaemic brain injury- injury due to shortage of oxygen and blood supply. In addition there is haemorrhagic injury in the extremely pre-term baby.

Many medical groups, our own group included, have been involved in long-term follow-up studies in order to improve our ability to obtain a prognosis, that is, to predict outcome from studies immediately after birth. One of the techniques we have used is cranial ultrasound. Newborn babies have an anterior fontanelle, the soft spot, through which it is possible to get good images of the brain with ultrasound. Even in very sick babies undergoing intensive care, it is possible to get good images of the brain. And a number of long-term prospective follow-up studies have shown that we are able to predict long-term outcome much more accurately than previously on the basis of ultrasound images. More high-technology methods, which I have been more particularly involved in, are also available. With nuclear magnetic resonance techniques it is possible to obtain very detailed information. Images of the brain can be obtained, as also phosphorus spectra which allows us to assess brain energy metabolism. There is also another technique, called near-infrared spectroscopy which enables infra-red light to be passed through the brain as a means of determining brain oxygenation and perfusion.

The reason for emphasising this is that as technology has advanced, so also has our ability to determine the severity of brain injury, and its likely prognostic significance within the first few days of life. There is no doubt that this trend will continue. This is a major research enterprise in which I and many of my colleagues are involved. The question is, as the information becomes more accurate and we are able to predict with a relative degree of accuracy the long-term outcome for any particular baby, how do we use this information in order to make decisions about intensive support?

The philosophical background

To step sideways and refer to some of the major philosophical background of these issues, I have been intrigued by a trend which is taking place among a group of philosophers. Basically, it involves redefining the newborn infant as a different category of being, compared with how babies have normally been viewed within medicine and society. John Harris from Manchester is a proponent of this view. He has said, "Nine months of development leaves the human embryo far short of emergence of anything that can be called a person." Peter Singer from Australia takes a similar view: "When I think of myself as the person I now am, I realise that I did not come into existence until some time after birth." Michael Tooley was the philosopher who initiated this concept of personhood. For Tooley, personhood is a question of having a 'continuing self'. A person is a being who is capable of understanding that they have a continuing self. The implication of this is that if you are not aware that you exist, then you have no continuing self. If you have no continuing self, then you have no rights, no individual rights, no ethical or legal rights of the kind that self-conscious persons in our society do. In particular you have no right to life.

Singer points out that there are many non-human animals whose rationality, self-consciousness, awareness, capacity to feel, and so on, exceed that of a week old, a month old or even a year old human baby. In fact, many domestic animals would be person's on Singer's criteria. For, as far as animal psychologists can tell us, they have a much greater self-awareness than a newborn baby, let alone an extremely pre-term baby.

This kind of thinking leads inevitably to the idea that ending the life of a newborn baby is merely preventing the existence of a person. 'The decision to kill a newborn baby is no more and no less the prevention of the existence of an additional person than is the decision not to procreate.' Contraception and infanticide are ethically equivalent according to Singer. That, at least, is the implication of that particular quote. Both practices represent the prevention of a person's coming into existence. The path along this line of reasoning is concept deriving from the utilitarian view of the world, namely that of the 'replacement infant'. If by killing a newborn baby we prevent a handicapped baby coming into existence, the parents can be encouraged

140

to have another baby, who we hope will be normal. Since the replacement infant will bring much greater happiness into the world, the loss of a happy life for the first infant is outweighed by the gain of a happier life for the second. The concept of the replacement infant is something that Singer and a number of like-minded philosophers have emphasised.

To step back historically, one of the quotes that I like comes from William Temple. 'If you don't know where you are going, it's sometimes helpful to know where you have been.' Interestingly the debate about the status and the philosophical significance of the newborn baby is not a new debate. It has been going on for more than two thousand years. If you go back to the Graeco-Roman Classical era, the most ancient text book of gynaecology, written by a Roman physician, Soranus, in the first century AD, has a chapter called 'How to recognise the newborn that is not worth rearing.' This chapter concerns a remarkably modern-sounding neonatal examination. 'The newborn should be carefully examined to ensure that it is perfect in all its parts, members and senses. That its ducts, namely the ears, nose, pharynx, urethra and anus are free from obstruction, that the natural functions of every member are neither sluggish nor weak, and so on. By conditions contrary to those mentioned the infant not worth rearing is recognised.'

To summarise, an interesting body of historical scholarship relating to that era, the Graeco-Roman ethical tradition viewed newborn babies as having potential value for the future, but little or no intrinsic value compared with adults. Thus, if a baby was sick or pre-term or abnormal in some way, its value for the future was reduced. Within the Graeco-Roman ethical tradition there was no general ethical duty to protect the defenceless and the vulnerable. Therefore, within that tradition intentional killing of abnormal babies was seen as both rational and morally acceptable. In fact, the Graeco-Roman classical philosophical tradition supported infanticide on eugenic grounds and on the basis of limited potential to contribute towards society.

It is interesting that within the Jewish nation, and then within the Judaeo-Christian tradition, a quite different perception of the newborn infant was current. Tacitus, who wrote frequently on the bizarre habits and beliefs of other nations, wrote with a faint air of astonishment that the Jewish people regard it as a crime to kill any recently born child. Philo of Alexandria, writing as an educated Jew wrote, 'Infanticide undoubtedly is murder, since the displeasure of the law is not concerned with ages but with the breach of the human race.'

The Judaic tradition came initially from the Torah. It sprang from the concept of the 'Imago Dei', the idea that every human being was a unique being made in God's image. And the intentional killing of a being made in God's image was regarded in some sense as a desecration of the unique image of God. To summarise the Judaeo-Christian ethical tradition, all newborn babies are unique beings who bear the image of God. Hence their status and value have nothing to do with their future potential. It is intrinsic. In addition, we must remember the Judaeo-Christian concern to protect the defenceless and the vulnerable within society, the child, as well as the slave and the orphan, the widow and the immigrant. It was considered a social duty to protect those who were defenceless and vulnerable. Within the Judaeo-Christian tradition intentional killing is always wrong.

Briefly to summarise, it seems to me that the same argument is going on today. We have two views of the newborn. We have one view which says that newborns have potential value but not intrinsic value. That view, I believe, can ultimately be traced back to the Graeco-Roman tradition. It implies that medical treatment depends crucially on the choice of the parents. Parental autonomy is the crucial value. There is no a priori duty to protect the defenceless. Intentional killing may be appropriate in some cases, and only limited resources should be applied if the future potential is limited.

On the other view of the newborn, the child has fundamental and intrinsic value. Medical treatment depends on the best interests of the child alone. The question of parental authority is secondary. There is an overriding duty to protect the defenceless from abuse. Intentional killing is always inappropriate, although futile treatment may be withdrawn. Resources should not be limited merely to those who have 'a good potential'.

What strikes me as a paediatrician practising in a pluralistic society- particularly in Central London, with an enormous range of ethical beliefs and traditions- is that there does seem to be a general core of parental intuitions. These emerge in conversations with parents when questions about the meaning of life, the world and the universe are discussed, as often happens when we are trying to debate the right course of action in the case of a particular baby undergoing neonatal intensive care.

To summarise, the majority of parents in my practice in 1997 would say: 'My baby is a unique irreplaceable member of my family; my baby is a person with a name and an identity; my baby must be treated by professionals with gentleness, with tenderness, and with respect.' I think that the word respect encapsulates what parents look for in the medical system. They look for respect, for a recognition of the dignity and the unique value of their child. 'My baby cannot be replaced.'

In contrast to Singer, I think that the concept of a replacement infant is not something that many parents accept. Most parents would say firstly- 'My baby cannot be replaced although I may have other, different, unique individual children in the future. Secondly, if my baby's outlook is hopeless, the most loving thing to do may be to stop treatment and to allow her to die.' In my experience, the vast majority of parents do believe that allowing a baby to die is not either morally or emotionally equivalent to deliberately killing her. Thirdly, the parents would say: 'If my baby does die, the permanent physical reminders of the uniqueness, the intrinsic significance of that baby are very precious, and the human status, value and significance of my dead baby should be recognised by the wider community.'

To sum up, it seems to me that parental intuitions are much closer to the Judaeo-Christian tradition which attributes intrinsic significance to the baby than to the Graeco-Roman view or the modern version expressed by Tooley, Singer and others, which hold that the baby is merely a being with potential for the future, but has no intrinsic worth.

Practical decision-making

How can we translate these ideas into practical decision-making? It seems to me that within the traditional Hippocratic and Judaeo-Christian tradition of medical

142

practice there are basically two indications for the withdrawal of treatment. First, the treatment is futile. Secondly, the patient is actively dying. The most helpful way of thinking about futile treatment is to consider the balance between the burdens and benefits of treatment. It is standard medical practice before any treatment is commenced to try to analyse the potential burdens versus the potential benefits of that treatment, and to ensure that the benefits outweigh the burdens. To give a treatment the burdens of which exceed its possible benefits is inconsistent with a humane practice of medicine. In fact, it could be seen as positively abusive. Neither is beginning futile treatment considered good medical practice.

Actively dying. With regard to the phrase 'actively dying', I translate that in practice to mean that a baby is demonstrating progressive irreversible deterioration despite maximum intensive support. In particular, this will involve lung-gas exchange, cardiac output and metabolic homeostasis. Most paediatricians would actually accept that it is possible to recognize the baby who is actively dying, who is spiralling downwards towards to irreversible death. In those conditions the withdrawal of intensive support so that the dying process is not prolonged seems entirely appropriate.

Futile treatment. A much more difficult question is the question of what we mean by futile treatment. I would classify futile treatment under three headings.

The first is the non-viable foetus. In current medical practice, babies who are of less than 23 weeks gestation are clearly not viable. The problem, just from a practical paediatric point of view, is that the assignment of gestational age is extremely unreliable, even with the highest technological input. The only situation where you can be certain of gestational age is where fertilisation has taken place outside the uterus, that is in vitro fertilisation. It is not at all uncommon for babies who are said to have a gestational age of 22 weeks, and therefore to be non-viable, in fact to have a gestational age of 24,25 or 26 weeks, which means that the outlook is completely different. Therefore I think the correct attitude is one of playing safe if there is any doubt. We teach our staff to initiate resuscitation, if there is any chance of success. This is on the understanding that treatment can always be withdrawn subsequently.

The second criterion is severe generalized brain injury of such severity that the possibility of a meaningful relationship in later life with parents is effectively absent, or profoundly curtailed.

The third criterion is an uncorrectable major malformation. Advances in paediatric care have meant that many malformations of the sort that Dr Nicholson has been describing are, in fact, correctable with modern treatment.[1] This completely changes the ethical issues. However, there are malformations that cannot be corrected. I am thinking particularly of a child who was born with no gut at all, no bowels, whose life had been sustained for a period by intravenous nutrition, but for whom there was no possibility of treatment that would provide a permanent life for that child. In such situations, it seems to me that the withdrawal of intensive support is appropriate- provided the burdens of treatment exceed the benefits.

Burdens and benefits

Of course, modern intensive care is burdensome. Potentially, it is an extremely unpleasant experience for babies. Hence, the removal of treatment which is excessively burdensome and unpleasant is far from being unethical. Indeed, one might argue that it would be unethical to continue treatment when the burdens clearly outweigh the benefits. It is certainly possible for neonatal intensive care to become a sophisticate form of child abuse, whereby babies are submitted to extreme technological interventions without any real prospect of improvement or cure. However, I- and I think most of my colleagues and most of the parents- do believe strongly that there is a clear difference between the withdrawal of intensive support, on the one hand, and euthanasia, defined as intentional killing, on the other.

Therefore, in answer to Richard Nicholson's earlier question about whether intention is important, my answer is yes. The intention of the medical and nursing team is paramount. If my intention is to kill, if my intention is to terminate a life, then I think it is an intention which is inappropriate in the context of traditional medical practice. If my intention is to withdraw treatment that is burdensome, then I think this is not unethical but good medical practice. Now, of course, there is a fine line between those two statements. This means that I am forced to accept some version of the so-called doctrine of double effect. Incidentally I very much dislike that phrase, the doctrine of double effect. It implies that the concept of double effect is an arcane, almost Jesuitical, concept dreamt up by Thomas Aquinas in the depths of his study and that it has no relationship to every day life. But in reality the concept of double effect is part of normal practice both in every day life and medicine. It underlies our reasoning when we give treatment such as chemotherapy which is potentially profoundly unpleasant, which causes marrow suppression, bowel disorders and so on. Chemotherapy does disastrous things to patients and may in fact kill them. But this does not mean that the oncologist who prescribes the therapy is guilty, intentionally, of murdering his patients. It is quite clear that the intention of the oncologist is actually to do something different, namely to treat cancer, although he foresees the side-effects of treatment. To say that intention is of no significance is to be light years away from 'common sense' practice, both medically and in the wider world.

Finally, I want to emphasise the fact that withdrawal of intensive support is not the same as withdrawal of care. There is a minimum level of care which all newborns deserve, including adequate analgesia and symptom relief, milk feeds except in exceptional circumstances and TLC, tender loving care. In fact, I regard providing terminal care to a newborn infant as really not different in kind from providing terminal care to a dying elderly patient.

Need for full discussion with parents

We have seen a huge advance in the palliative care of newborn infants. Thus I do not think that the tragic and very painful situations described by Dr Nicholson represent modern neonatal practice at its best. What is involved in the decision to withdraw intensive care?

First, adequate and full discussion with parents about the diagnosis and the mechanisms of brain damage, the prognosis and the degree of certainty, the treatment options which are available and finally a medical recommendation about a withdrawal of care. I believe that this is better than asking parents what they want to do. To my mind, we should give a medical recommendation. Treatment decisions are ultimately medical decisions. Life and death decisions are not decisions for doctors, treatment decisions are decisions for doctors, and the decision to withdraw treatment is ultimately a medical decision. I believe that the right approach is to put forward a treatment decision to the parents and to ask for their agreement. Can you agree to this course of action? This is effectively to offer the parents a veto.

It is important to discuss what is likely to happen if intensive care is withdrawn and to point out that very often we are not certain what will happen. I have several patients etched on my memory where I have rather confidently said that when intensive care is withdrawn this sequence of events will happen, only to be proved totally and catastrophically wrong. Therefore we must help people to understand that doctors are not omniscient, and that the consequences of the chain of events once treatment is withdrawn cannot always be predicted with 100 per cent certainty.

Secondly, it is important to give adequate time for the parents to discuss, and 'come to terms with' the withdrawal of support. They should also be given an opportunity for discussion with other family members and with religious leaders. Perhaps also a second opinion from an outside consultant may be very helpful. In my experience there are very few situations where a snap decision needs to be made. It is nearly always better to buy time to allow further discussion. I am very suspicious of snap decisions made immediately after birth about resuscitation. In my experience such decisions made very hurriedly, without full information may well be bad decisions. It is nearly always right to buy time for full discussion and, if necessary, involvement of outside people in those discussions.

Thirdly, it is most important to provide emotional support throughout the dying process. Again I emphasise the word respect. What parents are looking for is respect for the dignity, the uniqueness, the intrinsic value of their baby. I think this means open communication of feelings between staff and family, often including feelings of frustration and sadness which affect staff in these situations. For staff to express their emotions to the family is often extremely helpful. Moreover it is important to provide ongoing support, once the family are discharged form hospital. Helping babies to die at home is an option that we are increasingly keen to support. Babies may well receive better terminal care at home than in a neonatal intensive care unit.

We must also recognize the importance of physical reminders, memorials, services or rituals. Today, we put a great deal of emphasis on the importance of memorial services for babies who have died. We have an annual service for all the parents of babies who have died. We have found this to have made an enormous impact. It is an interdenominational Christian service. But we have found that people from many different faiths- and none- have come to this service, because it recognizes the unique value and significance of their baby. Photographs, footprints, mementoes, a book of remembrance, sometimes donations or the naming of equipment are all immensely important.

Finally, I must mention that in my experience and that of many of my colleagues, caring for the dying child is a uniquely stressful and emotionally demanding experience. Hence, in order to help babies to die well, we must provide support for the staff. This means making sure staff are adequately trained beforehand, and supported throughout this demanding experience.

The author John Wyatt is Professor of Neonatal Paediatrics at University College Hospital, London.

Notes

1. This paper was given at a Conference organised by the Centre for Bioethics and Public Policy (CBPP) in London in 1996. The references to Dr Richard Nicholson relate to comments made by an earlier speaker.
2. Further reading. Wyatt J. 'Matters of Life and Death'. *Inter-varsity Press*. Leicester. 1998. This book considers a wide range of healthcare dilemmas in the light of the Christian faith.

Chapter 11

Some Illustrative Case Reports in Children

This chapter, compiled by Gillian Craig, begins with four illustrative case reports, and ends with some examples of good practice in the care of children with learning disabilities.

1. Remembering Suzie

Susie was a child with a severe and progressive neurological disorder from which she died at the age of seven in 1963. Her mother shared her memories of Susie in a conversation we had thirty or more years after the child's death. Her story, which is quoted with permission, shows that a very severely handicapped child can be treasured as a person, and remembered as an important member of a family.

Susie was a classically beautiful baby, the third child in a family of four. She seemed normal at birth, but her parents realised there was something wrong by the time she was one. She didn't seem to want to do anything. They played her nursery rhymes that cheered her up, but when she was fed up with listening she would grab the machine and break the tape. She enjoyed playing with water, standing up at the sink. She was never able to speak but she learnt to walk and run around. At first her parents wondered whether she was autistic, but at the age of four she started to have fits and was admitted to Great Ormond Street Hospital for tests. Her mother recalled "They called us in and told it us it was neurolipidosis, an extremely rare condition. The illness would gradually stick the nerve ends together and she would gradually lose her faculties, her sight and hearing. She did eat a bit, soft things at this stage, but later on feeding was a problem and she lost a lot of weight. Sometimes when she was still walking she would grab the tablecloth when my back was turned and pull everything off the table breaking everything!"

Susie started to go to a special school each day with other disabled children. They were collected by mini-bus and sometimes her mother went too. The children seemed to enjoy themselves in a special care class but Susie lived in a world of her own. Eventually she gave up walking and had a little wheelchair. She sat in a corner of the kitchen and everyone waved to her as they came in. "Sometimes she would laugh and smile", said her mother - "those were rare times, rare as pearls, and we got a thrill out of this. More often she would be screaming, but she would settle down when my husband took her for a ride in the car.

"We took her to church in her wheelchair, and she would sit on my knee and grab the hat of the person in the pew in front. She went into Sunday School and I did drawings, holding her hand. I longed for her to say just one word but she never did. We lived from day to day, not thinking about the deterioration. Of all my girls she was the most beautiful - always chosen at auditions for advertisements in the early days of commercial television. To sit and watch her deteriorate was awful. The period of her life from when she started to have fits was quite difficult for all of us to handle. I needed great patience, and I was caring for three other normal children as well.

"One day, when we went on holiday, Susie went to Queen Mary's Hospital Carshalton for respite care and they kept her in. She was six and a half by then and she died when she was seven and a half. They started tube feeding in hospital as feeding had become difficult and dreadful for us to cope with because of her choking. I was frightened to see her tube fed at first as I hadn't been warned about this. I don't remember much more about that aspect - she wasn't tube fed for long, a year at the most. I would visit her every week and would go in at bath time and hold her. She could feel a caress but she could not see or hear me. My husband also visited her regularly, but he preferred to go alone.

"On one occasion towards the end of her life Susie was in an oxygen tent when I visited. The nurses took her out, sat her on my knee and went away, but she stopped breathing. For a second I wondered what to do, whether to do anything - then I called a nurse who gave her oxygen and she started to breathe again. It was still a shock when she finally died. They rang me at home and I went into see her. She missed out on life because of her disability.

"Even now, years later, I often think about Susie. It has given the other children something extra - they are more sensitive to anyone who is handicapped. My son gave up his spare time as a teenager to help disabled children. I have visions of my grandmother trying to look after Susie in Heaven! I still have a photo of Susie blowing out her first birthday candle!   She was very much a person despite her disability!"

2. The case of David Glass

This case illustrates how narrow and indistinct is the boundary between killing and letting die in medicine. It also illustrates the lengths to which a mother is prepared to go to save the life of her severely disabled, mentally incapacitated child. My information about the case is based on articles in the *Sunday Telegraph*[1] and *The Daily Telegraph*[2] in April 1999. At that time David Glass was a 12 year old, severely disabled English boy who was born with hydrocephalus. He was mentally handicapped, blind and suffered from spastic paraplegia – a term that means he had stiffness and paralysis of all his limbs. Despite his handicap he was greatly loved by his family. "This last fact" wrote Dominic Lawson of the Sunday Telegraph "seems to have caused some problems to the medical and legal professions".[1]

David was sent home from a Portsmouth hospital in October 1998 after a row between the family and doctors over how he should be treated. He had been admitted to hospital with a respiratory infection. The paediatrician decided to withdraw treatment and began administering diamorphine. David's mother Ms Carol Glass was told that her son was dying and that "nature should be allowed to take its course." . . . "I'm not sure" wrote Lawson, "how the administering of diamorphine can be described as nature taking its course, but then again, I'm not a doctor".[1] In any event, Ms Glass and other female members of the family did not want to see "nature taking its course", and the High Court were told they began "blowing raspberries in David's ears, banging his chest and rubbing his arms very vigorously, despite being asked not to do so". The witness, a paediatrician, complained to the Court that their action "had prevented him from dying".[1]

"How disgraceful", wrote Dominic Lawson. "Couldn't the Glass family see that their son was on the way out, and that it was, to quote one of the paediatricians "extremely cruel" to refuse to allow him to expire in a morphine-induced coma? Well, no they couldn't. And they were right, because David recovered, and when a representative of the Official Solicitor visited the child's home (some six months later) . . . he found him sitting up in bed, laughing and smiling, surrounded by his sisters. He was now being taken out to the shops and parks every day the High Court was told."[1]

The High Court in London was involved because Carol Glass sought a court declaration to clarify the legal position if David had to be admitted in future to a different hospital. Ms Glass had claimed that the hospital had no right, without a court order, to withdraw life-saving treatment from her son and that diamorphine could hasten his death. She sought to clarify the ground rules affecting how, and when, her son would be treated by doctors in the future.[2]

However, Mr Justice Baker Scott said the remedy of judicial review sought by Mrs Glass was "too blunt a tool" for the sensitive and ongoing problems raised by the case. "It would be too difficult" said the Judge "to frame in a hypothetical situation any declaration in meaningful terms, that did not unnecessarily restrict proper treatment by the doctors".[2] Should similar difficulties arise with David in future, the Judge felt it was "at least desirable, and I would have thought in everyone's interest, that the issue should be referred to a Family Court Judge before the situation became acute". In concluding, the Judge added that nothing should be read into his judgement to infer that it was his view the hospital trust acted lawfully or unlawfully.[1]

The Judge declared that "there are some situations that have to be left to the good sense of the clinicians".[1]"What that means of course", wrote Lawson "is that matters are left to those with bad sense and judgement. But perhaps it was difficult for the paediatrician treating David Glass to see the value of his life. Perhaps they could not see the point of an existence with so many limitations. Perhaps they subjected David to a cost benefit analysis and wondered how much more usefully they could fill the hospital bed that his twisted frame occupied. Thus it is that the medical profession, at the end of the 20th century conspires – from the best motives – against the weakest" .[1]

The General Medical Council found that the doctors involved had not been guilty of serious professional misconduct or seriously deficient performance and considered that the treatment complained of had been justified. The Crown Prosecution Service did not bring charges against the doctors involved for lack of evidence. Nevertheless the fact that a doctor caring for David Glass complained that the action of the family had prevented him from dying is significant, for to be protected under the doctrine of double effect a doctor must act with the intention of relieving physical or mental distress. To sedate with diamorphine and then complain if the patient survives suggests a rather different intention and one that is not lawful.

Criminal proceedings and a civil injunction were brought against some members of David's family by the hospital concerned and one of the doctors, as a consequence of a fracas that developed on the ward as the family fought to save David's life.[2]

The event described as a 'fracas' was a major rumpus and the police were called in. During fighting between members of the family and the doctors, two doctors and several police officers were injured and most of the children on the ward were evacuated. While the fight was going on Ms Glass managed to resuscitate David. His two aunts and his uncle were given jail sentences for causing the fracas that saved his life.

Surely all this distress could have been prevented by more sensitive handling and mediation? Yet as I write, there is still no formal mediation procedure in the UK short of the Family Division of the High Court, to which doctors and relatives can go in the event of a dispute. When a patient is actively dying or in imminent danger of death, that system is far too cumbersome to be of value.

Our Government and National Health Service would be well advised to heed the recommendations made by the House of Lord's Select Committee on Medical Ethics, who said:

> "Treatment limiting decisions in respect of an incompetent patient should be taken jointly by all those involved in his or her care, including the whole health-care team and the family and other people closest to the patient. Their guiding principle should be that a treatment may be judged inappropriate if it will add nothing to the patient's well-being as a person. In most cases, full discussion will ultimately lead to agreement on what treatment is appropriate or inappropriate..." [3]

Their Lordships were not satisfied that clearer guidance could be given, for "judgement must be made in relation to the condition, circumstances and values of the individual patient. Such matters cannot be defined or legislated for ..." [4].

The Appeal Court Ruling

Lord Woolf, sitting with Dame Elizabeth Butler-Sloss and Lord Justice Robert Walker in the Court of Appeal in London in July 1999, refused Mrs Glass leave to appeal against the High Court Judge's ruling. Lord Woolf said David was now back at home . . . and it would be "an inappropriate task for the court" to intervene under the circumstances. Should a similar crisis arise, the mother could take further legal action. [5]

General Guidance given by Lord Woolf
Lord Woolf made some general comments that indicate how the legal profession in England will approach similar cases in the future. According to *The Daily Telegraph*, he said that the considerations which could arise were "almost infinite" [5]. It was, in his view, "an inappropriate task for the courts" to try to make rulings in advance about such matters. The best situation was for the parent of a child to agree on the course which the doctors were proposing, having been fully consulted, and having understood what was involved. However, if agreement was not possible and the conflict was of a grave nature, then Lord Woolf said the matter should be brought before the court "so that the court can do what is in the best interests of the child concerned". The court would take into account the concerns of the parent and

the views of the doctors, and would take advice from other parties before making a declaration as to the legality of the action proposed by the doctors. Lord Woolf added, "An answer which will be given in relation to a particular problem, dealing with a particular set of circumstances, is a much better answer than an answer given in advance"[5].

Wider implications of Lord Woolf's remarks

Lord Woolf's comments support the line taken by the BMA in their guidance to doctors.[6] The indications are that providing that doctors and parents are in agreement about the proposals to withhold life-supporting treatment, the courts in England are unlikely to intervene. However, in cases of serious or grave conflict a judge could over-rule the proposals of a doctor by declaring them unlawful, or not in the child's best interest.

Lord Woolf's comments will bring some relief to parents with disabled children, who may be worried lest doctors withhold life-prolonging treatment against their wishes. Carol Glass was pleased that the judges had "made it clear that doctors have got to at least listen to the parents and, if it can't be resolved between parents and the medical staff, then go to court."[5]

Lord Woolf's comments have a bearing on advance directives in general, for if senior judges decline to interfere with medical decisions in advance, surely it is unwise for Parliament to make advance directives legally binding!

Many doctors in the UK will welcome the Appeal Court ruling, for it does not interfere with clinical judgement unless serious conflict arises. Hopefully, with sensitive handling, clear explanations and a willingness to listen to dissenting voices, serious conflict will be relatively rare. When difficulties arise, all parties will be able to discuss the situation in court and the judge's decision will be final.

Who pays?

If difficult decisions about treatment-limitation are to be taken to court the question arises, who pays for the court proceedings? Some 'no fault' arrangement that does not place a huge financial burden on doctors or dissenting relatives will have to be worked out.

How should we define futility?

Futility, in the context of medical treatment, is an exceedingly complex subject on which opinions vary widely. Some people felt strongly that the medical team caring for David Glass abandoned him and discriminated against him because of his handicap. Others would no doubt argue equally vehemently that the doctor's intention was compassionate. But compassion need not – and must not – kill.

It is not widely known that the Federal Government of the USA passed a Child Abuse Amendment Act in 1984 that applies to new-born children only. According to Prip and Moretti this Act "ostensibly aims to protect handicapped infants from 'discriminatory' behaviour on the part of the parents or health care providers, or both" [7]. The US Commission on Civil Rights commenting on this Act emphasised that- "*only the inevitability of death despite treatment, and not the persistence of disability despite treatment, renders the treatment futile*".[8]

This definition of futile medical treatment would certainly clarify thinking in the care of children like David Glass. His case demonstrates the need for a Child Abuse Amendment Act for neonates and children in the UK.

The European Court ruling

Eventually Carol Glass and David applied to the European Court at Strasbourg and argued that United Kingdom law and practice had failed to guarantee the respect for David's physical and moral integrity required by Article 8 of the European Convention on Human Rights, which guarantees respect for private life. The Court agreed and considered that the decision to impose treatment on David in defiance of his mother's objections gave rise to an interference with his right to respect for his private life, and in particular to his right to physical integrity. They also concluded that the decision of the authorities to override Ms Glass's objection to the proposed treatment, in the absence of authorisation by a court, resulted in breach of Article 8. The court awarded the applicants 10,000 euros for non-pecuniary damages, and 15,000 euros for costs and expenses. [9]

Thus, in her fight for the life of her son, Carol Glass, a brave and determined mother, has won a victory for parents.

"Letting a child die must be the hardest thing any parent can do"- said Andrew Grubb, Director of the Kings College Centre for Law and Ethics, in 1995. "Perhaps it is better for them (and society) that the court should take the decision that all life is worth living."

3. The case of child I

According to reports in *The Times* of July 13th 2000, child "I" was born prematurely with severe and irreversible lung disease and an abnormal brain. He spent nearly eight months in hospital and then went home to the care of his parents. Oxygen was continued day and night at home, and he had expert support and hospital supervision. Within six months he required inpatient intensive care again for respiratory failure, but recovered sufficiently to return home. Some months later he was taken back to hospital yet again. His parents tried to insist that he be ventilated, but the doctors disagreed and he was made a ward of court.

The High Court Judge, Mr Justice Cazalet had every sympathy with the parents, but ruled that it was not in the child's best interest to prolong his life unnecessarily.[10] This ruling worried anti-euthanasia groups, but many people would agree with the doctor's decision in this case. The outlook for the child and his parents was grim. With intermittent intensive care he might survive in a totally dependent state for a while. Without intensive care he was likely to die within a matter of weeks. Given the shortage of intensive care beds some rationing was regrettably necessary, for resources cannot be used indefinitely to preserve the life of hopelessly ill children. Nevertheless the ruling set a dangerous precedent and raised several questions about the attitude of the NHS towards patients and their families as was noted in a leading article in *The Daily Telegraph*. It was a sad "no win" situation. The court decision may limit the child's suffering, but it will cause great grief to the parents. The parents deserved understanding and compassion, but doctors cannot be forced to treat against their better judgement.

Badly Treated
A leading article in *The Daily Telegraph* of July 17th 2000.

Two recent court cases have pitted the medical profession against parents with a severely disabled child. And in both, the families have lost. In the first, Mr Justice Cazalet, a High Court Judge, ruled that a hospital was not obliged to resuscitate a 19 month old boy in intensive care should he need it. In the second, three relatives of a 13 year old boy received prison sentences for attacking doctors who, they believed, were allowing him to die. In each instance sympathy for the losers is unmitigated. The chief consultant in the infant's case argued that further artificial ventilation would cause him " distress, discomfort and pain" and lead to a death " neither peaceful nor dignified." And the assault on two doctors by David Glass's two aunts and his uncle in October 1998 was wrong. Yet the overall impression is that the wishes of the families were subordinated to those of the medical establishment.

The sense of injustice is particularly strong in the Glass case. According to the defence, the paediatricians at St Mary's Hospital in Portsmouth had decided that he should be allowed to die and wanted to administer diamorphine. The family disagreed, and the fracas ensued. David was discharged that evening to return home. Twenty one months later, his mother, Carol, says that he is "very well". It is difficult not to conclude that the intervention by his aunts and uncles saved his life. It is a warped idea of "intensive care" that tries to induce avoidable death.

A spokesman for the Portsmouth NHS Trust said the sentences showed "that violence against the NHS will not be tolerated." Yet that raises the question of what gave rise to the violence in the first place. The answer, as subsequent events have proved, is that two doctors mistakenly believed that nothing more could be done for David. Those closest to him, convinced that his life was worth preserving, have been vindicated. Yet Judge Roger Shawcross rejected pleas for suspended sentences, pleas made on the grounds that Mrs Glass's sisters and brother were essential in providing constant care, and refused an emergency bail application pending an appeal against sentence to the High Court. One cannot help suspecting that the Glass family, apparently working class and uneducated, have been treated without sufficient consideration of their deep feelings for David.

The two cases raise several questions about the attitude of the NHS towards patients and their families. Do those working for it see themselves as the servants of those whom they treat? Do they keep constantly in mind the clauses of the Hippocratic Oath which proscribe the administering of "deadly drug" and advice which may cause a patient's death? Do they take sufficient account of the views of those closest to patients who cannot speak for themselves? Ominously, the cases cited suggest that the answer is no.[11]

Addressing spiritual pain and anguish

The Daily Telegraph leader writer raised some important questions. There are indeed times when patients and their families are badly served, and badly treated by health care professionals. Many people working in the health service are drawn to medicine and nursing by an altruistic desire to serve suffering humanity in a general sense. Many continue to do so at great emotional cost to themselves. We do not see ourselves as supine servants, but as professional people, trained to use our skill and knowledge in a practical way. Doctors are trained to concentrate on diagnosis and treatment, nurses should concentrate on nursing care. Other people, such as hospital chaplains and social workers may be better placed to provide emotional and spiritual support to distraught families. The best that most health care professionals can do is to practice our profession with as much skill, gentleness and compassion as we can muster. Good doctors take time to listen to the views of parents and relatives, but some have a lot to learn. Too often in the health service, worried relatives are brushed aside and marginalized by busy doctors who need to concentrate on the medical problems of the patient. Resort to the law in cases of dispute should be a last resort, for it can increase the burden of suffering.

Inspired by the teaching of Dame Cicely Saunders, many people now recognise the spiritual dimension in the suffering of dying patients. The emotional needs of parents who have a stillborn child are also understood, and some churches have special services for such people. The spiritual and emotional needs of parents and families who struggle to care for disabled children like David Glass and child "I" must now be addressed. Every time such children are admitted to hospital their tired families will be in a heightened state of anxiety and apprehension. Bad news should be broken gently, and with compassion. It is natural to want your child to live, and to hope against hope that the situation will improve. It is natural to fight, metaphorically speaking, for your child's survival, but one must draw the line at physical violence.

Malcolm Johnson speaks of 'biographical pain,' and describes this as 'the irremedial anguish that results from profoundly painful recollection of experienced wrongs that can now never be righted…This happens when matters can never be put right by forgiveness or an apology.' [12] A society that has lost touch with formal religion must find ways to support those with biographical pain, says Johnson.[12]

Relatives who are badly treated may suffer with painful memories in later life. Call this what you will- biographical pain, spiritual pain, or post traumatic stress-[13] depending on the underlying cause. The practical point is that health care professionals must do all in their power to limit long-term emotional damage. When cure cannot be achieved and the end of the road is in sight, we must learn to tread softly lest we increase the burden on the patient's friends and family.

4. Playing God or choosing the lesser of two evils? The case of Jodie and Mary

At first sight the case of Jodie and Mary, conjoined twins born to parents from the Maltese island of Gozo, has little relevance to the hydration debate. On further consideration it reveals several important and potentially dangerous trends in medical ethics and medico-legal deliberation.

Jodie and Mary were born by Caesarian section in a hospital in Manchester, England, in August 2000. Their parents, devout Roman Catholics had travelled to England for the birth to give their children the best possible chance of survival. Malta has an agreement with Britain and sends 180 patients a year to the UK for specialist treatment. According to reports in The Daily Telegraph the twins were joined in the lower body and had fusion of the lower spine. They also shared a bladder and possibly other lower pelvic organs. Mary's heart and lungs were poorly developed and both twins relied on Jodie's heart and lungs for survival. Mary's brain was said to be rudimentary; she appeared unresponsive and required tube feeding. Jodie on the other hand was bright and alert and able to feed from a bottle. You could say for the sake of discussion that Mary represented a patient with a permanent vegetative state (PVS) or "near PVS", whereas Jodie was aware of her surroundings.

Without separation, the initial view was that both twins would die probably within months. An operation to separate the twins would cause the immediate death of Mary, but would give Jodie a 65% chance of survival to live a relatively normal life with residual disabilities. She would however require a series of operations to correct abnormalities and would spend months in hospital during the first five or six years of her life.[14,15] The parents were horrified by the stark choice that faced them and were deeply opposed to any intervention that would lead to the death of one twin. They wished to let nature take its course and leave their twin's fate in the hands of God. The doctors on the other hand were reluctant to lose two babies when there was a chance that they could save the life of one. They were on the horns of a painful dilemma, so the case went to the High Court.

An initial ruling by Mr Justice Johnson gave doctors permission to separate the twins, and this ruling was confirmed in the Court of Appeal on September 22nd 2000. The parents reluctantly accepted the Court of Appeal judgement and the case did not go to the House of Lords. At one stage surgical intervention seemed uncertain for there were rumours that the surgeons were reluctant to operate in view of the high level of public concern, and risk of failure. The case caused heated debate.

Legal aspects

Legal aspects received wide coverage around the world. My information is based mainly on reports in *The Daily Telegraph* of September 23rd 2000.[16] Joshua Rozenberg their legal editor reported the case in detail, outlining key points made by all three judges. The following points are taken from his report, with permission.

❑ *Lord Justice Ward* discussed the case in relation to the best interests of each twin, and argued that law and morality allowed the taking of life in self defence. The crucial question he said was whether circumstances could ever be extreme enough for the law to confer a right to choose that one innocent person should be killed rather than another. The case created an impossible position of conflict. The judge concluded that "The law must allow an escape by permitting the doctors to choose the lesser of two evils." Law and morality allowed the taking of life in self defence, and the doctors could therefore come to Jodie's defence. "Jodie is entitled to protest that Mary is killing her", said the judge.

- *Lord Justice Brooke* also constructed an escape route for the doctors, based on the "doctrine of necessity." He explained that as a matter of public policy this doctrine was normally rejected as a defence for murder on the grounds that such a defence would divorce the law from morality, and there would also be the problem of who would be the judge of what was necessary. However he argued that these objections did not apply in the twin's case for Mary was already "designated for death" and it was not obvious that saving Jodie's life would be considered immoral. He concluded that an operation to separate the twins would not be unlawful.

- *Lord Justice Robert Walker* argued in terms of the purpose or intent of the surgery proposed. He took the view that the purpose of separating the twins would not be Mary's death, though it would be the inevitable consequence. "She would die, not because she was intentionally killed, but because her own body could not sustain her life." The judge added "Continued life, whether long or short, would hold nothing for Mary except possibly pain and discomfort, if indeed she can feel anything at all." A separation would therefore be in the best interests of each twin. The judge concluded "The proposed operation would not be unlawful... Mary's death would be foreseen as an inevitable consequence of an operation which is intended, and is necessary, to save Jodie's life."[16]

Thus this case provides an interesting example of how the legal mind approaches agonizing medico-legal dilemmas. Note that the doctrine of necessity is not completely dead, although it is no longer recognised as a defence for murder. Note also that the judges, in particular Mr Justice Ward, were at pains to interpret the law for the benefit of doctors. Although it was stressed that the court did not have to value one life above another, the fate of Mary faded into the background in favour of Jodie. In purely pragmatic terms Mary was not viable as an independent human being, for she had too many congenital abnormalities to permit survival. Her fate was effectively sealed in the first days after conception when vital organs should have been formed, and cellular division should have separated her from her sister. Now her presence posed a threat to the life of her more normal sister.

Many people agreed with the judges' decision, but others were dismayed. There was particular concern that the deeply held religious beliefs of the parents were discounted. Given more time and gentle explanation they might have come round to the doctor's point of view. As it was the case became the focal point for conflict between pro-life and utilitarian agendas. Some lawyers denied that the case had set a dangerous precedent, others were quick to see the wider implications. Under present circumstances the law does appear to be willing to confer on doctors the right to choose that one innocent person may be killed for the sake of another.

Loss of a twin

A leading article in *The Daily Telegraph* of September 23rd 2000.

"There are two questions to be answered in the case of Jodie and Mary, the ill-fated Siamese twins. First, who should decide on the welfare of a child- her parents or the state? Second is it right to sacrifice one life- that of Mary, the weaker twin- in order to save another, in this case Jodie's? Insofar as such an extraordinary situation can have a right or a wrong answer, the Court of Appeal answered the questions correctly yesterday.

"The first question is answered by the law of this country: though the views of parents should usually prevail, the state was bound to make the decision. The parents were adamant that their children should not be separated. The doctors were not prepared to lose a life they were capable of saving. The opinion of the court was therefore sought; as Lord Justice Ward has said, "That is what a court is for". The body of family law is consistent when it comes to deciding how courts should deal with children: in Lord Justice Ward's words "the child's welfare (is) the court's paramount consideration... the parental view is not sovereign".

"When it comes to considering the twins' welfare, surgery is clearly in Jodie's interests: she will suffer problems arising from reconstructive surgery, but there is every possibility she will be of normal intelligence, capable of having children and surviving into old age.

"The Court of Appeal differed as to whether surgery would be in Mary's interests. Lord Justice Walker maintained that it would not be: keeping them together would be "to deprive them of the bodily integrity and human dignity which is the right of each of them." Lord Justice Ward's conclusion, that surgery would not be in her interests, is the preferable one. This is a laudable advance on Mr Justice Johnson's original High Court judgement which suggested that Mary's life was worthless.

"The only unsatisfactory part of the judgement deals with the justification for ordering the operation and so over-riding Mary's interests. Lord Justice Ward framed the decision in terms of self-defence; that the doctors were coming to Jodie's defence in order to save her from Mary's draining of her life blood. This does not ring true: the self-defence argument is an awkward attempt to graft legal precedent on to an unprecedented situation. Some will conclude that a new principle was created yesterday- one of state sanctioned murder, justified on the grounds that one life must be taken to save *another.* However this seems already to be recognised. The lives both of an unconscious mother and a terminally ill baby can be threatened in childbirth. In such circumstances, doctors can have a choice between saving one or the other, and it would be curious for the decision not to favour the mother. Admittedly this situation is not an exact parallel, and it is terrifying to think of the principle being applied widely. But it perhaps provides the best way of approaching the heartbreaking tale of Jodie and Mary.[17] "

© The Telegraph Group. September 23rd. 2000. Reprinted with permission.

Roman Catholics expressed grave concern

Senior clergy in Malta issued a statement that was published in *The Catholic Herald*. They said:

> "An adult person may, in an act of heroism, of his own free will sacrifice his own life for the good of others. However no authority may eliminate or sacrifice the life of a human person, not even to save another life.
>
> "It would be disastrous were the dignity of the human person to be evaluated according to criteria of utility, even if these were to favour another person. We would be undermining the dignity of the human person and introducing into society a harmful principle. It is God who gives life to man, and no one can decide to terminate it except God himself.... We are indeed sad that the legitimate will of the parents was overridden by the court." [18]

According to an editorial in *The Catholic Herald*, some of the medical facts were far less pessimistic than the public had been led to believe, for there was no life-threatening emergency that required immediate intervention. Estimates of life expectancy altered from an initial six months to an open-ended 'many months, even years.' Jodie's strong heart could support Mary for nobody knew how long. The editorial writer mentioned that in an American study of nine sets of conjoined twins where one was sacrificed to save the other, there were no long-term survivors. On the other hand it was noted that many conjoined twins 'have survived without separation, and have defended their right to do so.' It was also noted that the doctrine of double effect was not applicable in this case since in English law 'this doctrine can only be applied where the initial action and the consequences affect the same patient.' [19]

* * * *

Some comments from Dr Craig

Roman Catholics were concerned because they feared that the ruling set a legal precedent against the right to life. Looked at another way however you could say that that the case supported the right to life, for the hope was that one life would be saved rather than two lives lost.

My personal view is that it is somewhat unhelpful to talk in terms of eugenic infanticide or the deliberate killing of Mary. The doctors involved in these tragic cases are not ogres, but practical professional people who know what is feasible, and what is not. Their instinct is to save one life rather than let both babies die. Had the doctor's predictions of longevity been wrong in the case of Jodie and Mary, and had the twins survived together for 'many months, even years', Jodie would have been faced with the terrible prospect of life attached to an insensate tube-fed sister. She might have lived to regret that nothing was done at an early stage to spare her such a burden. Far better to attempt surgery sooner rather than later if it was to be done at all. There have been occasional survivors after 'sacrifice surgery' so a totally pessimistic attitude was not justified.

Taking a wide view, Jodie could be said to represent all the suffering members of humanity who could be helped with skill and determination at a cost. Mary represents the severely disabled, those who lack self-awareness, who are considered by some to be expendable. Yet all are inextricably bound together in the web of humanity and deserve to be treated with gentleness and respect. The end of this sad tale was that Jodie and Mary were separated in an operation that lasted 20 hours. Mary inevitably died, but Jodie survived. Jodie is now at home on the island of Gozo with her parents, and has a good chance of living a full and happy life.

* * * *

A documentary programme screened on BBC television in October 2000 filmed several conjoined twins. In the cases shown both twins were mentally normal and did not want to be separated. The Schappell twins of the USA who are joined by the head at frontal lobe level, are perfectly happy and take the view that "You do not ruin what God has made." The oldest surviving conjoined twins in the world, Masha and Dasha Krivoshlyapova, then aged 50, and living in Moscow said "We are a little collective, we share our grief and our fears." However the outcome is not always so happy for viewers were told that conjoined twins can be regarded as a monster, a curiosity, or a showpiece. Those with experience of the problem consider that a decision to separate conjoined twins is ethical and valid, for life joined at pelvic level is no life. It seems likely that as surgical skills improve, more and more successful separations will take place.[20]

There will be times when surgical intervention is essential and other times when masterly inactivity would be better. Sometimes doctors may have to choose the lesser of two evils and try to save one twin when they cannot save both. Whatever happens the health care professionals must guard against an overriding need to dominate and be in control. Difficult decisions are best made with loving parents or relatives, after careful and compassionate discussion with the most experienced doctors available. The law is an unwieldy, heavy handed and dangerous tool for decision making in these complex and difficult cases.

Caring for Children with Learning Disabilities

The care of children with severe disabilities is challenging and demanding work for the families and professionals involved. The work is multi-disciplinary requiring close co-operation between teachers and health care staff. Some children with swallowing difficulties need to be fed through gastrostomy tubes and need one to one care. Others may appear to be lacking in self-awareness, so risk having life-prolonging treatment withheld or withdrawn in accordance with current medical guidelines. Although many people devote their lives to the care of people with learning disabilities at considerable personal cost, some professionals treat them with disdain.

A doctor with specialist registration in Psychiatry writing to a Parliamentary Committee noted that medical ethics has shifted from principles laid down in the Hippocratic Oath towards relatively utilitarian positions. He said- "The relevance of this massive shift in medical practice now influences many areas of clinical practice. For example those with Learning Disability are often treated with disdain and receive poor medical care. I have personally had to fight for medical care for such people, when clinicians from other specialties have not seen their lives as of enough value to be worth treating with the same standard of care as other patients."[21] The case of David Glass illustrates this problem, for his relatives literally fought medical staff in order to save his life, and received a prison sentence for their pains.

Creating a responsive environment

Special skills are needed to communicate with children who have visual handicaps, hearing impairment and multiple disabilities. To an outsider the task may seem impossible, yet much can be achieved. Although some may appear to be lacking in self-awareness, skilled and dedicated teachers may find ways to communicate with them and respond to the smallest glimmer of awareness. Teachers who work in this field aim to create a responsive environment that is sensitive to the special needs of the children. Jean Ware, Director of Special Education at St Patrick's College, Dublin, writing in the Royal National Institute of the Blind publication "eye contact" in Autumn 2003 explained –

"A responsive environment is one in which people get responses to what they do, get the opportunity to give responses to other people, and have the opportunity to take the lead in interactions. Research shows that responsive environments are important because people both with and without disabilities learn to communicate through other people treating them as if their action had meaning. In a responsive environment people are more involved in social interaction, and people who experience a responsive environment learn more quickly. But for me what is most important about a responsive environment is that it embodies the respect and dignity with which all people, regardless of their age, abilities and disabilities ought to be treated." [22]

Therapy through movement

The foundations of the practice of sensory-motor therapy can be traced back to 1906 and the work of C.S.Sherrington and others. Various approaches have been developed over the years through the pioneering work of occupational therapists, music therapists and others. These include a neurodevelopmental approach, a neurophysiological approach, proprioceptive neuro-muscular facilitation, neuromuscular reflex therapy and a sensory integrative approach. In the sensory integrative approach using the Jean Ayres technique, each child has an individual therapy programme that may include sensory stimulation or inhibition aimed to 'normalise sensory-motor function.' Stimulation may be given by techniques such as brushing, vibration, stretching, visual and auditory stimuli. Calming influences include slow stroking, rocking, soft auditory stimuli, a gentle voice, reduced visual stimulation and the use of soft colours.[23]

Many people recognise the therapeutic value of movement and dance. With very disabled children the movement may be tiny, but it's significance great.[24] Dance massage -described as "dancing on the skin"- is regarded as "an interactive form of non-verbal communication that is especially helpful to people of all ages with sensory impairments and special needs."[25] Music also has an important part to play in the education of children and young people who are visually handicapped and have learning disabilities.[26]

160

Reaching the Inner Child through Movement and Voice

Maggie Craig, a specialist teacher working in Cambridgeshire UK, emphasises the need to respond to a child's attempts to communicate, rather than simply "do things to them". In the notes that follow Maggie suggests ways to reach the inner child through the use of movement, touch and voice.

Suggestions for interacting with John

John is a child with visual impairment, profound and multiple learning difficulties and severe cerebral palsy such that he can only move his head. My work has focussed on helping parents, carers and school staff to interpret and encourage John's endeavours to communicate. Finding a way of connecting with John will involve time, perseverance, and ingenuity. John does not respond consistently, and you will need to adapt your approach to his mood.

❑ **Find a peaceful distraction-free setting with no background music playing.**

❑ **Develop a familiar greeting specific to you alone.** I wear a tinsel bell bracelet on my wrist. I help John to feel it and then shake it gently as we say 'hello' and feel our way into the conversation. Do not rush this stage.

❑ **Combine voice, touch and movement to converse.** Be bold with the way you use your singing voice. Combined with touch and movement it can powerfully acknowledge John's different responses, however minute. Changes in the intonation of your voice and the type of touch and movement can speak words themselves. Mirror and reflect back his movements and vocalisations, picking up the essence of what he is doing. Respond with a variety of sounds and movements that he is unable to produce himself.

❑ **Notice his body tension.** Sometimes John's varying body tension gives clues to the way he is feeling. Responding to this with touch and voice can lead to a real sense of connection. Vary your distance, drawing closer to his face when the connection seems stronger, and retreating when you sense he needs space and a pause in the conversation.

❑ **Use props as a shared focus for your conversation** once you have successfully negotiated contact, and opened up the conversation. John sometimes enjoys his tiny vocalisations being responded to with a rhythm played on a deep drum, and a playful shake of his body or wheelchair. In quieter moods, he likes to feel a bead gourd rolling across his hand, combined with me singing. He also enjoys the feel of a rippling sari against his body (with added aromatherapy scent), linked with the rhythm of the drum, or in time with his vocalisations or head movements. His favourite instruments are Tibetan singing bowls. Sometimes he makes tiny noises, and we sing together over the beautiful sounds of the singing bowls.

John comes to life when he realises that someone is listening to him. Trust your intuition but be careful not to force your own agenda. Acknowledging John's quietness and closed off feel is often the way to get him to open up and express his more vibrant and joyful nature.

© Maggie Craig 2005.

How music and movement helped Stevie

The story of Stevie shows how important music and movement can be in the care of children with profound physical disability. The information is drawn from an article in the Sunday Telegraph of August 1ˢᵗ 2004. © Jonathan Chamberlain. Quotes are used with permission.

Stevie was born with a genetic disorder that affected her physically and mentally. At the age of six months she underwent an operation to repair a hole in the heart. All seemed well at first, but on the third post-operative day something happened and she sustained brain damage due to lack of oxygen to the brain. She survived but was left in a profoundly disabled state with severe visual impairment and epilepsy.

Stevie loved being bounced as a baby, and would reward her mother with a smile. Later as her mother "danced her up and down" she would respond with laughter. She also listened to music with intense pleasure. Her parents, who were living in Hong Kong, found the local Chinese tapes of children's songs exceedingly good. Her father wrote:

' When a tape finished, she would start to cry- not in pain, but as a signal for attention. "Eh, eh, eh!" Pause. Was anyone coming? "Eh, eh, eh". "What's wrong Stevie?" we would say as we came running. As if she could tell us. But it was always the music. The tape needed to be turned over.' [27]

Stevie knew when a tape was about to end, and would cry to indicate that she wanted it turned over. This showed her parents that their child had intelligence trapped inside her. Explaining the situation later her father wrote:

' Stevie is severely and profoundly handicapped. She can do nothing for herself. She can't sit up, roll over, speak, or even suck her thumb. But there is this light in her eyes. There is this way of *sensing* that she has. She questions things. She has this intelligence. I have no other word for it: she has intelligence. We can't measure it but it is there. Her eyes are luminous with her mental being…Stevie is fully human.' [27]

When Stevie was three her epilepsy became so bad that she was started on treatment with cortisone, which was extremely helpful, so much so that her parents arranged for her to go as a weekly border to a small centre for the handicapped where they hoped that a regime of exercise would be beneficial. She attended for two years, but did not respond to the regime and would come home to her cassette player with delight at weekends. So after two years her parents brought her home, engaged a domestic help to care for her, and concentrated on making her life as happy as possible.

Stevie suffered many episodes of pneumonia in her life, and was often admitted to hospital for treatment. Eventually, during one such episode at the age of eight she stopped breathing and died peacefully in hospital. Looking back on her life her father wrote:

"In the end, all I can say is that I was given the gift of Stevie, who by coming into my life brought me blessings, transformations and moments of immeasurably complicated emotion- love and pain and happiness and sadness. I can only hope that I, in turn, helped her in her journey through this life, and that, if there is a beyond- a place where the soul lives in the hereafter- that it is a place where she can blossom in wisdom and laughter." [27]

References

1. Lawson. The death of medicine. *Sunday Telegraph*. London, April 25th 1999.
2. Shaw, T. Mother loses battle over care for disabled son. *Daily Telegraph*. 23rd April 1999, p.8, columns 1-6.
3. Report of the House of Lords Select Committee on Medical Ethics. Para 255. Treatment   Limiting Decisions. *HMSO*, 1994.
4. Ibid . Para 256.
5. Shaw T. "Mother claims victory in fight over son's life. *Daily Telegraph*. 22nd July, 1999, p.15, cols. 5-8.
6. Withholding and withdrawing life-prolonging treatment. Guidance for decision-making. Section 15. Decision making for babies and young children who cannot consent for themselves. *BMA*. London, June 1999.
7. Prip W, Moretti A. Medical futility: a legal perspective. Chapter 13, p.136-153 in "Medical futility, and the evaluation of life-sustaining intervention. (Ed.) Zucker M and Zucker H D. *Cambridge University Press*. 1997.
8. US Commission on Civil Rights. 1989-90 as quoted by Prip and Moretti. (See ref 7 above; p.144).
9. European Court of Human Rights. Glass v United Kingdom. (Application No 61827/00). Judgement March 9th 2004, published March 11th 2004. Source Law Report *The Times* March 11th 2004.
10. Wright O and Peek L. Judge rules boy must be left to die. *The Times*. July 13th 2000, p 1 cols 1-3.
11. Leading article (anon), *Daily Telegraph*. July 17th 2000, p 21.
12. Johnson M. Committed to the asylum? The long term care of elderly people. The second Leveson Lecture, April 2002. *The Leveson Centre*. Temple Balsall, Knowle, Solihull B92 OAL (UK).
13. In the view of Craig, post traumatic stress can develop in relatives of dying patients who are treated badly. See "No water- No life: Hydration in the Dying." *Fairway Folio* 2005.
14. Hall C. How doctors plan to give sister a new chance of life. *Daily Telegraph*, September 23rd 2000. p4 cols 3-7.
15. Laville S. Parents begin to talk of the day they will take their daughter home. *Daily Telegraph*, September 23rd 2000, p5, cols 1-4.
16. Rozenberg J. 'Jodie is entitled to protest that Mary is killing her.' *Daily Telegraph*, Sept.23rd 2000, p4, cols 1-8. Quoted with permission. © *The Telegraph Group*.
17. Editorial (anon), *Daily Telegraph*, September 23rd 2000, p23.

18. Coppen L. Siamese twins verdict sets 'dangerous' legal precedent. *The Catholic Herald,* September 29th 2000, p7, cols 1-2.

19. Editorial (anon) Will our courts enshrine in law the doctrine of eugenic infanticide? *The Catholic Herald* September 29th 2000, p 7,cols1-2.

20. "Horizon" Conjoined twins. BBC Television. October 19th 2000. Series Editor John Lynch.

21. Kingsley D. Memorandum (MIB 731) Ev.320; 2.1.4.House of Lords, House of Commons, Joint Committee on the draft Mental Incapacity Bill. Vol ii Oral and written evidence. *HMSO*, 2003.

22. Ware J. Creating a responsive environment: First Steps. In *'eye contact'*; Autumn 2003: Vol 37 on Communication, pages 5-6. *Royal National Institute for the Blind*. E & E Division, Plumptre Court, 7, Poplar Street Fisher Gate, Nottingham NG1 1GP. [See also Ware J. Creating a Responsive Environment for People with Profound Learning Disabilities. 2nd Edition. *David Fulton*, June 2003. Available from RNIB (quote ED 401).]

23. Gretton Sue. The foundations and practice of sensory-motor therapy. Chapter 1, p. 29-34 in "Therapy Through Movement" Ed Lorraine A Burr. 1986. *Nottingham Rehabilitation Limited*. 17, Ludlow Hill Rd, Melton Rd, West Bridgford, Nottingham, N62 6HD.

24. Craig. M. Movement Sessions. *'eye contact'*; Vol 37, Autumn 2003, p10-11.

25. Rosenberg N. Dancing on the skin. Opening up communication using Dance Massage. In *'eye contact'*, 2003;Vol. 37; p. 21-22,

26. Ockelford A. Music moves. Music in the education of children and young people who are visually handicapped and have learning disabilities. *RNIB*. 224 Great Portland Street, London, WIN 6AA. Text © RNIB 1998. Songs © Adam Ockelford 1996.

27. Chamberlain Jonathan. For the love of Stevie. *The Sunday Telegraph*, August 1st 2004, Review, p1-2. Adapted from *Wordjazz for Stevie*. Available as an e book on www.longislandpress.co.uk/fightingcancer/wordjazz.html.© Jonathan Chamberlain 2004.

Part 4

Old People Matter

Introduction

Comments by Gillian Craig. Retired Consultant Geriatrician.

The last 10 to 15 years have seen major changes in the pattern of care for the frail elderly in the UK. In the 1980s most long term nursing care was carried out in long stay wards in National Health Service (NHS) Hospitals. These wards were staffed by doctors and nurses who were motivated to work with the elderly and chose to do so. However for reasons that were partly altruistic but largely financial, many long stay wards were closed in the mid to late 1980s and patients were moved into private nursing homes. The NHS was to pay a heavy price for this cost cutting exercise, since before long many hospital beds intended for the care of acutely ill patients of all ages, were occupied by the frail elderly. Now there is virtually no long stay provision in the NHS. To make matters worse, many nursing homes are now closing. Suddenly the Cinderella specialty of Geriatric Medicine has moved to centre stage. "Politics has become the politics of ageing" it has been said, for the burgeoning population of elderly people can no longer be ignored by politicians.

Closure of the long stay beds in the hospital where I worked as a Consultant Geriatrician left me with a sense of professional bereavement, but there was little that I could do to influence the situation. I drew attention to the need for Community Geriatricians, but my concerns were not heeded. Little has changed in the last ten years. A few community geriatricians are in post but the burden of care falls on general practitioners. Political and social factors continue to impinge on medicine to the detriment of patients. Few voices have been raised within the profession, but in 1994 the Bishop of Birmingham warned the British Medical Association that people must always come first. His comments are printed in this book.

Current interest in withholding and withdrawing life-prolonging medical treatment must be viewed in the context of demographic changes on the one hand and inadequate resources on the other. The underlying motivation of the Government and the medical establishment is utilitarian, and driven by economic imperatives. We live in dangerous times. "End of Life Care" is high on the agenda.

Worrying trends in patient care are illustrated by case reports in this book. Some of the cases mentioned are already the subject of public knowledge, but others are not. The problems illustrated are not uncommon. Most people nowadays know of a friend or neighbour, if not a relative, whose care has given cause for concern. In theory where serious concern is expressed about the withdrawal of life-prolonging treatment- in particular artificial or assisted nutrition or hydration- legal advice should be sought in accordance with professional guidelines. In practice, dissenting relatives rarely manage to influence events at ward level. As the law stands in England and Wales at present, if the patient is mentally incapacitated the Official Solicitor should be contacted and asked to represent the patient. When the

Mental Capacity Bill reaches the statute books, proxy health care decision makers will enter the equation: they already have legal standing in Scotland.

Although it is obligatory to refer patients with a permanent vegetative state to the High Court for a decision about treatment withdrawal, there is no such requirement for patients with lesser degrees of mental incapacity in the UK. To date, very few cases of treatment withdrawal in the elderly have reached the High Court during the patient's lifetime. The High Court case into questions raised by Lesley Burke was a rare exception. His case was exceedingly important in medico-legal terms for he sought reassurance that he would be kept hydrated and fed when he was no longer able to communicate his wishes to the doctors. Yet as noted elsewhere respected judges disagreed on crucial points of law. The Appeal Court Judges appeared to leave the decision to the doctors once Burke was dying and unable to communicate. This will leave a great many patients in limbo without legal protection.

If there is any doubt about the cause of death, or concern about possible neglect, the matter should be referred to the Coroner. In practice Coroners may be exceedingly reluctant to hold an inquest and have no authority to adjudicate in matters of medical ethics. In years to come with reform of the coronial system, complex cases that come to the attention of the Coroner may be referred to a High Court Judge for investigation. This happened in 2005 in the case of deaths at Kingsway Hospital Derby, for the inquests were delegated to the Deputy Coroner Sir Richard Rougier who was a retired High Court Judge. At present however many grieving relatives who deserve to be heard have no redress. There is a deep medico-legal chasm into which cases involving the frail elderly can fall and be forgotten.

Chapter 12

Case Reports Involving Elderly People

Compiled by Gillian Craig

The following case reports are intended to give readers some idea of the range of ethical problems that can arise in the elderly, when patients refuse food, or cannot take food because of swallowing difficulties, senile dementia, or brain damage due to strokes. The discussion is at a level that should be readily comprehensible to people with no specialist knowledge. I hope that the information given will prove useful to such people who may be required to participate in difficult end-of-life decisions in years to come.

Proxy health care decision-makers are an established part of the medical scene in the USA but have no legal standing in England and Wales at present, although the situation will change when the Mental Capacity Bill Act [2005] comes into force. In England and Wales at present doctors still have freedom to use their clinical judgement, but in matters of life and death it is considered good practice to involve close relatives and the whole health care team in decision-making.

A. Patients who refuse food or drink

Sometimes old people who want to die take matters into their own hands and refuse food and drink. This can be very distressing for the carers and family, but if the old person is not clinically depressed or mentally incapacitated, there is nothing that anyone can do about it. The following two cases illustrate this problem.

Case A 1

An elderly lady living in a major city in the UK was admitted with severe scurvy – a potentially fatal disease due to vitamin C deficiency. Sailors used to die of this in the old days on long sea journeys before it was discovered that lemons or limes would prevent it. Sadly this old lady did not want to be treated and told the doctor in no uncertain terms to go away. It transpired that she had been living on chocolate only for weeks. The nurses persuaded her to take one dose of vitamin C on the day of admission, but the following day she died. The case was referred to the Coroner who did not consider it necessary to hold an inquest. This appeared to be a case of suicide by starvation in a woman who knew what she was doing and was not overtly depressed.

Case A 2

An elderly lady who lived alone in rural England was transferred from an admission ward to a geriatric ward. She had no evidence of illness apart from some dehydration and raised blood urea. She was conscious and calm but refused to talk, and just lay there quietly watching what went on. A locum doctor set up a drip to rehydrate her. She pulled the first drip out, but it was re-sited and within a day or two her blood urea returned to normal and she looked a lot better. Still she refused to talk or drink.

The doctor called in a psychogeriatrician who made no headway either. The patient appeared neither depressed nor demented. The General Practitioner who was called in expressed the view that she should be allowed to die, but provided no insight into her behaviour. The ward sister tossed her head and was of the opinion that the old lady knew exactly what she was doing! The impression, based on no firm evidence, was that the patient wanted to die. No friends or neighbours were found who could shed light on the problem.

It was difficult to know what to do but the doctor decided to continue subcutaneous fluids. When the situation is in doubt one should presume in favour of life. Technically I suppose this action could have been interpreted as an assault, but on the other hand, to aid and abet a suicide is also illegal. I can only guess the end of the story for the doctor's short-term post came to an end. When last seen the patient was calm and comfortable on subcutaneous fluids. In her hand was a posy of flowers that the doctor had given her.

B. Patients who choke on food

Case B1.   Mrs O.

My information about this case is based on articles in *The Nursing Times* and *Daily Mail*.[1,2] The patient Mrs O was an 85 year old lady who was cared for in a nursing home in Lancashire under the supervision of her General Practitioner (GP). She died of bronchopneumonia and malnutrition in 1995, having had food withdrawn.

According to the GP, Mrs O had suffered several strokes and was severely demented. She tended to choke when eating and was at risk of developing bronchopneumonia. Her GP told a reporter "she could not communicate, so she could do nothing to stop the nurses feeding her".[1] She managed to swallow tiny amounts of food supplemented by a liquid food supplement. This suggests to me that she wanted to eat, for patients who refuse food clench their teeth and turn their heads away when food is offered.

In June 1995 the GP asked the nursing staff to stop her food. They were appalled and continued to feed her secretly with a feeding cup and syringe, until their supplies of liquid food supplement ran out.[2] Mrs O took 58 days to die, by which time, as the General Medical Council were told, her body was like something out of Belsen.[1] The case was referred to the Coroner.

An inquest found that Mrs O had died of bronchopneumonia as a result of malnutrition. One nurse described to the Coroner "the absolute horror in Mary's eyes" as the doctor issued the order to stop food. The nurse "strongly disagreed" with his instructions. "He seemed to be talking about euthanasia" she told the Court . . . "and I told him . . . that I would not be party to it."[2] The Coroner took into consideration the conflicting opinions of experts who believed either that the GP had "acted outside the bounds of good medical practice", or that his decision to withdraw the supplement was "entirely proper". "We could spend days discussing these ethical matters and not necessarily come to any substantive conclusions" said the Coroner.[2] The police subsequently investigated a charge of murder, but the Crown Prosecution Service decided not to press charges. The General Medical

Council gave the GP a token six month suspension from the medical register for his action.

The GP is said to have no regrets and would do the same again. He remains adamant that he did nothing wrong. "I didn't take the decision to withdraw food as an act of euthanasia as many people are saying", he told a reporter. "I did it to save her from more pain and discomfort and to prevent inhalation pneumonia".[1]

The GP did not apparently consider the possibility of feeding Mrs O by a nasogastric tube or gastrostomy tube (PEG), nor did he request a second opinion from a Consultant Geriatrician or Psychogeriatrician, although such people are available to advise and support GPs in the National Health Service and will visit patients in the community on request. Instead, as his counsel noted, he worked in a vacuum with no guidance from the medical profession or case law.[1]

Many people are said to have written to support the GP, recognising the dilemma that he faced. However, in my view he was wrong to stop the food supplements. If a person, however disabled is still capable of swallowing with skilled nursing care, food should not be withdrawn. Patients should not be left to starve to death in a civilised society. There are better ways of handling the situation.

According to the BMA guidelines of 1999, doctors may withhold sustenance from patients who are not terminally ill providing that they are unaware of their surroundings, cannot interact with others in any way, and cannot take control of any aspect of life. From the information available to me, it would seem that these criteria were not fulfilled in the case of Mrs O. It is generally considered to be unacceptable to provide hydration without nutrition on a long term basis in stroke patients with swallowing difficulties.[3]

The case of Mrs O brings into sharp focus the problem of medical supervision in nursing homes in the community. This is GP territory and hospital consultants can visit only on request. Unfortunately on some occasions GPs fail to seek advice from colleagues in the hospital service. The medical profession in general must recognise their responsibilities to the frail elderly in the community and find better ways to increase the flow of expertise across the hospital/community barrier. All doctors are now advised to seek a second opinion from a senior clinician before making irreversible treatment limiting decisions, with respect to the provision of food and nutrition by means of a tube.

Note. Quotes from reference 1 are reproduced by kind permission of *The Nursing Times* where the original article by Mark Gould was published on 14th April 1999.

Case B2. Deaths of psychogeriatric patients in Derby

As noted earlier – in Chapter 3 of this book, Michael Horsnell of *The Times* drew attention to the deaths of more than 40 patients on a psychogeriatric ward in a hospital in Derby.[4] The deaths had occurred over a number of years. It was alleged that some staff were hastening patients to their deaths by placing them on 'nil by mouth' regimes, claiming that they were at risk of choking. One source at the hospital thought that the regime amounted to euthanasia. The police took the allegations seriously and launched a full investigation in 1997.[4] The Coroner for Derby and South Derbyshire, Mr Peter Ashworth, took matters up and decided to hold an inquest into eleven of these deaths in 2004.

The inquest was taken by the Deputy Coroner, Sir Richard Rougier, a retired High Court Judge in January 2005. As noted earlier, Sir Richard Rougier took the view that whatever the reasons behind the decision to withdraw food, the underlying illnesses played "an inexorable progress" in the patients' deaths. He said that if "food and fluid were withdrawn at a time when they were perfectly capable of accepting it all because it was arbitrarily decided that is was time for them to die" it would amount to a policy that had been "totally unacceptable since the dark ages." On the other hand "If it should transpire that food and fluids were withdrawn in good faith and in the not unreasonable belief that it was in their best interests as the lesser of two evils, committing them to die in as much comfort and dignity as possible…it would be grossly unfair to record a verdict other than that of death by natural causes." (Source Britten N. *The Daily Telegraph* Jan.19th 2005 page 9.)

Having heard all the evidence Sir Richard Rougier concluded that the deaths were due to natural causes. This verdict is important for it could well set a precedent for the future.

Case B3.

A severely demented man was transferred to hospital from a nursing home after a stroke. He could not tolerate a naso-gastric tube and was alleged to be too weak for a PEG (another means of direct feeding rarely used in dementia). According to his daughter he could swallow but was not being fed. He did not like the food supplements offered but swallowed soup provided by his daughter. She however, was advised not to feed him because of the risk of aspiration. Hydration was maintained by a drip for six weeks while he slowly starved to death.

What would Sir Richard Rougier have made of his death I wonder? Although described as severely demented, this man responded to his daughter and could swallow soup. Therefore I suggest that he should have been given soup. Sometimes food is withdrawn prematurely because of value judgements made by ward staff. Ward staff and relatives need to talk matters through and come to an acceptable compromise. The risk of aspiration must be balanced against the risk of starvation. If one is only a possibility, and the other a miserable certainty, the way ahead should become clear.

General Discussion. The management of elderly patients at risk of choking.

If food and fluids are withheld to prevent choking or inhalation pneumonia the patient will inevitably die of dehydration within about a week. If hydration is continued by artificial/assisted means e.g. by giving fluids intravenously or subcutaneously, but food is withheld, the patient will slowly starve to death. There is no easy solution to the dilemma. The only sure way to prevent choking and continue sustenance in such patients would be to use tube-feeding. Some would approve of such action, but others would have grave reservations. Confused old people may pull out drips and tubes and find them very frightening. Attempts to prolong life in this way will sometimes be futile and inappropriate.

There is a case for suggesting that if a person with severe dementia starts to choke on food, the kindest course may be to continue to try to feed them with care and skill. Nourishment can sometimes be given using thickened liquids, or specially formulated liquid feeds that are available on prescription. Expert advice should be obtained from a doctor or dietician.

If bronchopneumonia due to inhalation of food or fluids occurs despite all reasonable precautions in a patient who cannot tolerate a nasogastric tube and is too frail for a percutaneous gastrostomy (PEG) it may be regarded as an inevitable terminal event and any discomfort can be relieved by morphine. Some competent patients may choose to take the risk of dying of inhalational pneumonia and continue oral feeding despite advice to the contrary.

Where the patient is demented and unable to take part in these difficult decisions, the issues should be discussed with close relatives, taking into account the risks, benefits and burdens and the patient's previously expressed wishes. If there is a valid advance directive, that should be heeded. When the Mental Capacity Bill reaches the statute books we will have authorized proxy health-care decision makers in the UK-their views should be heeded. At present where there is a severe and unresolvable disagreement between the parties and the patient is mental incompetent, legal advice should be sought, for the matter may have to be settled in court.

Some patients with dementia simply stop eating and drinking- they 'close up' to quote one experienced nurse. Maybe they realise that life is no longer worth living, maybe it is a consequence of their underlying disease process. Whatever the reason, it is a terminal event and death will supervene. At this stage some sedation to reduce any residual sense of hunger or thirst would be appropriate.

Relatives of patients with dementia may find the experience painful, for the person they once knew may be inaccessible or no longer there. They will need help and support during what is a living bereavement. Relatives and staff should continue to try to relate to the person inside the disabled body. We are learning all the time how to reach them, by a gentle touch or music for example. Sometimes flashes of the old person we once knew return to make the effort worthwhile. We must not give up on them.

It is important to recognise that the care of psychogeriatric patients is extremely demanding work. Society is only too ready to leave this work to others. Many hospital staff in the National Health Service are under intolerable stress and this will inevitably affect patient care. There may be too few pairs of hands to feed disabled people with the skill and patience that is needed. Staff who are doing their best under difficult circumstances deserve greater support, but starving patients to death cannot be condoned. NHS managers, politicians and society in general, must share some of the blame when old people are neglected and abused in our hospitals and nursing homes. Old age comes to us all in the end: we must ensure that the needs of old people are met.

C. Stroke Patients. Some general comments

What is a stroke?

A stroke is a general term used to describe the effect of sudden brain damage usually of a vascular nature. A stroke can render a person incapacitated without warning in a matter of minutes. The potential for recovery depends on the degree of brain damage incurred in the stroke, and whether the lesion recurs or progresses. If the stroke is due to a bleed for example, the bleeding may continue, causing the condition to deteriorate rapidly. On the other hand, if the stroke is due to a clot or embolus obstructing a blood vessel the level of damage will depend on which part of the brain that blood vessel supplies. It may be that only a small part of brain will be affected. Thus some strokes due to clots are devastating and cause death in a matter of days, but others cause relatively minor problems such as weakness of an arm or difficulty with speech. Strokes due to bleeds, clots and emboli are liable to recur.

Emboli are small solid particles that may be carried to the brain in the blood stream. They usually come from the heart in patients with an irregular heart beat, such as atrial fibrillation, or with infected heart valves, but emboli can come from or other sources such as atheromatous plaques [i.e areas of vascular disease] in cerebral arteries. Sometimes mini-strokes cause small areas of brain death (infarcts). If the insult recurs damage accumulates over time and may result in multi-infarct dementia. Thus minor strokes should be taken seriously, and the cause treated whenever possible, to reduce the risk of catastrophic brain damage.

Basic care and management of stroke patients.

The first point to stress is that stroke patients do sometimes recover against all the odds. Premature predictions about the imminence of death should not be made. Gloomy predictions sometimes prove wrong, so all concerned should leave room for hope and give life a chance.

It is dangerous to predict that a patient is dying and to withhold life-prolonging measures for that reason, since this makes the prediction self-fulfilling. When the outcome is uncertain one should always make room for hope.

If palliative care principles are applied to stroke patients, then the ethical principles relating to the use of artificial hydration in terminally ill patients should also be applied. Guidelines issued by the National Council for Hospice and Specialist Palliative Care Services in July 1997 require that the situation be kept under constant review, and the relatives concerns be addressed etc.[5]

It is essential to realise that a stroke patient is not like someone with incurable cancer- the situation is entirely different. By no means all stroke patients are terminally ill. With careful diagnosis and good treatment many recover to enjoy life for many years. Time must be allowed for rehabilitation and recovery. An attitude or guarded optimism should be adopted.

The need for hydration

A patient who suffers a major stroke may die within hours or days. Others remain unconscious for a while but then recover to a greater or lesser extent. If basic hydration is not maintained during the first few days the chances of recovery are reduced. If all treatment, including hydration, is withheld from the outset as sometimes happens, the outlook will be hopeless and death will inevitably occur in a matter of days. That is not a satisfactory situation for the patient and most relatives would object. The only safe approach is to maintain hydration initially by means of a drip or nasogastric tube if the patient cannot take oral fluids.

172

Once in a while you come across relatives who do not want the patient to be treated. That can cause difficulties if the views of the relatives and the doctor differ. The first duty of the doctor is towards the patient, whose views about treatment should have priority. Relatives may be in a position to indicate what the patient's views might be, if the patient is not in a position to express a view. Doctors should therefore consult the next of kin when possible. A doctor does however, have a right to treat without the patient's consent in an emergency, if the patient is mentally incapacitated. However, the doctor must only act in the patient's best interest. A valid advance directive, made by a patient when compos mentis, that is applicable to the circumstances pertaining, must be respected.[6] All possible care should be given to maximise the possibility of recovery, unless the patient has signed a valid advance directive forbidding intervention.

The need for nourishment

A proportion of stroke patients will die despite hydration but others may slowly recover. If they cannot take food orally within a reasonable time then after a fortnight at the most, the question of maintaining nutrition as well as hydration will arise. The problem for doctors at this stage is that they do not want to commit a patient with serious and possibly permanent disability to long term tube feeding. However stroke patients can continue to recover for at least six months, so premature decisions to limit treatment and avoid tube feeding should not be made, unless the patient has indicated that they do not wish to have assisted feeding of any sort. It is unethical to maintain hydration in the absence of nutrition for long. Decisions about tube feeding should be made sooner rather than later, for a patient who is starved will suffer and deteriorate mentally and physically and will inevitably die.

Withholding or withdrawing life-prolonging hydration and nutrition

If after several months the patient remains unconscious or lacking in self-awareness despite adequate hydration and nutrition, the outlook may well be hopeless and the question of withdrawing artificial hydration and nutrition will arise. Doctors working in the UK should pay due regard to guidance issued by the British Medical Association and the General Medical Council.[7, 8.] Relatives who object to treatment withdrawal should make their views known and would be wise to contact a solicitor without delay, for where there is disagreement the case may have to be decided by a Court. Decisions to withhold or withdraw tube feeding should not be taken lightly.

People who fear the possibility of tube-feeding for themselves or their loved ones may be comforted to know that 50% of people who are unable to swallow after a stroke die within one month, so the need for long term support is not great. Of those who recover the ability to swallow, most do so within one or two weeks, so the situation becomes clear quite quickly. It pays therefore to take an active and optimistic approach to treatment in stroke patients. The skill of the attendant doctors and nurses, and their general approach to the patient, will be paramount. Clinical intuition is more important in the care of stroke patients than rigid adherence to guidelines about management. 'Where there is life there is hope' is a good maxim to follow. Where there is a good rehabilitation team with caring gentle staff and a happy environment, the patient will have the best chance of recovery. Many of my patients did better on the geriatric rehabilitation ward than they did on the acute medical wards, for the pace of life was appropriate and the medical and nursing staff were tuned in to their needs. With the demise of so many geriatric hospitals, too many old frail people are subjected to the hustle and bustle of wards where they are not really welcome. Alternative health service provision is needed to replace the long stay and rehabilitation wards that have been closed. At present many frail elderly patients are cared for in nursing homes, but if they close the future for the elderly in the UK will be bleak.

In conclusion

When it comes to withholding treatment including artificial hydration and nutrition, the guidance of the British Medical Association or the General Medical Council should not be taken as the final word. Alternative guidance has been prepared by the Medical Ethics Alliance. They follow the advice of the House of Lord's Select Committee on Medical Ethics, who take the view that . . .

> "It should be unnecessary to consider the withdrawal of nutrition or hydration except in circumstances where its administration is evidently burdensome to the patient.[9]

The benefit/burden assessment is vitally important to the care of all patients who are unable to maintain their hydration and nutrition without assistance.

Some case reports involving stroke patients

Case C1. Starvation in hospital after a stroke

Mrs X, who was described by her son as a 'youthful elderly lady', was 83 years old when she died in a hospital in Scotland some years ago. Prior to the last year of her life she was up and about looking after her horses. She became ill with a chest infection, followed by a 'seizure' and was admitted to hospital one May morning. The details of the first summer and autumn of her illness need not concern us. She was discharged home to the care of her son one December day.

On discharge she was able to walk holding on to furniture or with one person holding her arm. She needed home helps to assist her with dressing and a district nurse visited occasionally. She was able to talk and had meals with her son in the evening. She even coloured some pictures in the week she spent at home. All seemed to be going well. Then one morning she had a major stroke, necessitating readmission to hospital.

Within hours of admission the Consultant decided not to resuscitate her in the event of a cardiac arrest. Her son, on hearing of this, said he wanted every possible step taken to ensure that she survived. The patient was said to be semi-conscious on admission and unable to speak. She received fluids in the form of 5% Dextrose via a drip initially, and was later fitted with a nasogastric tube through which, it is alleged, she was given virtually nothing but tap water for weeks on end. She could have been given nourishment through the tube but the health care team decided against this. Thus she was virtually starved until she died seven and a half weeks later.

Her son's repeated requests for her to be given nourishment were ignored. He tried without success, to get her transferred to another hospital, under the care of a Consultant whom he trusted. He was desperately worried and visited his mother daily, spending hours by her bedside. He was afraid to create too much fuss lest he be banned from visiting. He and other visitors gave her sips of cranberry juice that she seemed to swallow. There was a difference of opinion among the nurses as to whether she could swallow or not. The Speech Therapist is said to have thought she could not.

According to the son, his mother was often conscious for hours on end and would spend time looking at a photograph of a donkey placed on her locker. He continued to speak to her and drew intermittent responses. On one occasion she spoke a word, on another two distinct sentences. The son wrote 'I said to my mother she should have confidence and she must have thought I said "do you have confidence" to which she replied "not a lot", then added "don't bother me".'[10] This conversation demonstrated clearly that the patient was aware and *compos mentis*. The patient's son deserves praise for continuing to speak to his mother despite her lack of response. He was rewarded by two sentences that showed his effort was not in vain.

The son noticed that his mother was always very responsive when a certain nurse was on the ward. He also noticed that she was the only patient on the ward who had no Primary Nurse named as responsible for her care. Was this perhaps the nurses' way of avoiding responsibility? According to the son, one staff nurse who had initially been encouraging about progress was moved, against his wishes, to another ward. On his return he was edgy with a 'hunted look', and his comments at the bedside became discouraging such as "better off away", "no quality of life", "What a way to live". Another nurse made similar comments according to the son's testimony.

The son became aware that his mother "was in dangerous water in this ward". He wrote: " I felt she was at risk from those who were supposed to be caring for her … I had formed the impression that my mother had the will to survive…There is no doubt to my mind she would have done so, given the resources to do so ..."[10]

Inevitably the patient died, for no one can survive without nourishment. The cause of death was given as a cerebrovascular accident (Ia) and hypertension (Ib). Malnutrition was not mentioned on the death certificate and no post mortem was performed.

The case was eventually referred to the Procurator Fiscal who had the power to investigate the matter. He sought advice from a Forensic Pathologist, who was not a clinician. The pathologist considered that the patient had received every care possible and that the medical staff had acted in her best interests. This view prevented the Procurator Fiscal from proceeding further.

Discussion

The patient died before publication of the BMA guidance of June 1999 [7] but since she died in a teaching hospital it cannot be said that the doctors were working in a medical vacuum. Had a legal opinion been sought when the clinician's views were seriously challenged the patient's fate might have been rather different. In the light of professional guidance that is now available the management of the case would be open to criticism.

The British Association for Parenteral and Enteral Nutrition guidance of 1998/9 states:

> "...to continue artificial hydration without nutrition... over a period of weeks, leads to progressive malnutrition and is unacceptable policy. It has been suggested that the major reason for such an indeterminate policy may be to reduce anxiety among health professionals and the family. The possible relief of thirst must be weighed against the suffering involved in a prolonged process of dying..." [3]

Paragraph 91 of the General Medical Council guidance of August 2002 is also relevant for it states:

> "In holding discussions about cardiopulmonary resuscitation (CPR), you should make clear to the patient, the health care team and others consulted about the patient's care, that the provision of all other appropriate treatment and care would be unaffected by a decision not to attempt CPR."

The length of survival of non-obese adults, without food, is between 60 and 70 days. Mrs X managed to survive for 53 days despite her stroke. Since a nasogastric tube was in place she could have been given nourishment through the tube without difficulty, therefore the question of the doctor's intent in omitting to feed her should be addressed. Nurses and dieticians also have a professional obligation to ensure that the nutritional needs of patients are met.

Absence of speech in a conscious patient is not a reason for withholding treatment. Language may be a major means of communicating but "the limits of our language are not the limits of our world" as Habgood noted.[11] There is thought that is too deep to be expressed by language, there are feelings that can be conveyed by gesture, facial expression and body language. There are voices that can be heard, if not replied to. There is beauty that can be experienced through music or pictures (e.g. the donkey on the locker). All these means of communication are available for people who lack the power of speech. Good rehabilitation staff, given time to spend with patients, become adept at non-verbal communication and can teach the skills to relatives.

It is worth bearing in mind that in 1918 two people, Gibbons and Proctor, were sentenced to death for allowing a child to starve to death. The Judge told the jury "It is enough for you to find that they set up a situation that would inevitably in the course of time lead to death". That judgment still stands in English law.[12]

(Case reported with the son's permission)

C2. A stroke patient who was tube fed for six years

A thoughtful and interesting case report was submitted in evidence to Parliament when the draft Mental Incapacity Bill was under scrutiny. The patient had suffered a stroke and was tube fed for six years. The patient was not in a vegetative state, but she was paralysed and it was unclear how much she understood. The case is important because it shows that tube feeding can be worthwhile even in patients with limited awareness

The correspondent was a Professor and the patient was his mother. He felt that it was wrong to intend a patient's death through inaction, such as withdrawing nourishment. He told the Select Committee "Having spent so much time with my mother over those six years, I can say that quality of life is possible. Her family were able to show her constant affection, she watched television and the staff of her nursing home treated her as a person. She was aware and followed visitors around with her eyes." Her life was made more bearable with perfumes, ointments, videos etc. A day or two before her death his mother spoke. The son gave a very positive picture of the last six years of her life.[13]

C3. The case of Mr Y

An elderly man suffered a stroke and was admitted to hospital. His left leg was paralysed and he was unable to speak. On transfer to a geriatric ward he was unwell, sleepy but conscious. A doctor working as a locum in a junior role, reviewed his brain scan which showed some haemorrhagic transformation and mid-line shift. This being interpreted means that there had been some bleeding into the damaged area of brain, which had swollen, pushing the brain as a whole sideways across the mid-line so that the normal undamaged brain on the other side was being compressed. Many specialists treat such a situation with dexamethasone, a steroid that reduces brain swelling. Accordingly the doctor put the patient on dexamethasone. Within 24 hours he was much improved and mentally alert.

The Consultant arrived to do a ward round and stopped at the foot of the bed. The locum doctor explained the situation and drew attention to the patient's improvement on dexamethasone. "Oh we'll stop that!" said the Consultant looking offended. The patient meanwhile was listening to every word. The locum doctor suggested that the conversation should be continued later, and they adjourned to an office. En route the Consultant said that when he was a senior registrar the policy was that stroke patients were not treated in the first few days, the reason being that the worst affected would die, or words to that effect. The locum doctor took the view that active treatment was crucial from the outset, to maximise the chances of recovery. History does not relate the outcome in this case. One can only hope that the patient survived.

C4. Left to die

An elderly woman languished in a side ward in a small community hospital. She was conscious but unable to speak, and too weak to swallow. She had extensive deep vein thrombosis in her leg, abnormal liver function tests, and an irregular pulse due to atrial fibrillation. A brain scan had shown multiple small brain infarcts i.e. small areas of brain damage due to mini strokes, and she had been left to die, untreated and incompletely diagnosed. A locum doctor persuaded the Consultant to give her subcutaneous fluids for her dehydration and low dose heparin for her thrombosis. Her condition improved rapidly. Within a few days she was drinking, sitting out and speaking a few words. She was happy to be alive, but her recovery gave no pleasure to a member of the in-house medical team who pronounced it a "ghastly survival". How sad that he had not taken into account the views of the patient. She found life worthwhile and precious, despite her physical frailty.

C5. A Happy ending

An elderly woman, the mother of a Member of Parliament, suffered bilateral strokes, but recovered and asked for a quick relief if she had another. She did have another and was admitted to a nursing home. She was described by her daughter as being "still there as a spirit" and allegedly "on a drip only for three months." Then a doctor raised the question of a percutaneous gastrostomy. The daughter put the situation to her mother who said she most certainly wanted the operation. She survived for five more years during which she was a major source of inspiration to the family. The daughter spoke about this experience to a group of like-minded MPs and journalists and said-"All must be loved and supported to the end." Her talk was greeted with warm applause. Without a PEG the patient would have died.

(Case quoted with the daughter's permission.)

C6. An elderly widower

An elderly widower who lived alone, sustained a sudden cerebral haemorrhage early one morning. He managed to phone for help and was taken to hospital where his condition deteriorated rapidly. He was treated actively and received dexamethasone for raised intracranial pressure to good effect. Gradually his condition stabilised but he was left with a dense hemiplegia and severe speech problems. He could understand, but was unable to express himself except with an occasional word that was often the wrong one. This was intensely frustrating for him and difficult for visitors who did their best to communicate. There were times when some felt it would have been better if he had died, but this phase passed as the patient and his family adjusted to the situation. Swallowing was impaired, but with careful selection of foods he could take sufficient to sustain life.

The patient received physiotherapy, speech therapy and occupational therapy. His speech improved progressively over a matter of months and he hummed tunes that took his fancy when watching television. He learnt to stand with the support of one person but never regained the ability to walk or transfer from bed to chair unaided. After many months he returned home to his cottage in a wheel chair and remained there with maximum community support. He was fortunate to have loving relations who lived next door and could help at night if he needed them. Relief admissions were arranged on a regular basis to ease the strain on his caring family. Eventually the patient decided to move to a nursing home permanently but he remained an important member of the family. Every Sunday he was collected and taken home to lunch. He saw his grand children grow up, sang carols at Christmas, went to an occasional concert and kept a close eye on the football results. Of course there were difficult days and frustrating days but he enjoyed eight more years of valuable life before he died.

The human body has a great capacity for survival and repair. Many a severe stroke patient has lived to enjoy life, given appropriate care and support. We must not be too ready to give up!

(Case reported with permission of next of kin).

C7. Recovery after brain surgery

Mr S, a 43 year old man was admitted to a centre specialising in the care of severely brain damaged patients. He arrived having had extensive brain surgery and was only able to blink and move a thumb. Three years later, after extensive rehabilitation he could walk, talk, and eat small mouthfuls of food. He was continent and fully aware of his surroundings. He was glad to be alive, and said "...Everyone should be given the right to live. I always knew I was going to get better."[14]

C8-10. Three patients who did better than expected

Dr Clare Whitehead, a retired Consultant in Rehabilitation Medicine to West Berkshire Health Authority in the UK has 18 years experience of looking after people who have suffered brain damage from strokes or head injuries. She has expressed concern about the possibility of making the withdrawal of hydration and nutrition legal under some circumstances and advocates an active approach to treatment. The following case reports are taken from her memorandum to the Joint Parliamentary Committee that scrutinised the draft Mental Incapacity Bill in 2003.

Dr Whitehead explained: "People with an illness or injury, including brain injury, need to be given time to recover; and together with their relatives, come to terms with what has happened to them. Healing may continue slowly for months or even years. It is only too easy to hold onto low expectations of recovery when in fact the outlook may be more optimistic than expected." [15]

Three cases reported by Dr Clare Whitehead:

(a) A married woman in her 30s with husband and two children, was admitted to an acute medical ward unconscious having had a cerebral haemorrhage. She remained unconscious for several weeks and it was thought that the outlook was poor. When she recovered consciousness she was found to be hemiplegic with speech impairment. She made excellent rehabilitation progress and went home to her family with almost complete recovery.

(b) A man in late middle age was admitted for rehabilitation, being severely disabled from multiple cerebral infarcts (that is areas of dead tissue in the brain). He sustained many disabilities as a result, including impaired speech function and multiple disabilities of higher cerebral function.

He underwent inpatient rehabilitation for many weeks with definite but only slight improvement. He and his wife, who had advanced cancer, wanted him to be able to return home to enjoy being with her in the remaining weeks before she died. This slight improvement was enough for this goal to be achieved.

(c) On TV news recently we heard of a young man who had recovered consciousness after being in a coma for 19 years following a head injury! It seems that he is able to communicate meaningfully with his family members.

Source. Memorandum from Dr Clare Whitehead. Ev. 295, 4 a-c and 5. Draft Mental Incapacity Bill. Vol II: Oral and written evidence. HMSO 2003. © Parliamentary Copyright House of Lords and Commons. 2003. Reproduced in accordance with copyright conditions.

C11. The final indignity

This case report by journalist Ann Kent illustrates what happens when doctors do everything according to the book in a severe stroke case. From the information given it seems that the patient had a drip for 9-12 days after lapsing into unconsciousness following a stroke, then in the absence of benefit the drip was taken down and she had no fluids at all for 6 days. Then, since she opened her eyes briefly, she was tube feed for a few days until she developed pneumonia and died. Ann Kent was shocked by her experience.

The following case report by Ann Kent was published in the Daily Mail on February 15th 2000. It is reprinted with kind permission. © Daily Mail 2000.

"Aunt Molly was already on the way out, but why did the hospital not let her die in her own good time?"

'When journalist Ann Kent rushed to the hospital bedside of her Aunt Molly, the last thing she expected to be told was that a drip to hydrate her was about to be withdrawn. Though the once sprightly 87 year old was expected to live only a few weeks after her stroke, Ann was astonished that a hospital could order the removal of treatment that she felt provided comfort. Here, she asks why doctors are allowed to make the final decision-often without consulting the close family.

'What would you say if a doctor wanted to shorten the life of someone you loved, by withholding fluids? This was the situation facing my family when our Auntie Molly collapsed with a stroke.

'We were shocked to discover that doctors routinely decide whether to provide or withhold fluid, food or other treatments which could prolong a patient's life. And although relatives may make their views clear, the final. Life or death judgement belongs to the doctor.

'It started when a Scottish dancing class found itself locked out of its hall. Auntie Mollie walked back to her car to fetch her mobile phone, and collapsed.

'Molly was 87. But only chronologically. She had started dancing at the age of 70, when most people are considering hanging up their dancing shoes. She had recently amazed the family by announcing that she had taken up swimming again.

'In hospital, she lapsed into unconsciousness and we were told she was unlikely to recover. Her doctor set up a drip to provide her with vital fluids, but said this decision would be reviewed.

'A week later we were told by a nurse that Molly's drip was to be taken down because she was not benefiting from this treatment. We were astonished. Surely the giving of fluid was not a treatment, but part of the normal care of a patient, along with keeping her warm, clean and free from pain.

'How could you have a nursing care plan that withheld water, which is essential for human life? What seemed truly remarkable was the medical team's matter-of-fact approach.

'Until then I thought such decisions were made only in the most extreme high profile cases or when a patient is in such pain that it is cruel to prolong life. Molly looked as if she was simply asleep and showed no signs of discomfort. What was the hurry?

'I didn't realise that judgements to withhold liquids and liquid meals are everyday decisions for doctors throughout the UK, working with patients who are unlikely to survive. Because I objected the intravenous drip was left in place for a couple more days although the nursing staff tried to reassure me that it was not really necessary.

"I accept she is unlikely to recover, but it seems mean-spirited to deprive her of fluid," I said, embarrassed at the inadequacy of my words. Molly was a highly independent woman who had seldom seen a doctor, and now the health service was begrudging her extra time to die naturally. And then there was the question of suffering.

'Researchers can tell us little about what people experience while they are apparently unconscious. We do know they are often aware of what is being said- and sometimes of what is occurring around them.

'Withdrawing fluids causes dehydration. A domino effect sets in where organs fail, one by one, starting with the kidneys. Death occurs within three weeks, in which time the patient is likely to visibly shrivel.

'The assumption is that the patient is unaware of what is happening. Specialists in other hospitals confirmed that Molly's doctor was doing everything according to the book.

'Depriving someone of fluid will kill him or her…For someone as ill as Molly, giving fluids might prolong life, for a short while.

'The courts have stated that hydration and artificial nutrition (tube feeding) can be regarded as medical treatments.

'Last summer, the British Medical Association produced a report, Withholding and Withdrawing Life-prolonging Medical Treatment. It described artificial feeding and hydration (providing fluids) as treatments, which could be withheld if they did not lead to improvement or recovery.

'Although it stated that the family should be consulted, the final decision lay with the doctor in charge. Molly's hydration drip was removed after 12 days.

'Stubbornly, my physically strong, and young-for-her age aunt refused to die. After six days without fluid, she opened her eyes very briefly and seemed to squeeze a nurse's hand before she lapsed back into unconsciousness.

'Molly's 'recovery' was never repeated, although she was then artificially fed by tube for a few days. Nurses kept her clean and turned her regularly.

'Her nurse sat down with me and explained that withdrawal of fluids was normal practice in these cases. It was nothing to do with bed shortages. If Molly showed signs of restlessness or suffering, she would be given morphine.

'She did not see how illogical it seemed to turn a patient regularly to avoid bedsores, while depriving the same patient of fluid. "I can see I can't persuade you" she said with a smile.

'When Molly deteriorated, showing signs of a chest infection, her consultant ordered the removal of the feeding tube. There was to be no new hydration drip.

"Wouldn't Molly suffer from lack of fluid?" I asked.

"She is so deeply unconscious that she will not be affected," he said. "Hydration would simply prolong the inevitable. If it were my mother, I would not hydrate her under these circumstances."

'Within four hours of our conversation, Molly died of pneumonia, while nurses were turning her.

'So would she have suffered from withdrawal of fluids in the last three weeks of her life?

'Dr David Smithard, a stroke specialist and geriatrician in Kent, explained; "This is controversial. Some researchers think that if you don't supply fluid, the patient will suffer. But others say that if you don't put a drip up, then the body responds by producing its own natural anaesthetic.

"I don't have any hard and fast rules about this. Deciding whether or not to put up a drip for someone who looks as if they might die in a few days is one of the hardest decisions doctors must face."

'Dr Smithard says he takes relatives' views into account and would probably err on the side of those who wanted hydration and feeding to continue. However, he pointed out that sometimes it is the relations who are keener to stop treatment than is the doctor.

'Oin Redahan, Director of Communications for the Stroke Association, says: "What we want in this situation is for the patient's family to be consulted. Although in the end the doctor will take the final medical decision , emphasis should be given to what the family wants. It is difficult to know at what stage to say, enough is enough."

'Molly did not lie neglected on the trolley or hobble for months in agony waiting for a joint replacement. She was care for with efficiency and pragmatism.

'Some will think it does not matter what happens to an unconscious woman at the end of her life. But where is the compassion? What would you do if it were your Auntie Molly?

© Daily Mail. 2000. Reprinted with permission.

In conclusion

I have dwelt mainly on problem cases. Too often members of the public who complain are brushed aside, so that problems do not see the light of day. People in a position to influence events may then be lulled into complacency. However that situation is changing. Concerned relatives are now making their voices heard and are campaigning effectively for change, through organisations such as Alert and "SOS NHS Patients in Danger". The media and charities working for older people have also done much to raise public awareness of the issues in recent years. Concern about the care of elderly patients in the NHS is now a high profile issue.

In February 2002, Channel 4 television broadcast a documentary called 'The Age of Consent.' This was filmed in a teaching hospital in Nottingham with the full cooperation of the Consultant staff. Their aim seemed to be to show the public how the medical profession decides whether or not to resuscitate patients. Government policy now decrees that such decisions should be made in consultation with the patient where possible, and with key relatives. This policy does not meet with great favour in the profession for it is time consuming and undermines the views of those who prefer a more authoritarian approach. Treatment withdrawal and the application of 'futile care theory' is now common practice in the UK, but the Channel 4 documentary showed that relatives who make their objections known may be heeded.

The Mental Capacity Act [2005], when enforced in April 2007, will make advance directives legally binding, and will introduce proxy health-care decision makers in England and Wales. Members of the British public who are given this role may find themselves in the onerous position of having to make irrevocable decisions about withholding and withdrawing life-prolonging treatment.

References

1. Gould M. No regrets. *Nursing Times*. 1999; **95**: 10-11.
2. Anon. Why doctor ordered patient to be starved. *Daily Mail*. 14th May 1997.
3. Lennard–Jones J E. Ethical and legal aspects of clinical hydration and nutritional support. *British Association for Parenteral and Enteral Nutrition. 1998*.
4. Horsnell M and Foster P. Euthanasia claims sow doubt in families' minds. *The Times* 6th January, 1999; p.9, cols 1-5.
5. Ethical decision-making in palliative care. Artificial hydration for people who are terminally ill. *National Council for Hospice and Specialist Palliative Care Services*. London. July 1997.
6. Rozenberg J. Woman mentally fit to choose death. *Daily Telegraph*. March 23rd 2002, p 9.
7. Withholding and withdrawing life-prolonging medical treatment. Guidance for decision making. British Medical Association. *BMJ Books* June 1999. Revised version 2000.
8. Withholding and withdrawing life-prolonging treatments; good practice in decision making. *General Medical Council*. August 2002.
9. House of Lords Select Committee. Report on Medical Ethics. *HMSO* London 1994. para 257.
10. Personal communication from patient's son. Quoted with permission.
11. Habgood J. Being a Person. Chapter 8. Words and thoughts. p177. *Hodder and Stoughton* 1998.
12. R v Gibbons and Proctor (1918). Quoted by Gerard Wright QC at a conference in Eastbourne, England in 1999.
13. Ev 305-6. Draft Mental Incapacity Bill. Vol II. *HMSO* 2003.
14. From Medical Ethics Alliance evidence to The Joint Committee on the draft Mental Incapacity Bill in session 2002-2003. See Case 1, Ev 163, Draft Mental Incapacity Bill, Volume II, Oral and written evidence. *HMSO* 2003.
15. Whitehead C. Ev.295, 4 a-c and 5. Draft Mental Incapacity Bill Report. **Vol II**. *HMSO* © Parliamentary Copyright House of Lords and Commons 2003.

Acknowledgement

Parliamentary material is reproduced with the permission of the Controller of HMSO on behalf of Parliament.

Chapter 13

Feeding via a Percutaneous Gastrostomy Tube

Some factors that influence decision-making
in elderly stroke patients

Author Gillian Craig

This paper was first published in the Catholic Medical Quarterly in Feb 2005. It has been updated to take account of the Mental Capacity Act [2005] and the Appeal Court Ruling in the Burke case.

Introduction

It is generally accepted that to continue artificial hydration without nutrition over a period of weeks leads to progressive malnutrition and is an unacceptable policy[1], yet given the relative ease of maintaining hydration by means of subcutaneous fluids, and the relative difficulty of maintaining nutrition in patients who cannot swallow, this unacceptable policy is sometimes practised. The decision to insert a percutaneous gastrostomy tube (PEG) in elderly stroke patients can be fraught with difficulty if the patient is not in a position to give consent. Health care professionals and family members may have widely differing views about what should be done. Quality of life issues may be uppermost in some minds, self-interest in others. Some people consider tube feeding to be undignified- yet PEG tubes are invisible under the clothing and cause no discomfort to the patient. "Wouldn't it be better to let the patient go?" they ask. Some would advocate euthanasia were that lawful in the UK so we are treading on dangerous ground. The key person of course is the patient whose wishes should be paramount. But who knows what their wishes are if they cannot speak for themselves? Who knows whether previously expressed wishes remain valid? How many people have the patience or skill to communicate with the confused and demented? How many take the trouble to try?

Professional guidelines are available for doctors. Those issued by the British Medical Association and the General Medical Council relate to withholding and withdrawing life-prolonging medical treatment in general. The Medical Ethics Alliance have produced guidance of a more pro-life nature, and I have suggested a practical approach that some people have found helpful.[2] In this paper I will consider some factors that may influence the patient's wishes, the relatives views, and the doctor's opinion about the provision of food and water using a PEG.

A hypothetical scenario. What would your reaction be?

Imagine that you have just received a message that your beloved mother, sister or aunt has suffered a bad stroke, and is in hospital paralysed, unable to speak, somewhat confused and unable to swallow. She has shown no improvement but there is still a possibility of recovery. If she is given anything orally she will choke and could die of pneumonia. They have tried a nasogastric tube but she didn't seem to like it and pulled it out. Now the doctors feel she should have a PEG feeding tube, but this involves a small operation. You are needed to help them make the right decision. So you get out the car and drive to the hospital. On arrival you are shocked to see your relative so frail and incapacitated. Your mind is a whirl of conflicting thoughts.

Would you:

* Ask doctors not to use nasogastric feeding or fit a PEG ?
* Be worried but leave treatment to the doctors?
* Try to persuade the doctors to feed the patient?
* Assist by taking steps to persuade the patient yourself.
* Ask yourself "What would the patient want"?
* Discuss the risks and benefits calmly with the doctors and come to a decision.
* Agree while hoping that the patient would die before intervention was needed.
* Consider tube feeding in any form to be degrading.
* Consult other members of the family for their views.
* Consult another independent person, the hospital chaplain perhaps, or an ethicist.
* Seek advice from a solicitor.

If your instinct is to say " NO" to a PEG what are your reasons?

* Are you medically qualified or otherwise knowledgeable about these matters?
* Has a friend/relation had a bad experience with tube feeding?
* Do you know what your relative's wishes would be?
* Have you any legal authority to intervene in crucial medical decisions?
* Has the patient signed a valid advance directive prohibiting such intervention?
* Are you worried that she would not cope with a PEG?
* Have you considered what it feels like to starve?
* Are you afraid that the procedure would shorten life?
* Are you concerned about prolonging life with disability?
* Are you concerned about financial implications if life is prolonged?
* Are you are worried about future nursing home costs?
* Are you thinking of your inheritance?
* Are you putting your own needs above those of the patient?
* Are you truly considering the patient's best interests?
* What is your attitude to disability in general?
* What is your attitude to old age?
* Do you think it would kinder to let the patient die?
* Do you secretly advocate euthanasia?

Discussion

Who decides?

The attitudes of relatives and doctors can be vital for patient survival. Few people would admit to the thoughts that may go through their minds on these occasions, but anxiety and self-interest can influence proxy decision-makers. Inexperienced health care staff may not question the motives of relatives, and relatives may not question the motives of health care staff whose thoughts may not be entirely blameless either. In the brave new world of bed shortages and hospital closures, when elderly "bed-blockers" are not always welcome, it is not safe to assume that doctors will necessarily take an active approach to a PEG. The patient's best interest is only truly served when doctors and loving relatives work in co-operation. Very disabled people can often express an opinion if assessed with patience and skill.[3]

The key questions should be:

1. Is it necessary? 2. Is it feasible? 3. Can the patient tolerate the procedure? 4. What does the patient want? 5. Is the patient capable of making life or death decisions? 6. If not who decides?

The risks and benefits of PEG feeding

Some benefits

*   Fluids, nutrition and drugs go directly into the stomach.
*   Hydration and nutrition can be maintained.
*   Deterioration and death due to dehydration and malnutrition can be avoided.
*   Pain due to starvation and dehydration can be avoided.
*   A PEG is more difficult to dislodge than a nasogastric tube, as it has a retaining flap.
*   Most patients are unaware of a PEG once it is in place.
*   The PEG is out of view and is aesthetically more attractive than a nasogastric tube.

Some risks

*   Insertion carries a small risk of perforation or infection.
*   Insertion carries a mortality of 1-2% [1]
*   Most patients need some sedation that carries a small risk.
*   The endoscope may temporally obstruct breathing.
*   There is a 10% risk of aspiration pneumonia in the first few weeks.
*   Prolonged starvation carries a 100% certainty of death.

Proxy health care decision-makers are in a difficult position, for they have power, without knowledge or training. They may also have vested interests that colour their judgement and operate against the patient's best interests. Some of these have been alluded to above. People who stand to gain financially from a patient's demise should not be permitted to make irrevocable life and death decisions. Relevant conflicts of interest should be declared.

Doctors should not burden family members unnecessarily with life and death decisions, nor defer to them against their better judgement. If they do some patients will die unnecessarily and their friends and relatives may suffer psychologically as a result. There should be a system for monitoring the effects of end-of-life decisions on the decision-maker and other members of the family. If there is disagreement within the family, relationships may be permanently soured.

In England and Wales the role of proxy health-care decision-makers is changing. The Mental Capacity Bill was passed in Parliament in March 2005 and became the Mental Capacity Act. A Code of Practice will be added before the Act is adopted in April 2007. As the law stands at present, the views of the next of kin are rarely allowed to overrule the opinion of the doctor in charge of the case. If a patient is incapable of stating their wishes and there is serious dissent within the family, or between doctors and the family, a second expert clinical opinion should be obtained and legal advice sought. Good practice in the UK requires that all cases of PVS should be referred to a Court before provision of food or water via tube feeding is withheld or withdrawn. It is for Parliament and our judges to decide, in the light of the European Human Rights Act, where to draw the line in patients whose condition falls short of a permanent vegetative state.

In the USA it has long been the practice to appoint lay people as legal guardians with the power to make life and death decisions in health matters. High profile cases like that of Terri Schiavo show how dangerous this can be:-

Terri Schiavo was an American woman who collapsed at home in 1990 at the age of 26. She was admitted to hospital with serious brain damage, from which she never recovered. In 1998 her husband, who stood to gain financially from her death and wanted to marry again, petitioned for her tube feeding to be stopped with the result that she would die. Her parents opposed this. Eventually the fight was lost and Terri died in March 2005. [5,6]

Dealing with conflict

Doctors rarely take kindly to non-medical people who oppose their plans for a patient. Some react with irritation but the best talk the situation through. We have to tread a fine line between old-fashioned paternalism, excessive over-treatment and dangerous laissez-faire. We also have to try to understand the relative's point of view and treat the family holistically. It is very sad when family members disagree among themselves about what should be done. Some may be exhausted by caring and may wish the patient dead, while others simply want to be free to get on with their own lives. Whatever the reason patients cannot be abandoned because their family cannot cope. Alternative ways should be found to support the patient with the help of social workers and the health care team.

If tube feeding by PEG is advised, but is opposed by the next of kin, some doctors would say "OK, but we must review the situation in a week as the patient can't be left as he/she is much longer." Other doctors would defer to the relative against their better judgement and concentrate on other patients. Medical interest and involvement tends to be greatest in the early stages of investigation and treatment, and can ease off once the acute phase has passed. So it is best for people to try to co-operate and not antagonise the medical staff. Sometimes relatives need to take a polite but firm stand and insist on active treatment or a second opinion. Every case is different.

Each time a patient comes under the surveillance of a different medical team the doctors will take a fresh look at the situation. So when an old person moves from the admitting ward to a stroke unit or rehabilitation ward, their situation will be reviewed. This is a valuable safeguard for the patient, for situations can change. Some stroke patients regain the ability to swallow in time. Others who appear to be managing to eat a little may develop signs of malnutrition indicating that intervention is needed.

If there is disagreement within the medical team a relative who has been burdened with a difficult decision may receive conflicting advice. When the Mental Capacity Act is enacted in April 2007 and proxy decision makers are permitted in England and Wales, lay people will have the final word and the doctor's hands will be tied as happens in the USA. The medical issue should be whether a PEG can be provided without undue discomfort or risk, and whether there is any hope of recovery. However poor a patient's prognosis, potentially treatable factors should be treated, and all appropriate care given whether the patient has been labelled 'not for cardiopulmonary resuscitation' or not [7]. If there is a glimmer of hope patients should be given the benefit of the doubt. Neither doctors nor relatives, nor indeed judges should play God.[8]

The judgment in the Burke case has thrown professional guidelines into a state of confusion, and it is not yet clear how the law will stand when the dust settles. Nor is it yet clear how the Human Rights Act will impinge on medico-legal judgments. Unfortunately many interesting legal cases are languishing in the wings for want of the money needed to pay the lawyers. The legal route is one best avoided unless relatives wish to have years of their lives consumed in expensive controversy. The time to sort matters out is while the patient is still alive, by quiet discussion between the patient, the relatives and the doctors concerned, in the presence, if need be, of a trusted and independent mediator. When dissent becomes confrontation all are losers.

Nutritional policy and assessment

Most NHS hospitals have a nutritional policy that requires the regular monitoring of food intake. Guidelines are available from The British Association for Parenteral and Enteral Nutrition (BAPEN).[9] Patients at high risk of malnutrition should be referred to a dietician. BAPEN advise that "The selection of patients should be carried out by experienced members of the Nutrition Team. The prognosis of any swallowing difficulties should be discussed with a qualified Speech and Language therapist."[10] A speech and language test (SALT test) has become "de rigeur", but in some areas there is a shortage of qualified speech and language therapists so patients may have to wait. Skilled testing is crucial, for to feed a patient orally when they cannot protect their airway can be fatal. Nevertheless sometimes one has to rely on a simple gag test for practical purposes.

Patients should not be labelled "nil by mouth" and left without food or water for days or weeks on end while waiting for a swallowing test. Basic hydration should be maintained using parenteral fluids since death from dehydration can occur within a week. Tube feeding should be considered after a maximum of 10 days without food, and preferably earlier. A non-obese person who is hydrated but not fed can survive for up to 60 to 70 days.[11] If feeding is postponed malnutrition will cause slow but progressive deterioration. This deterioration can only too easily be used as a reason for non-intervention at a later stage. If tube feeding is likely to be needed for more than 14 days, BAPEN recommend that a PEG should be considered.[10]

Example. Waiting for a swallowing test.

A married woman aged 88 was admitted to hospital after a fall at home. She was unable to move her left arm or get out of bed. A stroke was suspected but there were complicating factors. She was designated "nil-by-mouth" although she had a normal gag reflex on admission. Oral medication was stopped on admission. The following day she had minimal left sided weakness, and her speech and memory were normal. Nevertheless she remained nil-by-mouth waiting for a formal swallowing test. She was given intravenous fluids for two days, but then the drip stopped running and according to the relatives was not resumed. She was still starving waiting for her swallowing test and a non-urgent CT scan when she suddenly died. almost six days after admission. The case was referred to the coroner who did not investigate matters. Death was attributed to a cerebro-vascular incident. Six years later the daughter was still heart-broken that her mother had not been fed.

(Case reported with the daughter's permission)

Assessment of nutritional state

When assessing a patient's nutritional state it is insufficient to rely solely on measurement of the body weight or the lack of visible emaciation. Patients can be malnourished and dangerously deficient in vitamins without weight loss[12]. Nutritional status should be assessed by dietary history, clinical evidence, biochemical evidence and anthropomorphic measurements such as body weight, mid-arm fat and mid-arm muscle mass [12,13]. A loss of weight of 5% in a month, or 10% in six months is considered a severe weight loss [12]. Oedema and excess body fluid in general, such as ascites or large pleural effusions should be taken into consideration as it can confound the issue and mask true weight loss. Height is important in evaluating weight, but due allowance should be made for loss of height in the elderly due to osteoporosis [12]. All these points should be born in mind when assessing nutritional status. Measurement of body weight alone is not enough.

Figure 1 shows data obtained at postmortem from an elderly patient who had swallowing difficulties after a stroke and died four months later amid concerns about her nutrition. The pathologist, relying on her body weight and the lack of emaciation, found no evidence of malnutrition. Yet calculation of her body mass index (BMI) making due allowance for the effect of some oedema, showed her to be malnourished according to World Health Organisation (WHO) criteria. Calculation of the BMI using the post mortem height (155cm) and weight (42.2kg) quoted by the pathologist, gave a result of $17.58kg/m^2$ signifying mild protein-calorie malnutrition according to WHO criteria.[14] If she had one litre of oedema fluid, her true body weight would have been 41.2kg [15] giving a BMI of $17.16kg/m^2$ this being almost in the moderate protein-calorie malnutrition range. Allowing for two litres of oedema and an assumed height loss of 5 cms due to osteoporotic vertebral collapse brought the BMI into the WHO severe malnutrition range. These results show how crucial it is to take all factors into account.

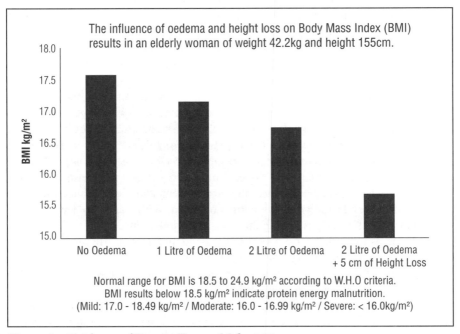

Figure 1 – Evidence of Protein Energy Malnutrition

Severe malnutrition can cause oedema, hepatomegaly, possibly some circulation effects, mood and behaviour changes, skin changes, hair changes, and other problems. Vitamin deficiency can develop slowly or rapidly, depending on the type of vitamin, but vitamin C and B (including folic acid) can become deficient over weeks or months. Folate affects homocysteine levels. High homocysteine levels are associated with a 2- to 40-fold increased risk of coronary heart disease [16]. Vitamin C deficiency causes scurvy, which caused the death of sailors on long voyages, until they learnt to take limes on board ship as a source of vitamin C.

Deterioration in a patient's condition can, all too easily, be used to justify further non-treatment. However this is a dangerous policy. Clinicians must not overlook the possibility that deterioration is due to treatable malnutrition. Deficiency of some of the B vitamins can cause mental confusion, irritability, apathy and dementia-like states, as happens in untreated pellagra caused by protein and nicotinic acid deficiency. Deficiency of the B vitamin aneurine can cause cerebral beri-beri – a disease that can mimic cerebral arteriosclerosis and causes death in a matter of weeks [17]. In some stroke patients, malnutrition, rather than progression of their stroke disease or dementia may be the cause of their deterioration and death. Food is a basic human need. To withhold food will cause death eventually, irrespective of the underlying condition.

The mental state factor

Existing professional guidelines issued by the British Medical Association and the General Medical Council give great weight to the patient's mental state. The BMA consider the lack of self-awareness to be a crucial factor.[18] The GMC guidance revolves around mental incapacity.[19] A patient's mental state is of course a determining feature when it comes to deciding whether they are capable of giving informed consent about any treatment. But those who cannot decide for themselves should not be valued less as people than those who are compos mentis. They should still be valued members of the human race.

Guidance that permits life-sustaining food and water to be withheld on the grounds of mental incapacity or the lack of self-awareness is open to serious criticism in law. The GMC guidance was declared to be unlawful in several respects by Mr Justice Munby in his High Court judgment of July 31st 2004 [20]. This ruling was overturned in the Court of Appeal in July 2005 (*R (Burke) v General Medical Council [2005] EWCA 1003*). The Appeal Court Judges ruled that in cases of dispute about the provision of ANH to a mentally incompetent adult, legal advice should be sought and a second expert clinical opinion obtained. With respect to decisions in a competent adult they said (in paragraph 34 of their judgment):

"…It seems to us that for a doctor to deliberately interrupt life-prolonging treatment in the face of a competent patient's wish to be kept alive, with the intention of thereby terminating the patient's life, would leave the doctor with no answer to a charge of murder".

A worrying aspect of Mr Justice Munby's judgment was his view that "Important though the sanctity of life is, it has to take second place to personal autonomy, and it may have to take second place to human dignity…" This leaves the door wide open to death by personal decree, and has been described as a "judicial gift to the Voluntary Euthanasia Society…"[20] Dignity and indignity are highly subjective factors, and dependent to a great extent on the attitudes taken by friends and relations. A person may value their life despite being in a situation that many able-bodied people would consider intolerable.

The potential for recovery

The potential for recovery is a crucial factor, and one that is difficult to predict with accuracy. As the law stands at present it is lawful to withhold or withdraw tube feeding from a person who is in a permanent vegetative state (PVS), but only with the permission of the High Court. At least a year is needed before making a diagnosis of PVS, and numerous cases have been reported of recovery of consciousness after this time in young adults who sustained brain damage as the result of an accident.

There is potential for recovery after a stroke too, if the patient is given the necessary time, so attempts to sustain life should not be stopped prematurely. The situation is somewhat different in patients who are affected by conditions that are untreatable and slowly progressive in a downhill direction. Yet if the mind remains clear many such patients value their life and wish to be supported and fed to the bitter end. Their wishes should be respected.

There remain patients who are suffering from a slowly progressive disorder that will in due course deprive them of their mental faculties and leave them in a condition that may seem undignified. I refer to unfortunate people in the terminal stages of Altzheimer's disease. Would such people wish to have their lives prolonged by tube feeding? Who can say? Very often in the late stages, these patients forget how to eat and choke on food given orally. They may become dehydrated as they forget to ask for a drink, or cannot reach the drink placed by the bedside. There may be some reduction in thirst sensation in the elderly, but if this is the case it makes it all the more important for carers to encourage the patient to drink. I have observed frail old people trying to drink from an empty cup, and have heard them cry out for a drink. There is no evidence that I am aware of, to indicate that thirst is entirely absent in severe dementia. In the USA patients with dementia are sometimes fed through a PEG, but in the UK this would be unusual. Most patients with dementia will pull out a nasogastric tube, because it frightens them, or is uncomfortable. Pulling out a nasogastric tube should not lead to the assumption that the patient does not want to be fed.

The advice of the House of Lords' Select Committee on Medical Ethics was good advice that should not be overlooked, for they said: "It should be unnecessary to consider the withdrawal of nutrition or hydration except in circumstances where the means of administration is of itself, evidently burdensome to the patient." [21]

Conclusions and recommendations

1. Malnutrition matters! 'To continue hydration in the absence of nutrition for a matter of weeks is unethical and leads to progressive starvation.'[1]
2. All patients, especially those at a high risk, should have their nutrition needs assessed on a regular basis, and appropriate action taken to avoid malnutrition. Vitamin deficiencies should not be overlooked.
3. No patient, whether mentally incapacitated or not, should be put at risk of death from slow starvation.
4. If a patient makes a valid decision not to have tube feeding, that decision must be respected.
5. Existing professional guidelines should be heeded but no doctor should be obliged to withhold treatment against their better judgement. Professional guidelines are readily available.[18,19]
6. It is relatively easy to maintain hydration by means of subcutaneous fluids, but nutrition can be a problem in patients who cannot swallow or cannot swallow safely. If a SALT test shows that oral feeding is dangerous, health care professionals continue oral feeding at their peril.
7. If the patient cannot tolerate a nasogastric tube a decision about a PEG should be made sooner rather than later, to avoid unnecessary deterioration in the patient's physical and mental state. All hospitals should have a clear policy on this.
8. It is dangerous to delegate responsibility for life and death clinical decisions to an untrained member of the public, but the views of dissenting members of the family should not be ignored.

9. There must be an effective independent medical and legal advocacy system to support and advise dissenting relatives- the present ad hoc arrangements do not suffice. Good independent legal advice and speedy access to an independent second opinion from a suitably qualified medical expert should be freely available during the patient's life.

10. In the event of a patient's death, the Court of Appeal have ruled that "there must be an effective investigation where agents of the State bear potential responsibility for the loss of life." [22] All such deaths should be reported to the Coroner whose responsibility it is to investigate and make a ruling on the cause of death.

Notes and References

1. Ethical and legal aspects of clinical hydration and nutritional support. A report by J.E.Lennard Jones for the *British Association for Parenteral and Enteral Nutrition*. 1999. ISBN 1 899467 25 4. p 33-34.
2. Craig GM. Respect for life. A framework for the future. *Catholic Medical Quarterly*. 2003; **Vol. LIV No 1**. (299): 13-15.
3. Boseley S. Car accident 'shows risk of living wills. *The Guardian* February 17th. 2000.
4. R (Burke) v General Medical Council [2004] EWHC 1879.
5. Smith W.J. Dehydration nation. *The Human Life Review*, Fall 2003: 69-79.
6. www.terrisfight.org. © Terri Schindler-Shiavo Foundation.
7. Withholding and withdrawing Life-prolonging Treatments: Good Practice in Decision-making. *The General Medical Council,* London, August 2002, para 91.
8. Andrews P. We must not play God. *British Medical Journal,* 2003; 326:634.
9. Standards and Guidelines for Nutritional Support of Patients in Hospitals. *British Association for Parenteral and Enteral Nutrition.* Ed.Sizer .
10. See ref 9 at page 29.
11. Shils ME, Olsen JA, Shike M Eds. In Modern Nutrition in Health and Disease 8th ed. Philadephia: *Lea and Febiger* 1994, quoted by Hoefler J in Managed Death, *Westview Press,* 1997 p 118.
12. Assessment of nutritional status and fluid deficits in advanced cancer. Sarhill N, Mahmoud FA, Christie R, Tahir A. *Journal of Terminal Oncology*, 2003, **2:1**, 29-37.
13. Bozzetti et al. Guidelines on artificial nutrition versus hydration in terminal cancer patients. European Association for Palliative Care *Nutrition* 1996, **12:3**, 169-172.
14. World Health Organisation normal range for BMI is 18.5 to 24.9kg/m^2.
15. One litre of water weighs one kilogram.
16. Health and Age and the American Geriatrics Society, General malnutrition. © 2002. Novartis Foundation for Gerontology. www.geriatricsyllabus.com
17. H de Wardener. See Chapter 10 Nutrition, at p335-339. The Practice of Medicine Ed Richardson J. 2nd Ed 1960. *J & A Churchill Ltd* London.

18. Withholding and Withdrawing Life-prolonging Medical Treatment. Guidance for decision-making. British Medical Association, *BMJ Books* 1999.
19. Withholding and Withdrawing Life-prolonging Treatments: Good Practice in Decision-making. *The General Medical Council,* London. August 2002.
20. Foster C. Right to survive. Solicitor's Journal. 2004, October 1st, p 1110-1111.
21. House of Lords' Select Committee. Report on medical ethics. London, HMSO, 1994:para 251-257.
22. Court of Appeal ruling of October 10th 2003 by Lords Justices Brooke, Waller and Clarke, in the Khan case. Reported by Rozenberg J. 'Dead girls' family wins ruling to question hospital'. *The Daily Telegraph,* Oct.11th 2003 p14 cols 1-3.

Chapter 14

The Problem of Ageism

1. Comments from Dr Gillian Craig

The public have been shocked by reports of mistreatment of the elderly in the National Health Service in recent years. *The Times* set the ball rolling with a front page-headline "Police check hospitals over 'backdoor euthanasia'" in January 1999.[1] Worrying reports about neglect of the elderly were also published by the charities Age Concern and Help the Aged [2,3], creating further media coverage of these issues.

In December 1999 *The Daily Telegraph* published allegations that elderly people are being neglected in our hospitals. Their front-page headline read "Elderly people 'left starving to death in NHS'." A consultant psychogeriatrician warned that patients were dying because of an unspoken policy of 'involuntary euthanasia' designed to relieve pressure on the National Health Service.[4] *The Daily Telegraph* staff were inundated with calls from the public recounting their experience. Many case reports were published throughout the week. Claims that care was being inappropriately limited were denied by the social care minister John Hutton, who dismissed them as "scaremongering". However, Dr Ian Bogle of the BMA told *The Daily Telegraph* that he believed that elderly patients did receive lower standards of care. He admitted that there was a problem of ageism in society as a result of the huge pressure on the system. Age Concern told *The Daily Telegraph* that one in ten people believed that a relative had been allowed to die because of a low standard of basic care. This statement was based on 'thousands' of responses.

The problem of poor care is not confined to hospitals, it can also be found in residential and nursing homes for the elderly. In September 2005 *The Daily Telegraph* published eloquent extracts from "Untold Stories" an autobiographical anthology by playwright Alan Bennett. When visiting his senile mother in a home for the elderly Bennett observed that: "Lacking one-to-one care, these helpless creatures slowly and quite respectably starve to death."

There are of course, many hospitals that still provide a high standard of care, but in general it is fair to say that many excellent geriatric departments have been destroyed by ward closures and reorganisation in recent years. Consultants have been slow to follow their patients into the community, as patients discharged from hospital become the responsibility of their General Practitioner.[5] The NHS can no longer cope with the demands of an ageing population within the financial constraints imposed by the Government. Without a good geriatric service, the NHS will inevitably grind to a halt. The BMA have warned repeatedly that funding is insufficient; finally following a week of extremely bad publicity the BMA voted to begin a major investigation into ways to privatise the NHS.[6] The public were outraged by the revelations in the press and it became clear that many people would gladly pay more taxes to ensure that care standards improve within the NHS.

The problem of ageism is a worldwide phenomenon. Prejudice against the elderly can be found in industrialised countries and in impoverished third world countries. Old people are no longer honoured in society. Traditional family loyalties and support structures are breaking down as children disperse around the globe in search of work and prosperity. Many children do go to great lengths to support aged parents, sometimes at considerable emotional cost to themselves, but too often the elderly are seen as an impediment to progress and a drain on the state purse. The global situation is discussed in a book 'Humanity comes of age'. The authors chart the creeping ageism promoted by some 'medical ethicists' who have proposed "that the governments deny older persons the right to expensive but life-saving medical procedures on the grounds that medical costs were getting out of hand."[7] Present trends towards treatment limitation, "end of life decisions," and involuntary euthanasia of the incapable must be seen in this context. It is a matter of urgency to address these issues and to tackle them at source. The contributing factors are deep set in society as a whole.

In the UK there have been major changes in the organisation of medical care for the elderly in the last decade. With the closure of long stay wards the NHS became dependent on private sector nursing homes for long stay care. Insufficient state finance was allocated to fund patients who qualify for government aid, with the result that many old people who are dependent on state support remain in acute medical beds. At the same time many private nursing homes have gone bankrupt for lack of referrals. A Royal Commission advised that the elderly should receive free nursing care even in private nursing homes, but the British Government were slow to act on this advice. This was a prime example of ageism driven by the desire to save money.

Management of health care has become an exercise in economics. There are indications that privatisation of public services is linked to global trade-expansion policies of international institutions such as the World Trade Organisation.[8] Big business has moved into the nursing home sector in recent years. The elderly may become expendable like tins on a supermarket shelf. Those past their sell-by-date may be discarded in the interests of business efficiency. One extreme example of this was reported in 1998 when a destitute old lady died in a nursing home. The local authority argued that her funeral expenses should be paid by the nursing home as her body was "business waste". They lost the argument when taken to court, but the case illustrates the views that can be expressed in our sick society. It is time to change this business culture, for ideas best suited to the world of commerce are degrading when applied to a health service. In the long run it will not benefit society to have hospitals that do not care for patients of all ages equitably, according to need. The sum total of human happiness is not increased by neglecting the elderly. The little old lady or aged man in the corner of the ward is someone's much loved relative and should be treated well.

The pressure of work in the NHS has increased dramatically in recent years as more and more patients pass through fewer and fewer beds. Consultant physicians have been overwhelmed with work and many feel angry and frustrated.[9] Under such conditions standards of care will inevitably fall and the risk of treatment withdrawal will rise.

As a consequence of the closure of hospital long-stay wards for the elderly, there is now a mismatch of skills and patients. Most of the doctors with expertise in geriatric medicine are hospital based, whereas most of the frail elderly are in the community. Restrictive practices within the medical profession and rigid adherence to the existing referral system from general practitioner to hospital consultant can operate against the interests of patients in the community.[5] Constructive change is hard to achieve, for the care of the elderly in the community receives little attention from the medical hierarchy and there is little support for the idea of Community Geriatricians.[10] Most consultants are only too happy to leave general practitioners to cope with the elderly as best they can. This is counter-productive, for higher standards of medical care in the community could reduce re-admissions to hospital and relieve pressure on acute sector beds.

Few physicians, surgeons or nurses these days can practice their profession without dealing with elderly patients, for approximately two thirds of hospital admissions are elderly. So resentment of the elderly is entirely out of place. Without them, most hospital doctors and nurses would be out of a job! Some training in the care of the elderly is now built into the undergraduate medical curriculum but by no means all doctors have postgraduate experience in geriatric medicine. This would increase insight and might help to reduce prejudice. Individuals who have difficulty relating to the elderly should be steered towards non-clinical roles in medicine, for as Sinason observed, "Human limitations bring out the worst and the best in individuals and society."[11]

In units all over the country there are still many dedicated doctors, nurses and paramedical health professionals who make a major contribution to the care of the elderly and do so with skill, patience and wisdom. They are the unsung heroes. Some inspired people are looking at ways to improve the quality of life in nursing homes through music and creative story-making; others are finding ways to address the spiritual needs of dementia sufferers. When medicine has no more to offer there is much that can be done to bring some peace and beauty at the end of life.

The needs of family members who care for the long-term disabled have been recognised through the work of organisations such as the Carer's National Association in the UK. Such carers now have rights that are recognised in law. It is time for society to recognise that professional carers have needs too, for without dedicated professionals the NHS will fall apart. There are already major staffing problems in some specialties and a constant stream of doctors and nurses leave the profession early. Administrators tend to respond by trying to recruit and train replacements rather than addressing the root causes of dissatisfaction. Stress in family carers can result in elder abuse in the home. Stress in professional carers may be a factor in elder abuse and ageism in our institutions. It is time to be kind to professionals – for they too are human.

Some people might well suggest that money spent keeping old people alive could be better spent in other ways, for example to benefit poverty stricken children overseas, or to house the homeless in our inner cities. There are many deserving causes in the world. There is however, no guarantee that the savings made would be spent wisely at home or abroad. The western world for all its wealth finds it very difficult to assist poorer nations with financial aid. Too often corruption somewhere along the line foils the best of intentions. Utilitarians may be willing in theory, to sacrifice one individual for the benefit of others but that philosophy when taken to extremes is highly dangerous. All human life has intrinsic value and dignity and should be treasured by mankind.

In the UK, still one of the eight richest nations in the world, we can afford to agonize about elderly patients who lack self-awareness. In other parts of the world children go blind for want of simple vitamins. The dying in the ghettoes of Calcutta may be fortunate to be given a wash and clean clothes to die in. We in the West must keep a sense of proportion in our demand for high quality health care. If a nation like Britain can be negligent towards its own citizens what hope is there for those in poorer nations? We must not lose sight of the need to address global inequalities in health care, but the immediate task for doctors in the UK is to put our own house in order.

In the year 2000 in an effort to defuse concerns about the NHS the Government announced a large pay award for nurses and the Prime Minister promised to increase government spending on health by billions of pounds. This could raise British spending on health from 6 - 7% of gross domestic product to the European average of 8% according to reports in *The Times*[12]. Finally in April 2002 the Chancellor of the Exchequer announced a significant rise in National Insurance contributions. The hope was that the money raised would provide the resources so badly needed to enable doctors to fulfil their obligations to their patients. The reality is that no amount of money will alter the situation unless the elderly are cared for by doctors with the necessary skills, patience, gentleness and experience.

By the autumn of 2005 it was becoming clear that no amount of money would save the NHS. There were reports of a £250 million shortfall in the NHS budget despite increased Government spending. Many hospitals planned to close wards, cancel operations and make doctors and nurses redundant. According to revelations in *The Guardian* of September 22nd 2005 the Health Secretary intends to allow private companies to take over some state-of-the-art operating theatres. There are also plans to transfer "significant volumes" of patients and staff from the NHS to private units. By 2009 the independent sector will provide about 10% of NHS operations, the aim being so it is said, to give patients more choice and better services. Worse still, there are plans afoot to transfer district nurses and some other community nursing staff to the private sector. Before long our NHS, once the pride and joy of the nation, will be no more.

Factors that contribute to ageism in the NHS

1. *General factors*
   - Demographic changes - an increasing elderly population.
   - More people live to experience degenerative diseases.
   - Medical advances increase the possibility of treatment.
   - Public expectations rise.
   - Financial constraints limit access to treatment.
   - Rationing and 'prioritisation' creep in.
   - Ward closures.
   - Management slow to appreciate needs of health care staff.

2. *Problems within the medical profession*
   - Medical students learn about rare and interesting diseases during their training. On qualifying they may resent having to deal with the relatively mundane problems that often afflict the elderly.
   - Low status accorded to those who care for the incurable.
   - Difficulties at the hospital/community interface.
   - Reduced power base for geriatricians as their specialty is merged with general medicine, and many geriatric hospitals close. Psychogeriatricians adversely affected by closure of long stay psychiatric hospitals. General reduction in hospital facilities for the care of the elderly.
   - Mismatch of skills and patients as long stay wards close, and patients move out into the community. Little interest in creating Community Geriatricians.
   - Territorial disputes between GPs and Consultants.

In conclusion

Left wing antipathy to the private sector has caused difficulties at the NHS/Private Sector interface. This, together with lack of finance for placements has contributed to delays in discharge of the elderly to private residential and nursing homes. Competition between social service and NHS budgets has added complications and caused much off-loading of responsibility.

The escalating workload and reduced facilities have caused an exodus of demoralised health care staff and there is now a shortage of nurses and doctors in the NHS. Elderly patients caught in the middle of this difficult situation can be resented and mistreated. Finally with limitation of life-prolonging treatment officially sanctioned by the BMA elderly patients with dementia or strokes are seen to be risk.

There is evidence of ageism throughout society and this is reflected in policy, practice and the delivery of services. The government tried hard to improve matters with "The National Service Framework for Older People" revealed in 2000, with plans for implementation in 2001. The charity Help the Aged was asked to convene an Older People's Reference Group, the aim being to propose standards that older people themselves would like to see established.[13]

The Health Advisory Service 2000 (HAS) have published standards for health and social care services for older people[14] as have the Centre for Policy on Ageing.[15] Analysis of these publications is outside the scope of this review. Suffice it to say that much thought has been given to these matters, and much paper has been generated. One can only hope that the outcome will be helpful.

A Chairman of the Commission for Health Improvement, took the view that the best way to encourage improvements may be to "hold up a mirror . . . a reflection of inadequate performance is a powerful incentive to change".[16] Many mirrors have been held up for those with eyes to see, and many glances have been averted. It is the responsibility of every citizen to ensure that these serious matters are addressed. Every action, every act of human kindness, however small, can help to change society. *"It is better to light one candle than to curse the darkness".*

2. Comments from Professor Sir John Grimley Evans

Professor John Grimley Evans, of the Nuffield Department of Clinical Medicine of Oxford University, headed the Department of Clinical Geratology at Oxford. Writing in the *Daily Telegraph* of December 7th 1999, he made the following comments, which were published at the height of the media furore, under the headline 'Euthanasia is a job for executioners not doctors.'[17]

Euthanasia is a job for executioners not doctors

'We hear increasingly of patients being given second-rate treatment or having beneficial treatments withheld, because they are above an arbitrary age. Prejudice against older people is common in British society but it influences health care more in some districts than in others. Deplorably, it is difficult for citizens to find out what is happening in their locality because they lack access to the necessary figures. The catalogue of complaints amassed by Age Concern published recently leaves little doubt that the problem is pernicious and widespread.

'Doctors and other health professionals are trained not to let personal prejudices affect the care they offer to patients. Most of those who institute or condone ageism do so because they think they are performing a public duty in keeping down NHS costs.

'A London meeting last week heard that the General Medical Council is unclear whether ageist practice should be regarded as unethical behaviour by a doctor, as would racism or sexism. Why should the GMC be in any doubt? It is no business of doctors to decree that some citizens are less equal than others.

'Ageism in the NHS has been condemned by ministers, but they missed an opportunity when targets for health care of older people that might have prevented ageist practice were struck out of the Green Paper on Our Healthier Nation.

'Ageism is morally wrong because it treats a patient not as an individual but as a member of a group. For an individual patient, benefit from a treatment depends on physiological condition. The risk of physiological impairment increases with age but there is wide individual variation in the rate of ageing.

'Many people in later life function within ranges normal for young adults; chronological age and biological age do not necessarily match. Specialists in intensive care find that if an adequate range of physiological functions are fed into an equation to predict outcome, age ceases to be relevant.

'Using membership of a group to withhold treatment from an individual would cause outrage if grouping was by social class or ethnicity, which are also associated with differences in health care outcomes.

'Grosser forms of ageist prejudice are being claimed, including accusations that elderly patients are being killed by starvation orders imposed by nurses. One hopes these will turn out to be based on misunderstandings, but the fact that misunderstandings can arise over such basic issues of patient care indicates a faulty system.

'End of life decisions about patients in hospital should be made at consultant level and consultants should be personally responsible for discussing them with patients and relatives.

'Issues surrounding food and fluids, forced feeding of patients with dementia or anorexia, whether treatment is prolonging life or spinning out the misery of a death, are particularly worrying matters that need to be thought out afresh each time they arise. But euthanasia, if it ever comes, will be a job for public executioners not for doctors.

'People aged over 65 comprise more than a quarter of the electorate but British politicians count on older people being too supine to vote tactically, as the elderly have done so effectively in America.

'By civilised European standards the NHS is under-funded to the tune of 25 per cent or more. While that continues, people who do not make their presence felt politically must expect to be left at the bus stop. Pensioners of the world unite!'

© *The Telegraph Group- Reprinted with permission.*

---

3. Death on the NHS

Comments made in an editorial in *The Daily Telegraph* of December 7th 1999.[18]

' Our reports that elderly patients have been left to starve in NHS hospitals is appalling but, in a gruesome way, not entirely surprising. The health service inevitably reflects the value of the society that sustains it. We are generally very keen, rhetorically at least, on children. If a hospital must spend a huge portion of its budget on a life-saving operation for a baby, we tend to approve. But our attitude towards old people is harsher.

'Death by dehydration in hospital is still mercifully uncommon. And, as we report elsewhere today, there are many hospitals where the elderly, like everyone else, can expect excellent service. But there is a difference between curing and caring. Even where medical treatment is reliable, older patients can still be subject to an array of indignities, ranging from the over-familiarity with which they are addressed to a lack of assistance with eating or dressing.

'The deliberate starvation of a patient is obviously in a different category from simple neglect. It may even be motivated by misplaced good intentions rather than callousness. But euthanasia and poor care are both rooted in the feeling that, once we are past a certain age, our lives have no real value.

'What is most worrying about our revelations is that this view of the ageing process seems to be becoming official policy. Routine testing for breast cancer ceases at the age of 65. The BMA has extended the circumstances in which it considers that the withdrawal of food and fluids may be justified. And, under a Bill now before the Scottish Parliament, patients would have the right to empower a guardian to order doctors, even against their medical judgement, to withdraw treatment.

'In an organisation with limited resources, there must obviously be some prioritisation. As we get older, we tend to require more treatment. There are obvious biological reasons for this. Our bodies are built to last to a certain age, and our component parts are designed accordingly. Why should nature fashion our hearts or lungs to last for 150 years when the rest of us will not? Thus, by the end of our lives, diseases come not as single spies, but in battalions.

'There may be circumstances in which it would be rational to offer, say, chemotherapy to an otherwise healthy 15 year old, but not to a 90 year old. But this is very different from deliberate termination. We enter hospital expecting to receive the best treatment that resources allow. How should we look upon our healers, knowing that, in certain circumstances, they might prefer us dead? In any case, many operations can transform the lives of elderly people. Someone in his eighties can still be granted long, productive years by a heart bypass or a hip replacement. If we expect doctors to decide who is and who is not worthy, we undermine the whole basis of medical ethics, and of trust between doctor and patient.

'Yet, as the NHS is structured, such decisions are routine. The nationalisation of healthcare has snatched from us the right to control our own treatment, and given it to state officials. When we enter an NHS hospital we put ourselves into someone else's hands. And, for those advanced in years, those hands may be none too gentle.

© *The Telegraph Group December 7th 1999. Reprinted with permission*

---

4. Some thoughts of Gautama Buddha

However much we try to eradicate ageism, a remnant will remain, for negligent attitudes to the elderly are as old as the hills. Gautama Buddha, in his discourses 500 years before Christ warned about this in a parable that carries a dire warning to those who do not value human life.

A man who cared for no one, and respected no one during his life, died and reached the underworld where he was questioned about his attitude to frail children and the elderly. He had of course seen them during his life but his attitude had been dismissive and negligent.

"Did you not see among men, a woman or a man, that was 80, 90 or 100 years old, senile, crooked as a rafter, bent, leaning on a stick?" . . .

"Did it not occur to you that you too were liable to old age, and would do well to strive for good?"

"I was not able"- replied the man, "I was negligent." . . .

"So out of that negligence you did nothing good?

Truly others will act towards you as befits that negligence.

That evil was done by you.

You will experience its fruit" .[19]

References

1. Horsnell M and Foster P. Euthanasia claims sow doubt in families minds. *The Times* 6th January, 1999; p9, cols 1-5.
2. Report. Turning your back on us. Older people and the NHS. *Age Concern, England.* 1999.
3. Report. Dignity on the Ward. Promoting Excellence in Care. *Help the Aged* and *The Order of St John Trust.* 1999.
4. Laville S and Hall C. Elderly patients 'left starving to death in NHS'. *The Daily Telegraph* 6th December 1999, p.1. cols. 1-4. See also p.10 cols 1-7 and coverage on 7th & 8th December 1999.
5. Craig G M. Problems in the delivery of medical care to the frail elderly in the community. *Journal of Management in Medicine.* 1995; **9**: 30-33.
6. Rumbelow M. BMA to seek new model for NHS funding. *The Times,* Dec.10th 1999, p.14, col. 7.
7. Paul S S and Paul J A. Humanity comes of age. 1994. *WCC Publications,* Geneva.
8. Price D, Pollock AM and Shaoul J. How the World Trade Organisation is shaping domestic policies in health care. *Lancet* 1999; **354**:1889-92.
9. RCP Report. Consultant Physicians Working for Patients. *Journal of the Royal College of Physicians of London.* 1998 ; **32**: No. 4, Supplement number ONE.
10. Morris J. The case for the community geriatrician. *British Medical Journal.* 1991; **308**: 1184.
11. Sinason V. Mental handicap and the human condition. p.12. *Free Association Books Ltd,* London, 1992.
12. Murray I, Webster P, Watson R. Pay soars as Blair 'panics' over NHS. *The Times.* 18th January 2000, p1, cols 1-3.
13. Dignity on the Ward. A campaign update - October 1999. *Help the Aged,* London.
14. Health Advisory Service 2000. Standards for Health and Social Care Services for Older People. *Pavillion Publishing.* UK. 1999.
15. Service Standards for the NHS Care of Older People. Co-published by the *Centre for Policy on Ageing* and *Health Services Accreditation.* London. February 1999.
16. On the critical list. *Health Service Journal.* 26th August, 1999, quoted by Help the Aged. (See ref. 13 above)
17. Grimley-Evans J. Euthanasia is a job for executioners not doctors. *Daily Telegraph.* Dec.7th 1999; p.14, cols 1-2. ©*The Telegraph Group.* Reprinted with permission. [Note. Professor Sir John Grimley Evans retired in 2003.]
18. Death on the NHS. Editorial (anon). *Daily Telegraph* 7th December 1999. p23, cols 1-2. ©*The Telegraph Group.* Reprinted with permission.
19. Gautama Buddha, *circa* 500 BC. Text adapted from "Something Understood". BBC Radio 4, 27th June, 1999. [Note that this programme was broadcast shortly after publication of the BMA guidance].

Further reading

- Grimley Evans J. Long term care in later life. *British Medical Journal* 1995; **311**:644.
- Black D and Bowman C. Community institutional care for frail elderly people. *British Medical Journal* 1997; **315**: 441-442.
- Hadley R and Clough R. Care in Chaos. *Cassell* 1996.
- Rosenthal TC, Horwitz ME, Snyder G and O'Connor J. Medicaid primary care services in New York State: partial capitation vs full capitation. *The Journal of Family Practice*.1996; **42**:362-368.
- Craig GM. The case for widening the referral system. *Journal of the Royal College of Physicians of London.* 1996; **30**: 80-82.
- Bright L. Care Betrayed. A discussion of the issues which give rise to abuse in homes. *Counsel and Care* London 1995.
- Department of Health "No Secrets: The protection of vulnerable adults - Guidance on the development and implementation of multi-agency policies and procedures." *HMSO* 2000.
- Securing Good Care for Older People. The Wanless Social Care Review. *Kings Fund, London.* March 2006.

Some sources of help or information for the public

Action on Elder Abuse. www.elderabuse.org.uk.
Age Concern England. www.ageconcern.co.uk
ALERT. www.donoharm.org.uk/alert (Anti-euthanasia)
Alzheimer's Disease Society, London. Tel 0207 306 0606
British Association for Parenteral and Enteral Nutrition
First Do No Harm. www.donoharm.co.uk
Help the Aged, London. www.help the aged.org.uk
http://www.internationaltaskforce.org (Anti-euthanasia)
Medical Ethics Alliance. www.medethics-alliance.org
NHS Clinical Ethics Committees: www.ethics-network.org.uk
Patients First Network: Helpline UK. 0800 169 1719
Right To Life. www.righttolife.org.uk
SPUC, London. www. spuc.org.uk. Tel 0207 222 5845
The Care not Killing Alliance: www.care not killing.org.uk
The Lawyers Christian Fellowship. www.lawcf.org
The Law Society. www.lawsociety.org.uk Tel 020 7242 1222
The Official Solicitor of the Supreme Court, London.
The Stroke Association. www.stroke.org.uk

Chapter 15

People Must Always Come First

1. A Bishop Addresses the BMA

The Right Revd Mark Santer addressed the British Medical Association in St Philip's Cathedral, Birmingham, England on July 3rd 1994. Bishop Santer was the Anglican Bishop of Birmingham at that time, but he has now retired. His address, as given, was as follows:

"What can a Bishop say to members of a professional organization like the BMA? As far as health is concerned, you are the experts. In your world I am only- but is the word "only" quite right?- only a layman, a patient (potential if not actual), a consumer (if you like that language), a more or less adequately informed member of the public. So what can I say on the basis of what I know as a theologian, or in virtue of my authority as a pastor and as a minister of the Gospel?

"Ethics, I suppose, is the area where you and I most obviously impinge on each other. Now when people talk about the ethics of medicine, they are usually talking about the kind of ethical questions that arise in relation to particular medical procedures- most obviously in connection with birth, reproduction and death.

"But there is another area of ethical concern which concerns me today: not medical ethics in the usual sense, but the ethics of social and political policy as they impinge on health and medicine. It is a part of the individualism of our age to suppose that moral questions only arise when we are talking about the lives or decisions of individual people. But there are also moral questions to be asked, and moral principles to be stated, about social and political issues- in this case about the availability and use of resources, about the way priorities are settled and decisions are made, about the health or disease of institutions....

"I the LORD am your healer," it said in our first bible reading. (Exodus 15:26) What does that say about our notion of health? What does it mean to speak of the Lord God as out healer, as the source of all human health and well-being, physical, mental and spiritual?

"In the New Testament the restoration of physical health is often linked (surprisingly to our ears) with forgiveness, with the restoration of broken relationships. That gives a perspective on health which is essentially social. It reminds us that the health and welfare of the individual cannot be separated from that of the community or society to which the individual belongs. And there is a further dimension. The link between health and the forgiveness of sins reminds us that no view of human health is complete which does not reckon with our relationship with God. We are created for life with God and with one another. Without God we are lost, and without one another we are lost. Any smaller view of what we are does not do justice to our human dignity or destiny.

"What this means is that any discussion of what is good for the health of the individual cannot be properly discussed without reference to what is good for society, nor the good of society without reference to the good of individuals.

"Let us take this a bit further. The Christian faith declares that human beings are made in the image of God... Interpersonal relations therefore have a sacred quality, because they reflect the life of heaven: they reflect the life of God. This has social and political consequences. Life in society is to be considered not as a mere convenience for individuals who may need it or want it. No, life lived in society, life lived in relationship with other people, is what gives to human existence on earth its true dignity as a taste or likeness of heaven.

"The category of the personal is primary. Of course we need institutions and structures. Once more than two or three people start living together, we need rules and conventions. But their purpose is to serve persons, and to serve their common good. Just as the Sabbath was made for man and not man for the Sabbath, so with everything else. Government, laws, political programmes, markets, administrative structures- none of them is sacred, none of them is of ultimate importance. In a properly ordered world, they exist to serve us, not we to serve them. People must always come first. So the dignity of persons and the quality of interpersonal relationships must always claim precedence over the needs of institutions or causes or programmes. As soon as we start treating people not as ends but as means or instruments, we in fact start rotting the foundations of a healthy society.

"And there is something else. The God in whose image we are made is good. So as human beings we find our fulfilment by sharing and showing those godlike qualities of goodness, justice, truth, compassion and mercy- all of them virtues which presuppose regard for other persons, and all of which require other persons for their exercise. You cannot be good, or just, or compassionate all on your own. To live a moral life, to live a godlike life, to live a truly human life, we need other people.

"The structures in which we live, whether they are small and comparatively simple like the family (but was there ever a simple family?) or whether they are large and complex like the NHS, have an inescapable moral dimension. Whether we like it or not, structures and institutions embody some kind of moral values, both in the way they are ordered and in the way they are run. Some families have rules and habits that help people to flourish. Others do not. It is the same with large institutions.

"These things do not just happen. It is not impersonal forces that shape and determine the ways that institutions are structured and managed. They are the products and instruments of persons accepting responsibility, making decisions, exercising power (or failing to do so)- all of it in accord with some idea of what is right and good, and all of it with an effect on other people. In the end we are all of us answerable to God for the exercise of the responsibilities and the use of the power which we have been given.

"Now what about the institution which concerns all of us here, either as practitioners or as consumers, customers or patients- the National Health Service? The very fact that words like "customers" and "consumers" should even come into my head shows how far we have travelled in recent years. You hardly need me to tell you anything either about the achievements of the NHS in the past forty-six years or about the symptoms of its present crisis. Its achievements were related to social and political ideals which were avowedly moral: health care for all, and equal access for all. The NHS has promoted and embodied a culture of generous service and unstinting care that continues to astonish those who receive it.

"But in a constantly changing society, no institution is invulnerable to change. Change is inescapable, even if seldom comfortable. You know far better than I do, the facts and questions that have to be faced. There are questions about resources- both how much of the national cake is to be allotted to health and how, once allotted, it is to be apportioned; questions posed by demographic change, or by changes in medical science and practice; questions about priorities- the claims of research and the claims of routine, the claims of the elderly and the claims of the young, the claims of acute medicine and the claims of primary care; questions about the relationship between mental and physical health and issues of unemployment, bad housing and poverty; questions about governance and accountability. One way and another these questions must be addressed and choices have to be made. There is no dispute about that, or about the fact that every one of these choices has a moral dimension.

"Change is inevitable, but not every kind of change is inevitable or desirable. It is no exaggeration (I speak as an observer) to say that the current wave of reforms in the National Health Service- and who would dare to say it is the last?- is proving deeply distressing to people who have a commitment to public service, who see their profession as a calling, who care profoundly for the quality of service they have been trained to deliver, and who observe the human consequences of what is happening around them. I well remember meeting a member of Mrs Thatcher's Cabinet, one of the wets, in the early eighties, when the policies of high interest rates and non-intervention were destroying industry and jobs on all sides. "I don't pretend to understand monetarism," he said over the dinner table, "but I see the effects."

"Well, it is like that now: we see the effects- effects that are symptoms of a system in distress. We have seen the hasty imposition of major change without adequate consultation or trial. Important facts about human behaviour have been ignored, such as that people do not function well if they sense that their professional expertise is being ignored, impugned or denigrated. (Do you remember that remark about doctors fingering their wallets?) The very speed of change itself has produced stress and distress in those involved in it. Hospital chaplains have spoken to me about the state of grief in the institutions where they work, of men and women who, after giving years of devoted professional service, find themselves losing heart. But if people who have given years of service to others feel themselves the victims of non-care and accordingly show symptoms of distress, what does that say about the health of an institution whose ostensible purpose is the promotion of mental and physical health and well-being?

"Judged not only on theory but also by effect, perhaps the most obviously questionable aspect of the reforms is the introduction of the language and habits of the market into what is properly understood as a service. The culture of competition has set doctor against doctor, hospital against hospital, colleague against colleague. Priorities and policies come to be determined not on the basis of human need, but in accordance with the accounting policies, themselves a human construct, of the NHS. These do not in fact reckon with all the costs. It may, to take a hypothetical instance, be cheaper for the South Birmingham Health Authority (which is where we happen to be) to buy certain services from hospitals in other districts, but who reckons up the costs of travel and inconvenience to patients and their families?

"This illustrates one of the most distressing defects of the market model. Despite all the rhetoric about patient choice, the patient is in fact not the purchaser. The purchaser is the District Health Authority or the fund-holding practitioner. The patient is reduced to the status of a unit of consumption and exchange. That, in the Christian view, must be wrong, because it is treating people as means and instruments instead of ends.

"Of course there are aspects of the NHS which are properly treated as a business, and of course there is the necessity at all times for financial responsibility and accountability. But still the business model won't do, above all because of the culture that it breeds. One has only to stop for a moment and ask, "Who is competing with whom for what? And who is supposed to be making a profit out of it?" to realize how inappropriate and therefore dysfunctional it is. It is dysfunctional because it excludes and distorts. It replaces what should be co-operation with competition, and it excludes from its reckoning precious elements that in fact help to give to the service its distinctive quality.

"Perhaps there are some practitioners who are only in it for the money. That is not my experience. The practitioners I know, of whatever profession, are fulfilling a vocation, they are offering a service of love and duty to their fellow men and women, and there is no price you can put on these things. The basic point is this: you cannot buy a gift. And yet it is those gifts of attention, care and compassion, which make all the difference to what it is all about, which is health and well-being.

"The basic issue can be put like this. Think of yourselves. Do you, in the end, see yourselves as having a commodity to sell or a service to offer? For whose sake are you in it?

"It is time to be positive. What do we need? First of all, we need to re-establish a publicly shared consensus on our purposes and objectives, a consensus that must have an avowedly moral basis. Necessary elements, from a Christian point of view, will include the continued acceptance by public authority of its duty to ensure adequate and proper provision for the health care of the nation as a whole; equality of access for all; dignity of treatment for all; and a particular care for the weak, the vulnerable and all who are structurally disadvantaged from fighting for their own interests. What we are talking about here is the institutional expression of the virtues of justice and compassion.

"Next, if policies are to be developed on the basis of a shared understanding of purpose and culture, there is a need for public discussion in which the facts of change and of financial choice and constraint are openly faced and acknowledged. Politicians and practitioners need to take the public into their confidence.

"Also, throughout the whole process of the discussion, formation and execution of policy, there needs to be proper recognition and acceptance of roles, responsibilities and competence. We need both to recognize other people's responsibilities, and to accept and not to abdicate from our own.

"Thus politicians have a proper responsibility, which needs to be recognised, for the determination of policy and the allocation of resources. Politicians also need to accept their duty to help to inform and lead public opinion and not to hide behind what they read in the newspaper reports or in their postbag. They should not shy away from telling people what it costs to run a decent public service.

"Administrators and managers also have a responsibility- their responsibility for enabling others to deliver the service as effectively as possible. Nobody is helped if the task of administration is despised or denigrated.

"Then again, there are the professionals like yourselves. Doctors, on the whole, are not trained in administration, and clinicians tend to look at the effects of policies on individuals rather than at the social or financial constraints that have led to those policies. So there is a need to acknowledge the competence of others. But we also need to accept the responsibility for naming and speaking of the things that we do know about. When a respected and compassionate practitioner tells me that there is human need in the community that he and his colleagues are not being allowed to meet, I listen to him, and so should the politicians and administrators- because in the end it is human need that counts. The famous bottom line is to be found not in the published accounts but in the human consequences.

"You as practitioners have a right to ask politicians to attend to the things that you say on the ground of your professional integrity. You also have a duty, of which I am sure you are sharply aware, of not confusing professional integrity with sectional interest. Your professional integrity is in fact something you hold in trust on behalf of society as a whole. It carries with it a duty of free and open speech, not so much for your own sake, but for the sake of the society you serve.

"I have one last point to make. Christians know that in this world we can never build perfection, only more or less imperfect approximations. We do the best we can, and we recognise the best that others can do, even when we know it can never be perfect and that even the best can always go wrong. But we also know that nothing that is good, however imperfect, will ever be wasted.

© Bishop Mark Santer 1994. Used with permission.

2. Eternal Wisdom In An Age Of Illusion

The following comments are taken from the 9th Annual Lecture for The Bahai'i Chair for World Peace, given in Maryland in April 2003 by Professor David Cadnam . The speaker drew on the teachings of several great spiritual traditions and explored the perennial philosophy that Aldous Huxley described as "divine Reality"[1,2] © 2003 The Baha'i Chair for World Peace. Extracts are quoted with permission.

"Language is important because it gives shape to our thoughts and therefore to our actions and thus to their consequences. You may recall that the Buddhist *Dhammapada* opens with this verse:

We are what we think.
All that we are arises with our thoughts.
With our thoughts we make the world.[3]

And again, in another translation:

> What we are today comes from our thoughts of yesterday,
> and our present thoughts build our life of tomorrow:
> our life is the creation of our mind.[4]

"If then, we wish to understand 'reality', understand who we are and how it is that we have come to be as we are, we have, it seems to me, to look not so much at our technological competence, our forms of government or, indeed, the state of our economy, but at *that which we hold to be true*. When all else is stripped away, what is it that defines who it is that we are? For "with our thoughts we make the world", "our life is the creation of our mind".[5]

"I suppose it would not be too much of an exaggeration to say that we enter the twenty-first century in the guise of Economic Man, *Homo Economicus*. That is to say that the characteristics that are most commonly used to define (perhaps I should say quantify) the nature of our reality are the characteristics of measurement and in particular the characteristics of costs and revenues. What we have become is a function of this most particular 'language'…This language, the language that has come to shape our world…is based upon the proposition that what is expressed as 'the *real* world' is confined to that which is tangible, concrete and fixed…[6]

"By contrast, the language of the perennial philosophy offers us a different reality, a divine Reality. Here, we cannot define ourselves entirely by reference to the material world…

"Do you, in truth, feel yourself to be no more than an entry on a balance sheet, a statistic in the calculation of national economic growth or do these ancient and timeless voices touch something else in you that you recognise as being true and of real worth?[6,7]…

"If we really do take ourselves to be defined as *Homo Economicus,* then the rules of the market place and the balance of accounts set the parameters of reason and of being…If on the other hand, we see ourselves as an expression of that which is Divine, then reverence for others now present and yet to come must cause us to temper our own desires with those qualities that are the teaching of all the great spiritual traditions- generosity, patience, simplicity, humility, harmlessness, compassion and so on, the very qualities that Huxley thought were necessary for those that would be able to understand and practise the perennial philosophy, those that are "loving, pure in heart, and poor in spirit."[8]

"It seems to me, then, that it is beyond doubt that the choice that we make about this matter of 'language' and 'reality' will lead us in different directions. The first, the language of convention, will continue to promote its own fantasy, promising ever-increasing consumption for all, and thereby reinforcing the environmental and social catastrophes that have already begun to take place- not least flood, famine, pestilence, violence and economic and political migration- ever waiting for the technological and political 'fix' that will redeem all…

"Those of you who are familiar with Buddhist texts will know the prophetic story of the Wheel Turning King who failed to give to the poor. Poverty led to theft, theft to violence and so on until at the lowest point, at the depth of degradation, just a few people had the insight and courage to turn away from this seemingly unstoppable tragedy and, once more, proclaim the ancient wisdom of generosity, wisdom and compassion until the well-being of all was restored [9]. Will there now, I wonder, be those that have the insight and courage to prick the bubble of our illusion and turn us away from such a calamity?

"We must pray that this is so; otherwise those that profess calamity may be prophetic... For Guenon, it is as if we may have to enter the dark and cold of Winter before the new shoots of another Spring can come to be. For he says " the passage from one cycle to another can take place only in darkness." [10]

"Despite this rather gloomy prognosis. It seems to me that the second path, the path of reverence and simplicity which is the path offered by the perennial philosophy, does at least provide us with the possibility of a more sustainable way- provided of course that we turn to it with resolve and without further delay...

"It seems clear to me, that in time- and not too distant a time- we must challenge the conventional definition of reality, before it is too late, abandoning the language of unbounded materialism and consumption and returning once more to the language and practice of the great spiritual traditions- the "divine Reality" of Huxley's *Perennial Philosophy*."

* * *

Cadman ended his paper by quoting William Penn, one of the earliest Quakers who said –

"A good end cannot sanctify evil means:
nor must we ever do evil, that good may come of it...
Let us then try what love will do..." [11]

Note. Cadman was speaking about world trade, but his comments about the need for simplicity and reverence could also be applied to medical ethics. We must respect and revere the divine spark that makes all human life special. We must also ensure a more equitable distribution of health care resources throughout the world.

References

1. Bushrui S. The Wisdom of the Arabs. *Oneworld*, Oxford, 2002.
2. Huxley. A. The Perennial Philosophy, *Chatto & Windus*, London 1946.
3. *The Dhammapada*, a new rendering by Thomas Byrom (New York: Vintage Books, 1976), p.3.
4. Source- *The Dhammapada*, Translated by Juan Mascaro, *Penguin Books*, England, 1973, p35.
5. Cadman D. Eternal Wisdom in an age of illusions: reflections upon a pathway. Ninth Annual Lecture, The Baha'i Chair for World Peace. Centre for International Development and Conflict Management. The University of Maryland. April 1999. [See p4 for quotes from the Buddhist text *The Dhammapada*.]
6. As ref 4 supra, pages 5.
7. Ibid page 6.

8. Ibid page 7.
9. Ref. Digha Nikaya, Division iii.26 as quoted by Cadman on page 8.
10. Rene Guenon, 'The Dark Age', The Crisis of the Modern World, *Sophia Perennis*, Fourth revised edition, 2001. First published in 1942.
11. William Penn, *Some fruits of solitude*, 1693. Quoted in Quaker Faith and Practice, 24.03.

3. A Life Affirming Approach

An Address By His Holiness Pope John Paul II

On March 20th 2004 Pope John Paul II gave an address that challenged the presumptions that underlie secular thoughts about the ethical use of hydration and nutrition in people with a vegetative state. Much that the late Pope said so eloquently is equally applicable to patients with lesser degrees of brain damage. If the Catholic view of the sanctity of life were more widely accepted the question of withholding and withdrawing sustenance from brain damaged patients would not arise. But sadly we live in an increasingly secular age, where respect for humanity is too often replaced by a brusque assessment of the level of disability and treatment withdrawal. This is a tragedy for patients, for the medical profession and for society. We owe a debt of gratitude to Catholics for shining a light in the darkness and standing firm.

Pope John Paul II was addressing participants at the International Congress on "Life-Sustaining Treatments and Vegetative State: Scientific Advances and Ethical Dilemmas" in March 2004. The conference was organized jointly by the Pontifical Academy for Life and the International Federation of Catholic Medical Associations The Pope's address was published on the Vatican web site, and was reprinted in the Catholic Medical Quarterly in May 2004. The Pope spoke as follows:

1. "I cordially greet all of you who took part in the International Congress: "Life-Sustaining Treatments and the Vegetative State: Scientific Advances and Ethical Dilemmas."

    " I wish to extend special greetings to Msgr. Elio Sgreccia, Vice President of the Pontifical Academy for Life, and to Prof. Gian Luigi Gigli, President of the International Federation of Catholic Medical Associations and selfless champion of the fundamental value of life, who has kindly expressed your shared feelings. This important Congress, organised jointly by the Pontifical Academy for Life and the International Federation of Catholic Medical Institutions, is dealing with a very significant issue: the clinical condition called the 'vegetative state.' The complex scientific, ethical, social and pastoral implications of such a condition require in-depth reflections and a fruitful inter-disciplinary dialogue…"

2. " With deep esteem and sincere hope, the Church encourages the efforts of men and women of science, who, sometimes at great sacrifice, daily dedicate their task of study and research to the improvement of the diagnostic, therapeutic,

213

prognostic and rehabilitative possibilities confronting those patients who rely completely on those who care for and assist them. The person in a vegetative state, in fact, shows no evident sign of self-awareness or of awareness of the environment, and seems unable to interact with others or to react to specific stimuli. Scientists and researchers realize that one must, first of all, arrive at a correct diagnosis, which usually requires prolonged and careful observation in specialized centres, given also the high number of diagnostic errors reported in the literature. Moreover, not a few of these persons, with appropriate treatment and rehabilitative programmes, have been able to emerge from a vegetative state. On the contrary, many others unfortunately remain prisoners of their condition even for long stretches of time and without needing technological support. In particular, the term 'permanent vegetative state' has been coined to indicate the condition of those patients whose 'vegetative state' continues for over a year. Actually, there is no different diagnosis that corresponds to such a definition, but only a conventional prognostic judgement, relative to the fact that the recovery of patients, statistically speaking, is ever more difficult as the condition of the 'vegetative state' is prolonged in time.

"However, we must neither forget nor underestimate that there are well documented cases of at least partial recovery even after many years; we can thus state that medical science, up until now, is still unable to predict with certainty who among patients with this condition will recover, and who will not.

3. "Faced with patients in similar clinical conditions, there are some who cast doubt on the persistence of the "human quality" itself, almost as if the adjective "vegetative" (whose use is now solidly established), which symbolically describes a clinical state, could or should be applied to the sick as such, actually demeaning their personal dignity. In this sense, it must be noted that this term, even when confined to the clinical context, is certainly not the most felicitous when applied to human beings.

"In opposition to such trends of thought, I feel the duty to reaffirm strongly that the intrinsic value and personal dignity of every human being do not change, no matter what the concrete circumstances of his or her life. *A man, even if seriously ill or disabled in the exercise of his highest functions, is and always will be a man, and he will never become a 'vegetable' or an animal.* Even our brothers and sisters who find themselves in the clinical condition of a 'vegetative state' retain their human dignity in all its fullness. The loving gaze of God the Father continues to fall on them, acknowledging them as his sons and daughters, especially in need of help.

4. "Medical doctors and health-care personnel, society and the Church have moral duties toward these persons from which they cannot exempt themselves without lessening the demands both of professional ethics and human and Christian solidarity. The sick person in a 'vegetative state', awaiting recovery or a natural end, still has the right to basic health care (nutrition, cleanliness, warmth, etc), and to the prevention of complications related to his confinement to bed. He also has the right to appropriate rehabilitative care and to be monitored for

clinical signs of eventual recovery.

"I should like particularly to underline how the administration of water and food, even when provided by artificial means, always represents a *natural means* of preserving life, not a *medical act*. Its use furthermore, should be considered, in principle, *ordinary* and *proportionate*, and as such morally obligatory, insofar as and until it is seen to have attained its proper finality, which in the present case consists in providing nourishment to the patient and alleviation of his suffering.

"The obligation to provide the "normal care due to the sick in such cases"[1] includes, in fact, the use of nutrition and hydration [2]. The evaluation of probabilities, founded on waning hopes for recovery when the vegetative state is prolonged beyond a year, cannot ethically justify the cessation or interruption of *minimal care* for the patient, including nutrition and hydration. Death by starvation or dehydration is, in fact, the only possible outcome as a result of their withdrawal. In this sense it ends up becoming, if done knowingly and willingly, true and proper euthanasia by omission.

" In this regard I recall what I wrote in the Encyclical Evangelium vitae, making it clear that 'by Euthanasia in the true and proper sense must be understood an action or omission which by its very nature and intention brings about death, with the purpose of eliminating all pain'; such an act is always 'a serious violation of the law of God, since it is the deliberate and morally unacceptable killing of a human person'[9]

"Besides, the moral principle is well known, according to which even the simple doubt of being in the presence of a living person already imposes the obligation of full respect and of abstaining from any act that aims at anticipating the person's death.

5. "Considerations about the 'quality of life', often actually dictated by psychological, social and economic pressures, cannot take precedence over general principles.

"First of all, no evaluation of costs can outweigh the fundamental good which we are trying to protect, that of human life. Moreover, to admit that decisions regarding a man's life can be based on the external acknowledgement of its quality, is the same as acknowledging that increasing and decreasing levels of quality of life, and therefore of human dignity, can be attributed from an external perspective of any subject, thus introducing into human relations a discriminatory and eugenic principle.

"Moreover it is not possible to rule out *a priori* that the withdrawal of nutrition and hydration as reported by authoritative studies, is the source of considerable suffering to the sick person even if we can see only the reactions at the level of the autonomic nervous system or gestures. Modern clinical neurophysiology and neuro-imaging techniques, in fact, seem to point to the lasting quality in these patients of elementary forms of communication and analysis of stimuli.

6. "However, it is not enough to reaffirm the general principle according to which the value of human life cannot be made subordinate to any judgement of its

quality expressed by others. It is necessary to promote the *taking of positive actions* as a stand against pressures to withdraw hydration and nutrition as a way to put an end to the lives of these patients.

"It is necessary, above all, *to support those families* who have had their loved ones struck down by this terrible clinical condition. They cannot be left alone with their heavy human, psychological and financial burden. Although the care for these patients is not, in general, particularly costly, society must allot sufficient resources for the care of this sort of frailty, by way of bringing about appropriate, concrete initiatives such as for example, the creation of a network of awakening centres with specialized treatment and rehabilitation programmes; financial support and home assistance for families when patients are moved back home at the end of intensive rehabilitation programmes; the establishment of facilities which can accommodate those cases in which there is no family able to deal with the problem or to provide "breaks" for those families who are at risk of psychological and moral burnout..

"Proper care for these patients and their families should, moreover, include the presence and the witness of a medical doctor and an entire team, who are asked to help the family understand that they are there as allies who are in this struggle with them. The participation of volunteers represents basic support to enable the family to break out of its isolation and to help it to realize that it is a precious and not forsaken part of the social fabric.

" In these situations, then, spiritual counselling and pastoral aid are particularly important as a help for recovering the deepest meaning of an apparently desperate condition.

7. "Distinguished Ladies and Gentlemen in conclusion I exhort you, as men and women of science responsible for the dignity of the medical profession, to guard jealously the principle according to which the true task of medicine is "to cure if possible, always to care".

"As a pledge and support of this, your authentic humanitarian mission to give comfort and support to your suffering brothers and sisters, I remind you of the words of Jesus: "Amen, I say unto you, whatever you did for these least brothers of mine, you did for me."[4]

"In this light, I invoke upon you the assistance of Him, whom a meaningful saying of the Church Fathers describes as Christus medicus and, in entrusting your work to the protection of Mary, Consoler of the sick and Comforter of the dying, I lovingly bestow on all of you a special Apostolic Blessing.

Address reprinted with permission from the Vatican

References

1. Congregation for the Doctrine of the Faith, Iura et Bona, p IV.
2. cf Pontifical Council "Cor Unum", *Dans le Cadre,*2,4,4; Pontifical Counsel for Pastoral Assistance to Health Care Workers, *Charter of Health Care Workers,* n. 120.
3. Encyclical Evangelium Vitae, n.65.
4. The Bible, St Matthew, Chapter 25, verse 40.

GOD does not act in conventional or political ways.
HE appears in unlikely places…
At the centre of the battle against evil…
In the ethics debate…
Holiness is to be found in the context of
unanswered questions.
We must be open to the possibility of God's presence,
For as Jacob discovered in Biblical times-
"Truly the Lord is in this place and I did not know it."

[Words spoken by the Venerable Dr John Holdsworth,
Archdeacon of St David's Cathedral, in a sermon given at
Trinity College, Carmarthen on July 25th 2004 and
broadcast on BBC Radio 4.]

Chapter 16

Living With Severe Neurological Disability

Comments from several sources compiled by Gillian Craig

---

1. Evidence of awareness in unconscious patients.

When Pope John Paul II spoke at the International Congress in March 2004 he was aware of the latest scientific research. More recent high technology brain scans confirm that there is significant brain activity in patients who appear to be unconscious. We must make room for hope.

Some patients with very severe brain damage have improved dramatically after years of apparent unconsciousness or minimal communication. One such was Sarah Scantlin who spent 20 years unable to communicate except by blinking her eyes in response to questions. Then she suddenly started to talk and phoned her family. While she was unable to speak or move she had listened to the TV in her room and knew all about the 9/11 disaster. Another was Donald Herbert a New York fireman who was in a near PVS state for 10 years, unable to see, speak or move. Then he suddenly spoke and asked to see his wife.[1]

A third such case, described as "The man who slept for 19 years" was Terry Wallis of Arkansas, who had an accident in 1984 involving a truck crash on a mountain road. He was in a coma, presumed to be a permanent vegetative state (PVS), but his family took him fishing and hunting, strapped in a car, as if he was normal. One day, in a nursing home, he recognised his mother and said "That's Mama". He woke from his coma thinking that his daughter was still a baby, but she was 19 years old. He was unable to walk, but thought of himself as able-bodied. He was taken to see a neurologist in New York and had a functional MRI scan of his brain. This was said to show that his language centre was normal. No one knows what "kick-started" his brain. Terry was 40 when his case was reported on TV in 2005.[2]

Advances in brain scanning techniques are stopping scientists in their tracks, for there is evidence that the brain of a patient in PVS can respond, in some respects, like that of a normal person.

In one study, published in 2002, three scientists from the Institute of Medical Psychology and Behavioural Biology at the University of Tubingen in Germany, with a scientist from the University of Padua in Italy, found evidence that patients in PVS have detectable cortical activity. A technique that measured event related brain potentials (ERPS) showed that the brain of a person in PVS can respond to human speech.[3]

In another study published in *Neuropsychological Rehabilitation*, and reported in *The Scientist* in September 2005, positron emission tomography (PET) scans showed that a patient in a PVS reacted to English sentences in the same way as a conscious subject. Functional magnetic resonance imaging (fMRI) on the same patient showed responses indicative of higher levels of speech comprehension.[4]

In another study, published in *Neurology* in February 2005, brain activity was studied by (fMRI) in two patients in a minimally conscious state. The researchers found "active cortical networks that serve language functions..." [5]

Dr Joseph Fins, chief of medical ethics at New York Presbyterian Hospital was reported as saying: "This study gave me goose bumps, because it shows...that these people are there, that they have been there all along, even though we've been treating them as if they are not." [6]

Colleen Clements, associate professor of psychology at the University of Rochester, N.Y., asked: "Has bioethics been making a terrible mistake to listen to advocates of either euthanasia or cost-cutting through patient termination?" [7]

The answer to that crucial question is almost certainly "YES!"

Sources

1. http://www.internationaltaskforce.org Update-Volume 20, Number 1. January 2006.
2. The man who slept for 19 years. Channel 4 TV. February 1st 2005. Producer Vivian McGrath.
3. Kotchoubey B, Lang S, Bostanov V, Birbaumer N. Is there a mind? Electrophysiology of unconscious patients. *News in Physiological Sciences*, 2002; Vol 17:1,p38-42.
4. Report in *The Scientist* December 9th 2005, according to www as at reference 1.
5. Schiff N.D. et al "fMRI reveals large-scale network activation in minimally conscious patients." *Neurology*, 2/05:514-523 as reported in reference 1 above.
6. *New York Times*, Feb 8th 2005, quoted in reference 1 above.
7. *Medical Post* September 20th 2005, quoted in reference 1 above.

2. Making room for hope

The following comments are taken from an article by journalist Christine Doyle, published in The Daily Telegraph of August 10th 2000. The article described the work of the Royal Hospital for Neuro-disability in Putney, London, UK.

'Karen Cusack is a familiar sight as she speeds her electronic wheelchair along the corridors of the Royal Hospital for Neuro-disability in south-west London. She pauses at one of the many intersections- which have angled mirrors to prevent collisions- on her way to "talk" to a patient who has Locked-in-Syndrome and who can only communicate by blinking. She is so enthusiastic, and visits so many patients, that at times she seems more like a member of staff than a patient with severe multiple sclerosis. Yet, four years ago, she was given 24 hours to live.

"My MS had progressed rapidly, and I had to give up my job with the Metropolitan Police. Then I had double pneumonia and, although I survived, I could not speak or move my limbs." With a dramatic turn of phrase- she is distantly related to one of the theatrical Cusacks- Karen, 34, says: "I'm not one of those people, who when they are 'dead', lie down."

She epitomises the eclipse that is the hospital's symbol. With some patients, it might seem at the outset that mental awareness or physical ability had been so "eclipsed" that progress is unimaginable. However, the Royal Hospital ethos is that even the most severely disabled patient can improve. There can be a quality of life beyond the eclipse. "With time, you might see awareness emerging," says Karen, "dimly, as through a mist."...

Many of the 300 residents are young people who have been severely brain damaged in road accidents or are victims of assault. Others have had catastrophic strokes or, like Karen, suffer severely from diseases that lead to progressive deterioration of their physical and mental abilities- such as multiple sclerosis of Huntingdon's chorea.

"If people are able to communicate or improve in any way we will help them to do so," says Dr Keith Andrews, the medical director. Some patients, for example, can make their wishes known only through a computer, which they control by blinking. For a young man being visited by Karen, this led to discovering a talent for writing poems. His "locked in" condition is similar to that of the late Jean-Dominique Bauby, who wrote about his emotions in 'The Diving Bell and the Butterfly'...

One major ethical and technical challenge for this hospital and others is how to tell if someone is irretrievably in a vegetative state; if their mind is functioning, but locked-in; or what level of awareness might be reached. One boy from the Hillsborough disaster emerged from a vegetative state after five years and can make responses, though he remains deeply brain damaged- all of which raise many questions about how to treat such patients.

Three years ago, in a widely publicised report, headed by Dr Andrews, researchers concluded that 42 per cent of patients said to be in a vegetative state were misdiagnosed. Dr Andrews, who lectures around the world on the issues raised by profound brain injury, says: "In truth, we rarely see a truly vegetative patient. Either such patients die, or there are movements that, after a year, cannot be put down to a purely reflex pattern. But we are not sure if the movements mean they are thinking. We are still struggling to learn more about this level of brain damage. Good tests are vital.

"In the misdiagnosis study, we found that 60 per cent of those who were misdiagnosed were either blind or very severely visually impaired. Yet often, when looking for signs of response, doctors emphasise the importance of seeing if a patient's eyes will follow an object consistently."

Unsurprisingly the hospital is at the forefront of research. Occupational Therapists in the Profound Brain Injury Unit have developed a special testing kit, which offers a structured window into the brain. It is called Sensory Modality Assessment Rehabilitation Technique (Smart), and is used to assess meaningful responses to sight, smell, touch, hearing and taste. The kit contains such things as feathers, bottles with different smells or tastes, "yes" and "no" cards, a buzzer and a hefty manual. This is not a one-off test, but is carried out several times a day, often for months. One patient had been assessed elsewhere and been diagnosed as being in a vegetative state. Through Smart, it was found that he could make tiny movements of his thumb, which led to him being able to select letters of the alphabet. After seven isolated years, he was able to write to his wife.

220

Such cases are prompting new ways of describing levels of brain damage. In America, a group of specialists known as the Aspen Consensus Group is drawing up guidelines to a grey area they have called the "minimally conscious state." (MCS). Dr Andrews explains: "It is beyond the vegetative state, but the patients have not reached the level where they show any evidence of thought. They might never do so, which raises questions about withdrawing tube feeding. But it could be a transition stage to becoming more mentally alert. It is rather like looking into a stream flowing into the river. We know when it is a stream, but when does the stream become a river?"

Comment from Dr Craig

The wonderful care given to brain damaged patients by Dr Andrews and his team at the Royal Hospital, shows up the relative lack of care given to many brain damaged patients, especially elderly stroke victims, in some other institutions. Surely all patients whose level of awareness is in doubt should be entitled to careful assessment of cognitive function before life-prolonging treatment is withdrawn? Sadly this is not the case at present.

We need more places of sanctuary for people with profound brain damage. Ideally given adequate resources, both human and financial, high quality care should be continued indefinitely, providing of course that it was felt that the individual concerned would wish to remain alive. Sometimes even when loving care is available, a person may find life in a disabled state a burden too great to bear. Allowance should be made for such tragic cases, allowing inappropriate treatment to be withdrawn. But sometimes, people want to live even when the odds seem stacked against them. The following case illustrates how essential it is to try to communicate with brain injury patients to ascertain how they feel about matters of life and death. For trapped inside a paralysed body, unable to speak and apparently lacking all awareness may be a "locked-in person" who desperately wants to live.

3. A car accident victim who wanted to live.

Miss X once told her family that if she was ever in a permanent vegetative state she would not want to live, but when she found herself paralysed and unable to speak she changed her mind. Thanks to skilled assessment the message that she wanted to live got through before tube feeding was withdrawn. The case shows the dangers of 'living wills' and demonstrates the need to assess a person's level of awareness and ability to communicate before making irrevocable end-of-life decisions.

The case of Miss X was reported in the journal *Brain Injury* by Professor Tom McMillan in 1996 [1], with follow up reports by McMillan and Herbert in 2000 [2] and 2004 [3]. Sarah Boseley the Health Correspondent of *The Guardian* brought the case to public attention in 2000.[4]

The following information is drawn from articles in Brain Injury. An abstract from McMillan and Herbert's paper of 2004 gives a valuable summary of the case and is reprinted with permission. Note that the word 'tetraplegic' means paralysed in all four limbs, and 'anarthric' means unable to speak at all.

Further recovery in a potential treatment withdrawal case 10 years after brain injury.

T.M.McMillan and CM Herbert.
Brain Injury, 2004, vol 18, No 9, 935-940.

Abstract. A young woman was rendered tetraplegic and anarthric as a result of a traumatic brain injury in 1993. Two years later she was considered to be in a minimally conscious state and became the subject of legal debate in the UK with regard to withdrawal of artificial feeding and hydration. Before injury she made a verbal advance directive that she would not wish to continue living if ever becoming severely disabled. Neuropsychological assessment found statistically significant evidence for sentience and expression of a will to live and the application to Court was withdrawn. Further meaningful recovery occurred between 7-10 years after injury. She now lives in the community with 24 hour care. She speaks, initiates conversation and actions, expresses clear and consistent preferences and has a spontaneous sense of humour. She uses an electric wheel chair, eats solid food and drinks through a straw. Her mood is variable and sometimes low. This case demonstrates the need for careful consideration of advanced directives and for specialist neuropsychological assessment in people with severe cognitive and communication difficulties. It supports the view that routine assessment and follow-up of people thought to be in minimally conscious states is important. In addition, it shows that recovery with reduction in disability and significant implications for quality of life can continue for at least 10 years after extremely severe traumatic brain injury.

Additional information drawn from McMillan's papers in *Brain Injury*

As a result of the car accident the patient sustained a fracture in the right fronto-parietal region of the skull (ie the front and side of the skull on the right) with an associated blood clot that pressed on the brain. She suffered a cardiac arrest and required urgent decompression of the brain. Next day a CT scan showed evidence of severe raised intracranial pressure so a large volume of brain had to be removed as a life-saving measure. She was in coma for 19 days. At five months she was thought to be depressed and had a trial of anti-depressant medication to no avail. At 10 months a decision was made to withhold antibiotics in event of an infection. She was described as aware but "only a little beyond a vegetative state." She needed a feeding tube initially.

Eighteen months or so post injury all medical experts gave an opinion that further substantial recovery was not likely. The patient was unable to speak or write and communication by other strategies was thought to be unreliable with the possible exception of communication by pressing a buzzer to say "No" or "Yes." Several medical experts gave the view that, because her level of responding was little beyond a vegetative state, her quality of life must be low, and termination of voluntary feeding should proceed. However Professor Tom McMillan was asked for his opinion. Using a three step test he established that the patient wanted to live. The Health Authority withdrew its application to remove the feeding tube three days before the court hearing

When reporting this case in *Brain Injury* in 1996 McMillan suggested four principles for the future.

❑ "Where there is any possibility of a locked in state and the issue of cognitive ability or will to live is in doubt, an expert and independent neuropsychological assessment is essential and should be mandatory."
❑ McMillan advised about various safeguards for such testing.
❑ "If there is any suspicion that the patient is responding randomly because of any acute or reversible medical complication, medication or fatigue, then no opinion should be given."
❑ "It is essential that assessment should take into account the often invaluable experience of occupational, speech and language therapists in terms of use and positioning of the response device and also in positioning the patient. The patient should ideally be tested over several days and preferably several days each week over several weeks…."

Over the next ten years with good rehabilitation and care the patient continued to improve as summarized below.

Evidence of steady improvement in the patient's condition over 10 years

3 years post injury Ms X was transferred to a nursing home.

4 to 6 years post injury she was feeding orally and talking. Neuropsychological assessment showed she could learn new information and retained some for at least 12 months. She could move her right arm and right forefinger but still had no functional use of any limb. She could eat and drink but could not maintain her weight by this method so received supplementary nourishment via a gastrostomy tube. She was determined to communicate by talking rather than through communication aids.

5 years post injury she was being fed with a soft diet by a carer and no longer needed a PEG. She could stand and transfer with the help of one and was having weekly physiotherapy. There was evidence of improved mental function on testing.

6 years post injury. She could tolerate travel and was being taken shopping. She enjoyed aerobics with a group of people with disabilities. She enjoyed music, had a mischievous sense of humour and was champion of the Trivial Pursuits League in her nursing home. There was hope of a long-term placement in an adapted home, living with her mother and additional care staff but this was dependent on the outcome of a civil compensation case.

On 10 year follow up she had moved to a modified bungalow and was able to walk 16 metres with 2 helpers. She could brush her hair using her right arm, was independent in an electric wheel chair and was able to feed herself with a spoon and finger foods.

McMillan and Herbert concluded:

"The view of others is subjective and open to bias, especially in the arena of treatment withdrawal, which is often emotionally charged. Quality of life is essentially subjective and strongly influenced by personal, cultural, religious and societal views. Some have suggested that quality of life will be low in people who are minimally conscious, particularly if they are depressed, in pain, highly dependent and have insight, but arguably these matters have to be considered in law on a case-by-case basis if withdrawal of treatment is being considered, as demonstrated by the case (we have) reported." [3]

(Source. McMillan & Herbert. Brain Injury 2004, 18, p935 and 936.)

References

1. McMillan TM. Neuropsychological assessment after severe head injury in a case of life or death. *Brain Injury* 1996; **11**: 481-490.
2. McMillan TM and Herbert CM. Neuropsychological assessment of a potential 'euthanasia' case: a 5 year follow-up. *Brain Injury*, 2000;**14**:197-203.
3. Further recovery in a potential treatment withdrawal case 10 years after brain injury. T.M.McMillan and CM Herbert. *Brain Injury*, 2004, vol.**18**, No 9, 935-940.
4. Boseley S. Car accident 'shows risk of living wills'. *The Guardian* February 17th 2000.

All quotes from *Brain Injury* are used with permission.© Taylor and Francis Ltd. The web site for Brain Injury is http://www.tandf.co.uk

4. Coming home to die. Heartbreak battle over for coma girl's mother

Miss D was a car accident victim. After years of struggle following brain injury Miss D became depressed and wanted to die, then lapsed into a coma after a fit. Her poignant story was told by journalist Nick Hopkins in the Daily Mail of March 24th 1997 as follows:

'Her parents had prayed so long for her home coming, but not one like this.

When their daughter is released from hospital today there will be no excitement at seeing her in familiar surroundings, no talk of recovery. The 29 year old coma victim will return home with all the dignity that can be mustered. Her sorrowing parents will see her fade away for lack of food and water until her heart is too weak to carry on.

Last Friday the couple won the right to die for their daughter, who for legal reasons can be referred to only as Ms D. Sir Stephen Brown, President of the High Court Division, ruled she should be released from a 'living death'.

Since then pro-life campaigners have condemned the family. The anti-euthanasia group Alert called the ruling 'shocking and horrifying.'

But for the student's parents, it was a decision taken out of love after doctors confirmed there was no prospect of her ever recovering.

All their lives they had adored her, fought for her, wept for her, the eldest of their three children and their only girl.

The first testing time came when as a young child she developed hydrocephalus-water on the brain- a potentially lethal condition and one that can leave victims brain-damaged.

But with considerable care, she was nursed back to full health with no signs of permanent injury.

Miss D grew into a talented all-rounder, sailing through her O- and A-levels and excelling at sport, including tennis and skiing. She was also beautiful. 'She had lovely dark hair,' said a neighbour. I would think how striking and athletic she was.'

Her 53-year old parents....watched with pride as Miss D went to university and talked about training as a teacher. But in her second year at college she had the first of two appalling misfortunes which were to ruin the rest of her life.

A car crash put her in intensive care for weeks and in hospital for six months. She went home partially paralysed and confined to a wheel chair. Her speech and memory were both impaired. The medical prognosis was gloomy. She would never fully recover, said doctors. But Miss D's mother had no intention of giving up. 'She devoted herself entirely to her daughter's welfare,' said a friend. 'She was determined to do everything she could.'

The family's four-bedroom detached house was transformed to accommodate the invalid, a swimming pool was built so that she could exercise and a live-in carer joined the household.

The family included Miss D in everything they could- outings, holidays, trips to friends- hoping contact with people could help her. 'It took years, but slowly she improved,' said a friend. 'Her mother's energy was extraordinary.' But as Miss D's awareness increased, she became depressed and talked of suicide. In one of the most poignant moments of the court hearing, her mother passed the judge a note in which her daughter had written; 'Thank you once again for everything. I do say the biggest thank-you that I have ever said before... so please let me go.' In August 1995, Miss D was out of her wheelchair and walking. But three weeks later she had a seizure and fell into a coma. Doctors warned she might never recover.

Again her mother refused to accept defeat. 'Every morning she would go to hospital and sit at the bedside, holding her girl's hand and talking to her just hoping something would register,' said the friend. 'She has been like an angel looking after her all these years, but in the end the time came to let her go.'

Yesterday Professor David Chadwick, a neurologist who looked after Miss D, said the family went through 'a tremendous soul-searching before deciding to ask the court that she be allowed to die. Miss D cannot feel anything. If she could there would have been no question of the court granting this application. What is inhumane is that her mother will have to watch her daughter slowly fade away. After all the mother has done, it isn't fair that she must suffer this too.'

Copyright the Daily Mail 1997.Used with permission.

Comment from Dr Craig

This case raises many important points. Every commentator will have their own view on the rights and wrongs of the court decision. For my part one of the most telling features was the fact that as awareness increased in the years after the initial car accident Miss D became depressed and talked of suicide. She pulled through to the point where she was out of her wheelchair and walking, but then had a seizure and fell into a coma. What would she have wanted had she been able to communicate? My feeling is that the parents and the judge made the right decision. To talk of best interests in this case is meaningless, merely a verbal formality, a "stamp" used by officialdom to bring deliberations to an end. Miss D's best interests would have been best served by complete recovery, but that sadly, was not a realistic prospect in this world. Her poignant note, which was to all intents and purposes an advance directive, said it all. She did not want to be treated. Her wish was granted. May her soul rest in peace.

"I am thirsty". An article by Cardinal Thomas Winning.

The late Cardinal Thomas Winning, leader of Scotland's Roman Catholics at the time, found the case of Miss D deeply disturbing and warned that the nation was sleepwalking towards catastrophy. The following comments are taken from a forthright article the Cardinal wrote in the Daily Mail of March 27th 1997. His dire warnings about the consequences for the seriously sick have proved prophetic.

'Tomorrow, Good Friday, when we hear those words of Jesus on the Cross, from St John's account of the Passion, my thoughts will turn to the woman known to us only as 'Miss D'...the High Court judgement which determined that she should die signposts an issue which should not be shirked.

Her heartbreaking condition led Sir Stephen Brown, President of the High Court Family Division, to pass the death sentence by declaring; 'I am driven to the conclusion that it is in the patient's best interests to withdraw the artificial feeding that is keeping her body alive.'

Who says we are not sliding down the slippery slope leading to the elimination of anyone deemed to be in a state of 'living death'? What will be the long term consequences for all of us by making that journey?

Already, as far as the courts are concerned, people in a so-called persistent vegetative state (PVS) may be eliminated- even though many specialists in neurology and neuropathology admit that not a great deal is known about the condition.

Yesterday's news that Andrew Devine- the Hillsborough survivor cared for by his parents since 1989- is recovering from PVS should surely provoke a rethink of what we are tolerating in silence.

Using disputed medical knowledge as a basis for establishing ethical criteria is bad enough; what is infinitely worse is the relentless ongoing stretching of the culture of death typified by last week's court case. For, and this is what is particularly alarming, everyone involved agrees that Miss D is clearly not a PVS patient. She responds to stimuli, reacts to threatening gestures and can follow objects moved before her eyes.

Without doubt, her family is deeply anguished as they watch her pitiable condition. Nobody with an ounce of compassion can feel anything but sadness for them. Her death will bring them a measure of relief.

Which brings us to a key question about current attitudes to the seriously sick: should the trauma experienced by their relatives determine that they should be put down?

And if this principle is accepted, where does it leave senile dementia sufferers, or people afflicted with terminal cancer whose worsening condition must also be traumatic for their watching families? Why allow them to linger when a final, immediate solution is available quickly, quietly and clinically?

Miss D is to be denied food and water to bring about her death. Can it be right to regard basic nourishment as an extraordinary medical treatment, especially in an age when tube-feeding is commonplace in every hospital?

Indeed, if it is right to starve a person to death by a slow process of dehydration- a strategy that can take up to 14 days- how can it be right to prolong the watching family's agony for a second longer than is necessary when a single lethal injection could instantly bring them the relief that they seek?

This is the awful logic of court and medical judgements which are largely influenced by the desires of third parties and which are utterly devoid of objective norms or principles. It is a logic which could, eventually, overtake us.

There is another frightening aspect to the slippery slope of euthanasia- and we are sleep walking towards it more speedily than we might imagine. Death, especially when hastened, lightens the financial burden of care carried by the NHS- a factor that should not be lightly dismissed as scaremongering when the financial costs of treating the incurably ill and caring for the senile are growing concerns.

Indeed, are we that far from asking why the family, or even the patient, should have a decisive say when there are massive financial implications for the state?

The danger of moving from a so-called right-to-die mentality, which is already being assiduously promoted, to a duty-to-die attitude, is a real one.

To see how quickly this can infect the moral fibre, just look at the Dutch experience. It was, after all, only in 1973 that the first voluntary euthanasia societies were formed in Holland. Now the Dutch euthanasia toll runs to thousands a year…

Britain's history of legalised abortion is also an instructive warning that hard cases make for bad laws- to the point of opening flood gates which lead to social and moral catastrophy.

Just over 30 years ago, emotive instances of misery experienced by pregnant women were cited as justifications for legalising the killing of the youngest among us. Subsequently, the siren voices shifted neatly to defending a 'woman's right to choose' to kill.

Consequently we have witnessed almost four and a half million abortions, overwhelmingly on social grounds, and a grotesque quality control targeting of the handicapped.

Today the pain of families of those said to be afflicted by PVS is being highlighted. However deep one's sympathy for them, the danger on the horizon is that we may have to come to terms with the social reasons for killing the sick…

There is more to the recent spate of court decisions than meets the eye. A debate is needed, and it needs to take place in the political arena, too, since- sooner or later- some politician will again grasp the nettle and push the agenda in a direction which will have us trembling at the prospect of growing old or falling sick.'

Copyright the Daily Mail 1997.Quoted with permission.

5. Experience of gastrostomy feeding over a period of 12 years. The case of James Rogers.

This article by Ann Rogers, describes how she cared for her son James for 12 years.

On 1 January 1987 my only son James was travelling to Daventry as the front seat passenger in a car driven by one of his friends. In an overtaking manoeuvre, the driver lost control causing a head-on collision. James was severely injured and was rendered unconscious on impact. He was taken by ambulance to Northampton General Hospital (NGH) where, on arrival, he was intubated. It then became necessary to rescuscitate him three times. In addition to a severe head injury he had sustained life-threatening injuries. After a few hours he was transferred to the neurosurgical unit at the Radcliffe Infirmary at Oxford, where a CAT scan was carried out. A diffuse cerebral injury was revealed by the scan and we were subsequently informed that there was no treatment available that would improve this condition. A pneumothorax was diagnosed at Oxford and this was treated. After four days, he was transferred back to Northampton General Hospital. Up to this time he had been fed intravenously.

Once James condition had been stabilised in the intensive care unit he was transferred to a trauma ward where initially the intravenous feeding continued. Later, when he became able to digest food, a nasogastric tube was inserted. Almost from the outset, I could see that this was going to prove unsatisfactory. Despite his condition, James managed to remove the tube during the night and it had been found lying on his bed in the morning. My nursing experience made me aware that infections and ulceration of the nose and pharynx can result from prolonged use of nasogastric feeding. Furthermore the constant presence of a tube in this position is both uncomfortable and undignified. I therefore decided that that the nasogastric tube must be removed and a better way found to provide nutrition for my son. As I was attending the hospital every day to assist in James' care, I set myself the task of feeding him orally. I found this procedure very time consuming and it caused a great deal of coughing as James' reflexes were reduced and the hospital food not always of ideal texture. Despite this it was clear that he enjoyed the variety of flavour and the satisfaction of taking food more or less by the normal process. I continued to persevere for the full term that James remained at NGH.

In the December of that year, we obtained a place for James at the newly opened brain injury treatment centre at the Royal Hospital and Home, Putney. I rented a flat near to the hospital so that I could continue to play a significant part in James' nursing care. On the subject of feeding I had hoped that Putney would support me in my efforts to feed James orally. However it soon became clear that this was not to be the case. After making several observations of my feeding procedures, the nutritionist at Putney warned that in her opinion there was a strong risk of aspiration, because of the way that James tended to choke on his food. Although I had fed him orally for ten months, without any sign of chest infection, I was persuaded to accept their opinion that a change to gastrostomy feeding would be in his best interests.

I was introduced to the leading surgeon in this field and remember the feeling of elation that the insertion of the necessary feeding tube could be carried out in such a simple way. I was also excited to think that this less time consuming and convenient feeding method would allow more time for therapeutic work which we were still hopeful would improve James' condition. The tube end was neat and discreet, tucked inconspicuously under his T-shirt. He immediately started to gain weight and his life became more pleasant and ordered. A regime of night time feeding was started, giving greater flexibility to the range of activities that could now include visits to the garden and to the pool for hydrotherapy. It also provided a simpler method of administering the anti convulsive drugs that he needed for the epilepsy resulting from his injury. The gas that builds up in the gastric system could be easily released by venting the tube. It was quite easy to keep the site of the stoma clean by normal hygiene methods during bath time. It was pleasing to be able to give a little food, of suitable texture, by mouth to allow James to continue to experience the pleasure of taste. This would not have been possible if the naso-gastric tube had remained. The nursing staff were relieved of the time consuming work involved in oral feeding. We were able to adjust his fluid intake to correspond with the warmer weather and to variations in urine concentration. During his stay at Putney the tube needed exchanging for a new one and once again this procedure proved to be perfectly straightforward and without problems.

From February 1991 we cared for James in accommodation at our home, built in such a way as to provide for his severely disabled condition. With a team of nurses and carers, we continued with the methods of managing his condition that we had learnt at Putney, making improvements as we became more confident. We also continued with PEG feeding and the daily maintenance routine proved to be quite straightforward and well within the capabilities of a reliable carer.

We established excellent relations with the gastric clinic at NGH and on the occasions that a tube needed replacing, this was done smoothly and on a day visit basis. As further development in tube design came about, it became possible for us to replace the tube at home, thus removing the necessity for a journey into hospital and relieving the clinic and the surgeon of this work.

James survived 13 years after the accident that changed his life so dramatically. Despite the fact that some neurologists had diagnosed him as being in PVS, others saw, as we did, that there was much more to this part of his life than mere vegetative existence. The members of his care staff grew very fond of him and surprisingly they were able to recognise the sort of friendly compassionate person that typified the seventeen years of his pre-accident life. During the thirteen years in which my husband and I helped our son through his difficulties, we naturally made many sacrifices, socially and recreationally and to the detriment of my husband's business. Despite this, we are absolutely sure of the abiding worthwhile nature of the time we spent. In the five years that we have now lived without James we have not faltered once in this conviction.

When it was finally decided after all the processes of law had operated that the administration of food and fluid should be regarded as 'treatment' and could therefore be denied to patients in certain circumstances, I became very concerned. My fears centred on the thought that if James should live long enough to survive my husband and myself, his life might be terminated in a very different fashion. Instead of leaving us, as he did in March 2000, peacefully and comfortably in his own home surrounded by the loving care of his family and carers, he could have been subjected to the cruel and undignified process of death by starvation and dehydration.

© *Ann Rogers 2005.*

6. Lucid but paralysed. The case of Miss B who wanted to die

This article is based on reports by Joshua Rozenberg, Legal Editor of The Daily Telegraph and Celia Hall their Medical Editor. All quotes from these articles are used with permission and are copyright. © *Telegraph Group Limited, March 2002.*

A High Court ruling in March 2002 enabled a lucid but paralysed woman, known only as Miss B, to insist that her life-supporting respirator be turned off, against the wishes of the doctors caring for her. The case came to court because the doctors were concerned to establish that the patient was competent to make such an irrevocable decision. The Judge, Dame Elizabeth Butler Sloss, President of the High Court Family Division, ruled that she was competent. The ruling served to underline the well established legal principle that people with the necessary mental capacity can choose to accept or refuse medical treatment. Dame Butler-Sloss stated "A mentally competent patient has an absolute right to refuse to consent to medical treatment for any reason, rational or irrational, or for no reason at all, even where that decision may lead to his or her death." That right would prevail over the natural desire of doctors to keep a patient alive, she said. The law was clear, but its application was "infinitely more difficult to achieve."[1]

The patient in this case was a 43 year old unmarried social worker, who had risen to be head of a hospital social work department. In August 1999 she developed symptoms due to a ruptured blood vessel in her neck. Doctors warned that a malformation of blood vessels in her spinal column could result in serious disability. She therefore wrote out a living will expressly stating her wish not to receive treatment if she was left suffering from a life-threatening condition, unconscious, or with permanent mental impairment. Initially her condition improved and she was able to return to work. However in February 2001 further bleeding left her with complete paralysis from the neck downwards, and dependent on a respirator in an intensive care unit, where she remained for over a year.[2]

The doctors respected her and liked her, and felt unable to comply with her request that the respirator be turned off. An anaesthetist explained to the court that the patient had been offered a chance to leave the hospital and go to a rehabilitation unit but had refused. "I don't think an intensive care environment is the place for a patient to make a decision such as this…" said the anaesthetist- "The patient is just asking us to kill her and that is something we would not wish to do." The consultant in charge of the case tried desperately to find ways to make the patient happy and give her some enthusiasm to go on living.[3]

Robert Francis QC, Counsel for the NHS Trust drew attention to the dedication and skill of the medical team caring for Miss B and said "These doctors are working at the very frontier of life with people at risk of death, and they are struggling to keep them alive." He noted that there was "conflict between their ethical obligations to do their best to save a patient's life…and a patient's wish that life-saving treatment should be stopped." He explained that the patient was suffering from the most severe degree of physical disability imaginable. It was analogous to extreme pain or phobia that could render decision making difficult. She had been in an intensive care unit for a year among patients who were terminally ill, which he suggested "must make it near impossible to believe that life could be different in terms of quality elsewhere."[4]

Mr Francis suggested that the patient's relationship with, and attitude towards, doctors and other carers- and her anger and intense feelings about the way she was being treated- could render her unable to balance matters in her mind. Dame Elizabeth Butler- Sloss found that argument unattractive and took the view that the patient's anger and its effect on her relationships could not be treated as a loss of capacity. The Judge understood the woman's frustration at not having her request to die respected and accused the doctors of being "very paternalistic".[2]

One psychiatrist took the view that Miss B was not suffering from depression or any psychiatric illness. She was "undoubtedly a very accomplished and mature individual" he said. He had been "impressed" with her and "struck with the poignancy and disparity between the liveliness I saw in her and her wish to die." He thought that the fact that she was in an intensive care unit might influence her decision. The woman's "difficult" childhood and adolescence and her attitude to some of her carers might also be a factor. For example when the patient experienced pain she closed her eyes and repeated the words "rag doll, rag doll", exactly as she had acted when she suffered what he described as "severe adversity" at the hands of an adult during her childhood. A second psychiatrist assessed her mental state as being "on the extreme of considerable competence." There had been some confusion between her values and those of others attending her. "To put it perhaps much too simplistically, she values the prospect of remaining on the ventilator and the disabilities associated with it as being worse than being dead."[5]

After taking oral evidence at the patient's bedside, and from the doctors treating her, Dame Elizabeth returned to her court in central London. Proceedings at the bedside were relayed to the court by closed circuit television, and subsequent hearings in court were relayed to the bedside to enable Miss B to follow proceedings. The initial hearings lasted three days after which Dame Elizabeth reserved judgment for several weeks, explaining that it was a "particularly difficult case."[2]

The judgment

In her judgment on March 22nd 2002, Dame Elizabeth Butler-Sloss found herself "entirely satisfied" that the patient was competent to ask for an end to her ventilation. She ruled that any hospital caring for her was allowed to administer "appropriate drug treatment- including pain relieving drugs- and palliative care to ease her suffering and permit her life to end peacefully and with dignity." The judge stated that "unless the gravity of the illness has affected the patient's capacity, a seriously disabled patient has the same rights as a fit person to respect for patient autonomy." She added "There is a serious danger, exemplified by this case, of a benevolent paternalism which does not embrace recognition of patient autonomy."

Dame Elizabeth Butler-Sloss criticised the unnamed hospital for allowing the case to drift, and marked the finding that it had treated its patient unlawfully by ordering it to pay her a nominal £100 damages for unlawful trespass. It was also ordered to pay costs for both sides, estimated at over £100,000.[1] The hospital trust expressed regret for "any distress unintentionally caused" to its patient and said it would not appeal against the ruling.

Dame Elizabeth said of Miss B "She is clearly a splendid person and it is tragic that someone of her ability has been struck down so cruelly. I hope she will forgive me for saying, diffidently, that if she did reconsider her decision, she would have a lot to offer the community at large." The woman's identity was protected by a court order, but the judge said that she was born in Jamaica and had lived in Britain since the age of eight. She had an unhappy childhood but overcame many difficulties to achieve a social science degree, followed by a master's degree in public policy and administration.[6]

Discussion

Commenting on the judgment Dr Andrew Cohen spokesman for the Intensive Care Society, was reported as saying "Our aims and objectives are to care for patients, to improve the duration and quality of life if possible, and if not, to care for them in death. Doctors are human beings as well. The dividing line between assisting suicide and withdrawing a treatment which will result in a patient dying is one that a lot of people will find difficult to come to terms with." [7]

It would be inappropriate to speculate in any detail on the reasons why Miss B was so determined to die, but many complex factors could have influenced her attitude to her disability, and her relationship with those who were trying to help her. Her physical weakness and dependence on others may have revived painful memories of the "severe adversity" that she experienced in childhood. Perhaps too little was made of this point that the first psychiatrist alluded to. Would psychotherapy have helped her? We will never know. Nor are we told what social support Miss B had at home as an unmarried professional. A trouble shared is a trouble halved, but a trouble endured in isolation can be overwhelming.

As a senior hospital social worker the patient was well aware of her rights, and must have been used to making decisions about other people's lives. This may have added to her anger and frustration when her request to be allowed to die was not heeded. The fact that she was Jamaican and her carers white could have added to the situation of conflict in her mind. The doctors caring for her were concerned that her distressing circumstances might have influenced her judgement. They hoped, not unreasonably, that a change of environment with rehabilitation outside an intensive care unit would be beneficial, but the patient rejected their plans.

In his book 'Love, Medicine and Miracles' Dr Bernie Siegel talks about the healing partnership between doctor and patient, and notes that 'the ambience of the clinical environment influences the attitude of both doctor and patient.'[8] An intensive care unit is not an ideal place to find peace of mind and inner strength. Therefore the doctors caring for Miss B were right to try to persuade her to spend time in a rehabilitation unit. It could also be argued that they were right to drag their feet about turning off the respirator, for ample time should be allowed for reflection before irrevocable life or death decisions are taken.

Moreover, Siegel states that- 'Among patients with spinal-cord injuries, those who express strong grief and anger make more progress in rehabilitation than those with a more stoical attitude'[9]. Thus had Miss B agreed to try a rehabilitation unit she might have responded and found life worth while.

It is not unusual for patients to wish themselves dead in the immediate aftermath of some devastating illness, but most come to terms with their situation in time with the loving support of family and friends. Miss B was unusual in her determination to have her life ended. She had decided before her devastating bleed, that she did not want to live in a disabled state, and her opinion did not change. It was indeed a very difficult case for all concerned.

This sad case will have dangerous repercussions for many desperately ill patients who value their autonomy more highly than their life. The final outcome was that Miss B was transferred to another hospital, where the staff complied with her wishes. A few weeks after the judgment the respirator was turned off at her request, and as a consequence she died.

7. Lucid and paralysed: but life can be worth living

Articles in this section describe the experience of some people who were struck down by devastating neurological disability, but came to terms with their situation and found life worth living.

The case of Christopher Reeve

Christopher Reeve used to be hail, hearty and handsome. He was well known to the public in his role as James Bond. Sadly one day his life changed. He had a riding accident, broke his neck, was paralysed from the neck down and relied on a respirator for life. His experience contrasts with that of Miss B in many ways. Like her there were times when he wanted to die, but laughter, the support of his family, and the love of his wife gave him the will to go on. Reeve made the following comments about his situation in a radio programme on disability in 1999. On the need for independence he said "Please help me, but don't patronise me- I want to make the decisions about my life." On the importance of not giving up he said "Don't just sit staring out of the window. There are breakthroughs coming that may help. Every little gift of movement helps. Just breathing on my own would be a reason for celebrating with fireworks!" (At that stage he could manage without a respirator for 15 to 90 minutes only.) Lack of solitude was a problem. Reeve found it difficult to adjust to the fact that he could no longer be alone, but this was not possible as the ventilation machine was liable to break down, and he was also subject to episodes of high blood pressure[10]. He died in 2004.

The man from Sarajevo

A young physicist living in Sarajevo was paralysed by a bullet in cross fire as he walked to University one day. He was left with very limited movement and unable to walk. Nevertheless he carried on bravely with life, within his limitations saying "I am my mind, I am not my body!" With a positive attitude like that, physical disability disappears to vanishing point.

A young American woman

Some years ago Channel 5 TV screened a documentary that featured several people with devastating neurological disability. One was a young American woman who was bed-bound, paralysed, mentally aware and dependent on a respirator. She was cared for at home by her devoted mother. Before tragedy struck she used to love to wear beautiful dresses and to go dancing. In her disabled state she imagined herself dancing again. From time to time she expressed the wish to die. On one such occasion, featured on TV her mother indicated a willingness to turn off the respirator. "Do you want me to turn it off now? " she asked. "No, not yet!" came the reply. This exchange left an indelible impression of human courage and maternal devotion in adversity. Loving care and respect for autonomy can be very costly.[11]

The story of Joni Eareckson

In July 1967, when she was seventeen, Joni Eareckson dived into Chesapeake Bay near Baltimore, USA and broke her neck sustaining a fracture dislocation between cervical vertebrae four and five. Since then she has been quadriplegic, confined to life in a wheelchair. There was a time after the accident, when she desperately wanted to kill herself such was her mental and spiritual torture. Her helplessness made her angry and despondent, but she was physically unable to commit suicide[12]. At one stage some months after her accident her bitterness was 'a raging torrent that could not be ignored.' She was forced to make a decision. Either she could allow herself to continue 'wallowing in anger and bitterness' or she could abandon this course and hand the situation over completely to God. There was no middle way, so Joni (pronounced Johnny) chose to leave matters in the hands of God [13]. Nevertheless peace of mind was hard to achieve in the early years following injury. Time was needed to mourn her loss and gather courage to face the future.

The broken neck had caused spinal cord damage so that there was no movement in muscles supplied by nerves below the level of injury. Joni was able to move her shoulders and had some movement in a biceps muscle, but no control of her hands, lower arms, trunk or legs. She was also dependent on a catheter. However she could smile, read a book and talk, and learnt to draw really well holding a pencil between her teeth. Her vision and hearing were normal and her intellect was unimpaired. She could also breath without a respirator, so her situation was not so dire as that of Miss B or Christopher Reeve. Like them she was completely dependent on carers, who washed her, dressed her, moved and lifted her, and supported her in every possible way. It was a far cry from her carefree life before the accident.

On her discharge home after two years in hospital Joni was deeply depressed, and seemed to have nothing to look forward to in life. Salvation came in the form of Steve Estes, a tall, lanky, sixteen-year-old boy with faith, energy and spiritual maturity far beyond his years. He 'radiated confidence, poise and authority (and) spoke convincingly of the Lord and the simple, quiet strength that faith in Christ brings to life...' wrote Joni[14]. Steve lifted her spirits and enabled her to come to terms with the situation through faith in God. Joni learnt to view her suffering as an opportunity and used her wheelchair 'as a platform to display (God's) sustaining grace' in countless speaking engagements[15]. Eventually she came to see her accident as a blessing saying- "It took a broken neck to back me into a corner and get me thinking seriously about the lordship of Christ" [16]. She went so far as to say that her paralysis had "drawn me close to God and given a spiritual healing which I would not trade for a hundred active years on my feet..."[17]. Her fears that the accident would ruin her chances of marriage proved groundless, for in the course of time, in the 1980's, she married and her name is now Joni Eareckson-Tarda.

Joni became an inspiration to countless people, and was greatly helped herself by the work of C.S.Lewis 'The Problem of Pain'[18] and a book by Packer 'Knowing God'[19].

Joni used a quotation from C.S.Lewis to explain the situation- "God whispers to us in our pleasures, speaks in our consciences, but shouts in our pains: it is His megaphone to rouse a deaf world."[18]

8. Living with motor neurone disease

People view the prospect of suffering from motor neurone disease with particular dread. From time to time individuals, backed by pressure groups such as the Voluntary Euthanasia Society, press for a change in the law to permit assisted suicide. Such cases receive intense media coverage, whereas individuals who endure with patient courage often go unnoticed.

Motor neurone disease is a condition of unknown aetiology that causes progressive damage to the nerves that transmit impulses from the brain to muscles. There are two types of motor neurone anatomically- upper and lower. The upper set connect the brain to cells in the spinal cord, called anterior horn cells. The lower neurones connect anterior horn cells to muscle fibres. Damage to the motor neurones causes muscles to become weak and wasted: they may also be stiff and painful. In the course of time most voluntary muscle function may be affected so that the patient will lose the ability to move, speak, swallow and breath, but intellectual activity, vision and hearing remain unaffected. The median length of time from diagnosis to death is said to be 2.5 years, but the range is very wide, and some patients live more than a decade[20].

Many problems can be overcome for a while and most symptoms can be relieved with skilled care. Individuals can be offered a gastrostomy tube for feeding purposes when the need arises, and non-invasive ventilatory support is sometimes considered. Electronic voice synthesisers can be helpful to enhance communication when the voice gets weak. General support and advice is available from the Motor Neurone Disease Society in the UK.[21]. With the support of friends and family, and skilled medical and nursing care the final years of life need not be too distressing, and most patients die peacefully in their sleep. However all too often fear can dominate life. Sadly, the prospect of death from suffocation or choking, or a life of prolonged dependency can drive some people to thoughts of suicide.

The case of Diane Pretty

The last two years of Diane Pretty's life were dominated by fear to such an extent that she tried to obtain exemption from prosecution for her husband, should he assist her to commit suicide. Her request was refused by the British Courts, so with the backing of the Voluntary Euthanasia Society she took her case to the European Court of Human Rights in Strasburg where her case was also rejected. Lawyers acting for Mrs Pretty tried to stand the Human Right's Law on it's head, claiming that the right to life also implied a right to die, but their arguments were rejected by judges in Strasburg. The European judges ruled that "To seek to build into the law an exemption for those judged to be incapable of committing suicide would seriously undermine the protection of life, which the 1961 Suicide Act was intended to safeguard, and (would) greatly increase the risk of abuse."[22]

The case received wide coverage in the media, attracted considerable public sympathy and opened up the euthanasia debate yet again. Senior Anglican clergy in the UK supported the judgment. A statement to the Voluntary Euthanasia Society made on behalf of the Archbishop of Canterbury, said "To cut across the journey towards death with the violent and intrusive act of killing at what may, for all the onlooker knows, be the most inappropriate time, would be to commit an act of folly and arrogance."[23]

The European Court judgment in the Pretty case was announced on April 29th 2002. Ironically this was also the day on which the death of Miss B was announced, drawing inevitable comparisons between the two cases. It was noted that in Miss B's case doctors were forced to stop artificial respiration at her request, with the result that she died, whereas in the case of Diane Pretty her husband was not allowed to actively assist her to commit suicide. The two cases highlighted the somewhat tenuous but important legal distinction between lawfully withholding life-prolonging medical treatment and unlawfully causing intentional death by a deliberate action. Few people appreciated that Mrs Pretty could, at any time, have asked that her feeding tube be removed, or that food and fluid administration by this means be stopped- but she chose not to die in this way.

Suicide is not a crime in Britain, but it is unlawful to assist a person to commit suicide, such an action being punishable by up to 14 years in jail at present. After the verdict Mrs Pretty persisted in the view that the law had taken her rights away, but her husband admitted that he was pleased in one respect "because it means I will have my wife with me for a little bit longer." A few days after the judgment Mrs Pretty was admitted to a hospice for terminal care. She died there peacefully on May 11th 2002, at the age of 43, and was honoured to have an obituary in *The Times*.

The case of Pamela Vack

Pamela Vack is a lady who is thought to have atypical motor neurone disease. Her case is a complicated one and it has taken doctors in various teaching hospitals several years to arrive at this diagnosis. The clinical picture was complicated by cervical spondylosis and Meniere's disease, and at one stage a diagnosis of multiple sclerosis was entertained. Much to Pam's chagrin, her joy and strength of faith in God through all her troubles was misinterpreted as 'euphoria'. Specialised tests of muscle function were beginning to show problems at an early stage, and protein levels were said to be raised in spinal fluid, indicating organic pathology, but with the passage of time these tests seemed to be overlooked. As happens so often when the physical diagnosis is uncertain, psychological explanations for her disability were mooted, but Pam refused to accept such suggestions. Her disability has been slowly progressive over the course of some 15 years. She is now said to have considerable muscle wasting with generalised sensory and motor neuropathy, and upper motor neurone signs, especially in the legs. These days Pam uses a wheel chair although she can walk a short distance with two sticks. She copes courageously with the support of her husband, and is said to emanate peace and calmness.[24] She paints in oils and watercolours, visits her local Motor Neurone Disease Day Centre for physiotherapy, and encourages other patients by her example.

Pam has written a book about her experience, which was published in 2001[25]. The book 'Facing the Lion' describes how the stalking lion of long term disability can, only too easily, breed hopelessness and despair and threatens to tear faith to shreds. At times during her illness Pam felt utterly isolated and estranged from her doctors, and sought help from alternative sources. Frustration mounted as doctors persisted in their attempts to give her troubles a psychological label, which she resisted. This experience will no doubt be familiar to many patients! It was a relief when various tests seemed to confirm the physical diagnosis that she had long suspected. Pam is now under the care of skilled and experienced doctors who have her trust.

In coping with her illness Pam has learnt the importance of laughter, and the fellowship of loving supportive friends and family. She has found a creative outlet in art and has had the satisfaction of selling paintings through commercial outlets. Her religious faith has been a source of great strength and inward peace. She has learnt to let go, and to let God carry the burden for her. She has also learnt to redirect negative thoughts into more positive channels. Learning to receive help, rather than to give it, has not been easy. Taking to a wheelchair was a difficult decision, for she dreaded appearing weak and tried to keep up a brave face. With great honesty, towards the end of her book, Pam admits that she has shed tears of mourning for her lost strength, and has fears for the future. She now needs help and assistance and dreads the possibility of losing the ability to communicate. Already her voice is noticeably weak, and she can no longer sing. The road has been hard, the vale of despond deep, the mountains are often steep to climb, yet Pam goes on with quiet courage and faith in God.

* * *

Living with disability: some helpful advice

- ❏ Seek fellowship, laughter and the love of friends.
- ❏ Cultivate inner strength.
- ❏ Find creative outlets, e.g. writing/painting/music/poetry.
- ❏ Concentrate on what you can do, not what you can't.
- ❏ Take one day at a time.
- ❏ Don't worry about the future but make reasonable contingency plans.
- ❏ Don't make major decisions when depressed.
- ❏ Be thoughtful for carers.
- ❏ Be gentle with yourself.
- ❏ Seek professional help from people you can trust.
- ❏ Make room for hope.

People like Pamela Vack and Joni Eareckson and countless other unsung heroes, have shown by their quiet courage that neurological disability need not be an unmitigated disaster. The human spirit can triumph over adversity.

Joni was inspired by a poem written by a French noblewoman Madame Guyon who was imprisoned in 1688. Remember when physical disability seems intolerable, and your room like a prison, that your soul is free! Roam in the imagination. Make room for hope!

> My cage confines me round;
> Abroad I cannot fly;
> But though my wing is closely bound,
> My heart's at liberty;
> My prison walls cannot control
> The flight, the freedom of my soul.
> *Madame Guyon.*[26]

References

1. Rozenberg J, Woman mentally fit to choose death. *The Daily Telegraph* March 23rd 2002 p9 cols, 1-8.
2. Hall C. 'We can't pull the plug on a conscious woman we have known for a year.' *The Daily Telegraph* March 7th 2002 p4, cols 1-7
3. Horsnell M, Lister S. Right to die case judge attacks medical conceit. *The Times* March 9th 2002 p8, cols 1-3.
4. Rozenburg J. 'Right to die' woman angry at lack of choice. *The Daily Telegraph* March 8th 2002 p7, cols 1-4.
5. Rozenberg J. 'Right to die' woman must wait for a ruling. *The Daily Telegraph* March 9th 2002 p12, cols 1-3.
6. Rozenberg J. Paralysed woman has the right to die, judge rules. *The Daily Telegraph* March 23rd 2002 p1, cols 1-3.
7. Derbyshire D. Miss B's plea clashed with principle of care that guides doctors. *The Daily Telegraph* March 23rd 2002 p9, cols 1-8.

8. Siegal B. Chapter 2, The healing partnership, p49 in Love, Medicine & Miracles. *Arrow* 1988.

9. Siegal.B. As ref.8. Chapter 4, The will to live, p104.

10. No triumph-No tragedy. BBC Radio 4. January 5th 1999.

11. Channel 5 TV (UK) "Raising the dead." December 27 and 28th 2000.

12. Joni Eareckson with Joe Musser. Joni, p47-49, *Pickering & Inglis edition.* May 1978.

13. Joni Eareckson and Steve Estes, A Step Further; pages 75-77. P*ickering & Inglis* 1979.

14. As reference 12, Joni, p135.

15. As reference 13, A Step Further, p140.

16. Ibid, Chapter 7, Breaks us and makes us; p66.

17. Ibid, Chapter 14, Prayers and Promises, p 158.

18. C.S.Lewis, The Problem of Pain. *Macmillan Publishing Co., Inc.* New York 1962; p93, as quoted in reference 12, p74.

19. Packer J.I. Knowing God. *Hodder and Stoughton Ltd.* London, 1975.

20. Pearce V. Symptom relief is desirable. *Health and Ageing.* June 1997 p34-38.

21. Motor Neurone Disease Association, PO Box 246, Northampton NN1 2PR. Fax 01604 278020.

22. Gibb F. Diane Pretty loses battle for right to assisted suicide. *The Times* April 30th 2002, p7 cols 1-8

23. Bowder B. Diane Pretty loses fight to be helped to die. *Church Times*, May 3rd 2002 p5 cols 1-3.

24. Skinner N. A true ambassador for Christ. *Catholic Herald*, Sept 15th 2001 p15.

25. Vack P. Facing the Lion. *WinePress Publishing PO.Box 428 Enumclaw, WA 98022, USA..* 2001.

26. Guyon 1688. See reference 13 above at page 112.

Chapter 17

The Threat of Euthanasia

In 1984 Dr Helga Kuhse, a leading campaigner for euthanasia, speaking at a Right-to Die Congress in Nice said "If we can get people to accept the removal of all treatment and care- especially the removal of food and fluids- they will see what a painful way it is to die and then, in the patient's best interest they will accept the lethal injection."

Now the Voluntary Euthanasia Society are fighting tooth and nail to persuade Parliament to pass a law that will permit a doctor to help a suicidal patient to die. Their figurehead at Westminster is Lord Joffe, a peer in the House of Lords, who introduced The Patient (Assisted Dying) Bill in the House of Lords in 2003. It was defeated but reappeared as The Assisted Dying for the Terminally Ill Bill [HL] in 2004. Meanwhile their Lordships appointed a Select Committee to consider the arguments for and against this legislation – their report was debated in October 2005 and a revised Bill is now before the House of Lords. And so the "death brigade" in the UK marches on. One thing is certain- they will get no support from the Anglican Church for there was a resounding "No" vote against assisted suicide when the matter was debated at their Annual Synod at York in the summer of 2005.

In recent years the British medical establishment have made strenuous efforts to take an apparently neutral stance in this crucial debate. According to a report in *Right to Life News* a small group in the Royal College of General Practitioners took a neutral stand, but had to reverse this stance following demands from grass roots members.[1] They were compelled to issue a press release declaring that- "We would not want euthanasia campaigners to exploit our neutrality for their own agenda."[2] In December 2004 the Royal College of Physicians published a discussion paper in their journal *Clinical Medicine* setting out arguments for and against assisted suicide. Professor Raymond Tallis, then Chairman of the College Ethics Committee argued the case for euthanasia, but Professor John Saunders who succeeded him as chairman took the opposite view.[3] In the summer of 2005 the vote at the BMA Annual Representatives Meeting was cunningly manipulated, with the result that BMA policy moved from a position of opposition to physician-assisted suicide, to one of neutrality.[4]

Following the BMA vote FIRST DO NO HARM – a British offshoot of the World Federation of Doctors Who Respect Human Life commissioned an on-line opinion poll to assess the response of family doctors to the change in BMA policy. 70% of the 501 respondents disagreed with the neutrality policy and felt that the BMA should express a view on doctor-assisted suicide.[5]

The Report of the Select Committee on the Assisted Dying for the Terminally Ill Bill [HL] was debated in the House of Lords in October 2005.

Dr Anthony Cole observed and recounted events as follows:

"The House of Lords have just debated the report of the Select Committee on Lord Joffe's Assisted Dying for the Terminally Ill Bill. The debate attracted 70 speakers who were more or less evenly divided on the measure, which had actually been dropped, but a new bill is anticipated soon. This is widely expected to be similar to the Death with Dignity Act of the US State of Oregon, which allows doctor assisted suicide for terminally ill patients. There is ample parliamentary time for a new bill to proceed through the upper house and although government has declared itself "neutral", it is widely thought that it harbours covert support for the Bill.

"The arguments advanced by the proponents of assisted suicide and euthanasia have changed noticeably. There now seems to be agreement that modern palliative care can relieve terminal pain and suffering and that few request suicide, once appropriate care is given. There is, however, a group of persons who wish to have control over the manner and time of their deaths whatever treatment may be available. This they lay claim to by asserting an absolute autonomy, the manner of their death being just another of life's choices which should not be denied them by society. Those who oppose them, have their motives called into question. It was claimed during the debate that they were religiously motivated and attempting to impose their beliefs on a secular society. There were sharp exchanges with Anglican bishops who were arguing for a principled, rather than absolute autonomy.

"Though the debate was impassioned and went well beyond midnight, a great deal of controversy can be anticipated if the proponents of assisted suicide continue with their efforts as they have said they will. What is more, they have indicated that theirs is an incremental approach with a desire to achieve their full agenda by degrees. Three proposals seem to be emerging. The first is non medically assisted suicide, the second a medically assisted suicide measure, and thirdly combined euthanasia and assisted suicide.

"At the heart of the debate is a claim to the so called "right to die", and there are those who are sufficiently determined to pursue this without regard for the consequences for the elderly or other vulnerable groups. The argument resolves itself into one of the **will** of the strong minded regardless of the weak, who are currently protected by society. If this line continues the debate is likely to turn increasingly ugly."

Source. Cole A. Editorial, *Ethics and Medicine*, Issue 1, Volume 9, November 2005. On line at http//www. medethics alliance.org © A.Cole 2005. Reprinted with permission.

The Rt Revd Lord Habgood, a former Archbishop of York, alluded to the debate in the House of Lords when reviewing a book – "The Ways of Judgment" – for the Church Times. His review shed light on the difficult relationship between theology and politics in our sectarian society.

"In a recent debate in the House of Lords on a contentious ethical issue, it soon became clear that direct arguments from scripture or Christian tradition carried little weight with the majority of peers; in fact, they were more likely to generate opposition. There seemed, however, to be equally little awareness of the degree to which unspoken theological assumptions underlay not only most of the arguments, but also the whole political exercise in which we were engaged.

"Reading O'Donovan after that debate was a helpful lesson in identifying the level on which a political theology can, and should, operate.

"In a previous book, The Desire of Nations, he explored the way in which Jewish and Christian political concepts found expression in European civilisation. The Ways of Judgment approaches the same subject from the other end, by exploring political concepts, their roots in Jewish and Christian tradition, and the distortions to which they have been subject.

"The point he is making is not that such religious concepts should be directly applicable to contemporary political issues, but that they have, in fact, played a large part in shaping both our political structures and the content of political debate. Against this background, the main political task, as he sees it, is the practice of judgement in the pursuit of truth and effectiveness.

"While there is no simple path from theological insight to political action, theology can shed light, for instance, on false and destructive ideas of what it is to be human. To start, as does much contemporary thinking, from the isolated autonomous individual is to ignore the primacy of communication as the basis of our personhood, and to distort our relationships by failing to see that what is "mine" is in some sense also "ours". Both insights have profound political implications…"[6]

© Church Times Feb.17th 2006. Used with permission.

Following the debate in October 2005 Lord Joffe wasted little time before placing the Assisted Dying for the Terminally Ill Bill before the House of Lords again. He is pursuing this matter relentlessly, and has been given many platforms from which to promote his views during the year. As Dr Cole noted, the issue of assisted suicide is being presented as a matter of choice, just one of a range of options. For example at a conference organised by Worcestershire NHS Department of Palliative Medicine in February 2006 the theme was Ethical and Legal issues in Palliative Care and Lord Joffe was an invited speaker. The conference brochure stated:

"Patient autonomy has not always been seen as the key factor within healthcare. However in recent years ensuring that patients have choice and are involved in decisions regarding their care has become identified as 'best' practice. The speakers at this conference will discuss areas in which patient choice has a stronger ethical impact, where health professionals beliefs are challenged and decisions tread a fine line between an individual's best interest and society's best interest."

The Government views on choice are set out in a paper entitled "Building on the Best. Choice, Responsiveness and Equity in the NHS." This was presented to Parliament in December 2003 by John Read, when Secretary of State for Health. The first chapter states at paragraph 9:

" …We must place real power- the power of making real choices about health care and exerting real influence over those choices- in the hands of all users of services, especially the otherwise disadvantaged."

The trouble is that this freedom of choice does not work out in practice. Take for example the case of Mr Lesley Burke, as recounted earlier in this book. All he wanted was a guarantee that he would receive food and water by tube feeding if his condition deteriorated to the point where he could no longer speak or swallow. John Read wrote to the Appeal Court Judge to point out the cost implications. Mr Burke did not get the declaration that he sought. So choice becomes no choice if you want to be fed, but if you want to refuse tube feeding your wish will be respected.

Some years ago a debate about palliative care and euthanasia would have been unthinkable. When the subject was raised at a conference at the Royal College of Physicians in 1999, not a single delegate said a word. Now the subject has moved centre stage. Those who consider it immoral for a doctor to assist a suicide or kill a patient must make their voices heard above the clamour of the "death brigade".

The Brunel University Survey

Seale C. National survey of end -of -life decisions made by UK medical practitioners. *Palliative Medicine*, 2006; **20:1**, pp.3-10

In 2004 Professor Clive Seale of the school of law and social science at Brunel University, carried out an anonymous postal survey of 857 GPs and hospital specialists to estimate the frequency of different end-of-life decisions in medical practice in the UK. The survey was published in *Palliative Medicine* in January 2006. The participating doctors were asked about the last death they attended. Professor Seale then extrapolated the results on the basis of the annual death rate in the UK. The results created a media furore when they were made public in January 2006. It was reported that the research suggested that nearly 3000 patients were helped to die by doctors in the UK in 2004. The total deaths due to voluntary and involuntary euthanasia in the year amounted to 2865 or approximately eight a day. The survey results are shown in Table 1.

No doctor in the survey reported a case of doctor-assisted suicide. 2.6% of participating doctors said that changing the law would benefit patients, and 4.6% felt that UK law had interfered with their preferred management of patients. Our voluntary euthanasia and physician-assisted suicide rates were significantly lower than those in the Netherlands and Australia. Our non-voluntary euthanasia rates were lower than in Belgium and Australia. Non-treatment decisions were made more often in the UK than in most other European countries.

Table 1   End-of-life decisions in the UK in 2004

Percentage	Deaths	Cause or mode of death
100%	584,799	deaths from all causes in UK.
0.00%	none	physician-assisted suicide (PAS).
0.16%	936	voluntary euthanasia.
0.33%	1929	non-voluntary euthanasia.
32.8%	191,811	symptom relief with possible life shortening effect.
30.3%	177,192	non-treatment decisions.

Media Reports

* Boseley S. Euthanasia: doctors aid 3000 deaths. *The Guardian*, January 18th 2006.
* Lister S. Doctors 'hasten one third of deaths by using pain relief'. *The Times*, Jan. 18th 2006.
* Doughty S. Doctors 'help' 2 in 3 to die. *Daily Mail* Jan.18th 2006.

References

1. Anon. *Right to Life News*, Issue No 44, August 2005. www.rightolife.org.uk
2. See Cook M. How a minority in the BMA got their way on euthanasia. August 9th 2005. http://www.spiked-online.com © spiked 2005.
3. Tallis R, Saunders J. Assisted dying: considerations in the continuing debate. *Clinical Medicine*, 2004; **5:6**, p543-547.
4. Cole A. The BMA drops its opposition to doctor assisted suicide. *Medical Ethics Alliance Newsletter*. Summer 2005, page 3.
5. First Do No Harm. The Doctor's Federation, PO Box 17317, London SW3 4WJ. www. donoharm.co.uk E-mail enquiries@donoharm.co.uk
6. Habgood J. Where we get our civic ideas from. *Church Times* Feb 17th 2005 p.23. **Note** "The Ways of Judgment" by Oliver O'Donovan is published by Eerdmans. ISBN 0 8028 2920

Assisting Suicide

A paper by Wesley J. Smith on a movement that could get out of hand.

This article was first published in New Directions in February 2002. It is reprinted with permission. © Wesley J.Smith 2002.

It is hard to tell the truth about assisted suicide. Actually, the difficulty isn't in the telling, it is in getting people to hear, or more precisely, to listen.

Most people are about as enthusiastic about pondering the issue of assisted suicide as they are about working out the details of their own funeral. The subject hits too close to home, involving as it does, the ultimate issues of life: the reality of human mortality; fears about illness, disability, and old age; the loss of loved ones to the dark dampness of the grave. Thus simply getting people to pay close attention to assisted suicide- to truly grapple with its threat- is often a challenging task.

This is almost as true of people who are religious and/or pro-life, whose faith informs them that death isn't the end but the beginning, as it is about those who identify more overtly with the popular culture. In my work as anti-euthanasia activist, I have often appeared in front of pro-life and religious organisations to speak about assisted suicide, as well as in secular settings. More often than not, event organisers tell me that the audience is one-third to one-half of what it would have been had the programme been about other issues of concern. This has happened so many times now that it is a clear pattern.

I don't take the empty chairs personally. I understand the emotional dynamic at work. Life is difficult and worrisome enough without visiting the painful issues assisted suicide conjures. It is difficult, even for deeply religious people, to listen, to hear, to heed, and to care enough to become involved. Unfortunately, avoidance of the assisted suicide issue is a luxury that those who believe in the infinite value of life can no longer afford.

The most effective weapons in the pro-assisted suicide arsenal are fear-mongering, distortions, euphemisms, half-truths, lies, and damn lies, along with constant chanting of the mantra, 'choice.' These are easily spread in the contemporary media that generally eschew depth and context and thrive on 30-second sound bites shallowness and the soap opera values of tabloidism. The best defence to this propaganda onslaught is to be constantly about the business of spreading truth. After eight years in the moral struggle against the medical culture of death, I can state confidently that the more people learn about assisted suicide, the less they support it. The key to victory then, is education, education, and education.

Aiding and Withholding

Too many people support assisted suicide because they have watched in horror as loved ones were hooked up to medical machines and kept alive against their desires when they were in the last days of life. The threat of such abuse is fading as the economics of medicine moves inexorably towards slashing the level of services in an effort to cut costs. Still, for many non-ideological supporters of assisted suicide, 'being hooked up to machines' is the prime concern.

I can't tell you how often in my experience supporters of assisted suicide turned into opponents once they learned that they have the right to refuse unwanted medical treatment – even if refusing care will probably lead to their deaths. If a dying person doesn't want a ventilator or kidney dialysis, they don't have to have it. If they want to die at home instead of in hospital, they can. No one need commit suicide because of fears of falling prey to high tech medicine.

Eschewing unwanted treatment is the philosophical foundation of the hospice movement – which helps people die without killing them. In hospice, nurturing the patient and controlling his or her pain and other symptoms are the prime goals. Hospice does not seek to extend life but to help dying people live out their days in comfort and dignity and to care for them in a womb-like embrace of unconditional love. Hospice works so well that it is almost a *cliché* for the dying person to declare that their dying experience has been a 'blessing'. Here, then, is true death with dignity – and nobody hooked up involuntarily to machines.

Controlling the pain

Assisted suicide advocates often try to create a false moral equivalency between medically controlling pain and so-called mercy killing. Their argument goes something like this: since some people's deaths are hastened by the powerful medications often required for effective palliation; and, since pain control is considered moral and ethical based on the ethics principle of 'double-effect'; then assisted suicide should also be viewed as moral and ethical since the intent of the assisted suicide is similarly to alleviate suffering. There's only one problem with this argument. It completely misapplies the principle of double effect.

Double effect recognises that there are occasions when a person may intend to do a good thing while recognising that a bad thing *might* occur despite all their good intentions. Even if the bad outcome then occurs, so long as the original intention was good, then the action is deemed morally and ethically acceptable.

If properly applied pain control accidentally hastens a patient's death, the palliative act remains ethical because the bad effect – death was not intended. On the other hand, assisted suicide *intentionally causes death*, not the alleviation of suffering. Thus killing utterly fails to fall within the double effect principle because it explicitly intends a bad result. Thus, assisted suicide is an immoral and unethical act and a profound violation of the 'do no harm' values of Hippocratic medicine.

The terminal and the terminated

Most assisted suicide advocates do not want to limit death doctor services to people who are terminally ill. Advocates are well aware that popular support for assisted suicide evaporates when the legalisation criteria involve chronically ill, elderly, depressed or disabled people. This presents an acute political problem for them: they want a broad licence for assisted suicide but know they can't promote it openly because they will lose substantial public support. Thus, they will use words such as 'incurable' or 'hopeless' illness when describing the kinds of afflictions that would justify medicalized killing.

The use of these words is meant to make the reader or listener think 'terminal', when they mean something quite different. For example arthritis is an incurable illness, but it is not generally terminal. The same can be said about diabetes, multiple sclerosis, spinal injuries, and a plethora of other disabilities and afflictions that are part of the human condition.

The true agenda of the assisted suicide movement came into rare focus in October 1998 when the World Federation of Right to Die Societies – an organisation consisting of the world's foremost euthanasia advocacy groups- issued its 'Zurich Declaration' after its biennial convention. (Among the signatories to the document was Dr Michael Irwen, one of the leaders of the British euthanasia movement.) The Declaration urged that people 'suffering severe and enduring *distress* [should be eligible] to receive medical help to die.' (My emphasis.) Finally, the actual goal of the assisted suicide movement is revealed: deaths on demand for anyone with more than a transitory wish to die.

Use and Abuse

A time-tested mantra of the assisted suicide movement is that abuses will be prevented by protective guidelines. But this promise of protection is as empty as the repeated assurances that assisted suicide will be restricted to people who are actually dying. One need only look to the experience of the Netherlands to see what scant protection restrictive guidelines actually give.

Euthanasia has been practiced openly since 1973 in the Netherlands, and the practice was recently formally legalised. If doctors follow the legal guidelines enacted by the Parliament when they kill their patients, they will not be prosecuted. Among these guidelines are the necessity of repeated patient requests, unbearable suffering for which there are no reasonable alternatives, and the requirements of doctors to obtain second medical opinions. These have remained essentially unchanged for many years.

In actual practice, the so-called protections are ignored or have been expanded by court decisions that are now utterly ephemeral. A recent study published in the *Journal of Medical Ethics* about euthanasia in the Netherlands, reveals that the Dutch policy is 'beyond effective control' since 59 per cent of doctors do not report euthanasia or assisted suicide to the authorities as required by law. Worse, the categories of people who doctors kill have expanded steadily since euthanasia entered Dutch medical practice. Today, in the Netherlands, not only are terminally ill people who ask to be killed euthanized but so are chronically ill people. (For example, an anorexic young woman in remission was assisted in suicide because she was worried about returning to abusing food, and the doctor was not prosecuted.)

Doctors also kill depressed people. This resulted from the prosecution of a psychiatrist who had assisted the suicide of a grieving mother who wanted to be buried between her two dead children. The Dutch Supreme Court validated the psychiatrist's decision; ruling that for purposes of judging the propriety of euthanasia, suffering is suffering and it does not matter whether the suffering is physical or emotional. Not only that, Dutch babies born with disabilities are killed by doctors at the request of parents, even though babies, by definition, cannot ask to die. According to a study published in the July 26th 1997 edition of the British journal, the *Lancet*, 8 percent of infants who die in the Netherlands are injected with drugs by their doctors 'with the explicit aim of hastening death,' amounting to 80-90 killed infants a year.

Finally, Dutch doctors practice involuntary euthanasia. According to several Dutch studies conducted during the last decade, more than 1000 who do not ask to be euthanized are killed each year by Dutch doctors because the *doctor's values* dictate that their deaths should be brought about- and this number does not include the many hundreds who are killed each year by intentional overdoses of morphine. As far as I know, no physician has been jailed for this practice.

The price of life

In the end, assisted suicide would be less about 'choice' than about profits in the health care system and cutting the costs of health care to government. This is the conclusion of no less than Derek Humphrey and pro-euthanasia attorney, Mary Clement, who in their book *Freedom to Die*, admit that cost containment may become their ultimate *raison d'etre* for physician assisted suicide (PAS), that is, killing as a financial benefit to society:

> ' A rational argument can be made for allowing PAS in order to offset the amount society and family spend on the ill, as long as it is the voluntary wish of the mentally competent terminally ill adult. ... There is no contradicting the fact that since the largest medical expenses are incurred in the final days and weeks of life, the hastened demise of people with only a short time left would free resources for others. Hundreds of billions of dollars could benefit those patients who not only *can* be cured but who *want* to live.' (Emphasis within the text.)

Imagine a health care system in which profit incentives favour killing as the best 'treatment' for cancer, motor neurone disease, multiple sclerosis, spinal injury, Alzheimer's disease, and many other medical conditions that eventually impact us all. Imagine the potential for abuse and coercion in a health care system in which killing is seen as a way to broaden accessibility to health care for others in society. The result could lead to a profound devolution of our culture and our moral values.

The time has come for good people to come to the aid of their culture. Legalising physician-assisted suicide would be to return us to equivalent practices of ancient societies that exposed disabled infants on hills and left the elderly and infirm by the side of the road. Beating back the tide is not only essential to this country but to the world.

Wesley J. Smith, an attorney for the International Task Force on Euthanasia and Assisted Suicide is the author of Culture of Death: The Assault on Medical Ethics in America, *published by Encounter Books in 2000. He wrote the above article while on a lecture tour in the UK in 2002.*

Paradise Lost: The Devolution of Medical Practice

An earlier version of this paper by Gillian Craig was first published as a guest editorial in Ethics and Medicine in January 2000. © Craig GM.

Many British doctors will have been shocked by an editorial "When learned doctors murder" that was published in *Ethics and Medicine* in 2000.[1] The author C. Ben Mitchell, a Professor of Christian Ethics referred to the devolution of medical practice, and warned of the dangers of using euphemistic language to make murder seem respectable. His warning was timely, but the word murder does not trip easily off the tongue when speaking of medical practice…

James Hoefler, an American associate professor of political science has written a sinister guide to foregoing treatment at the end of life. He talks quite openly about dehydration, describing this as "a time-honoured, foolproof alternative to tube feeding for terminally ill patients who are prepared to die". He also discusses dehydration as an alternative to physician-assisted suicide. "The key" to managing death, suggests Hoefler, is "knowing when to shift the focus from curing to caring...If we really care we will think long and hard about whether to impose artificially provided nutrition and hydration".[2] Few doctors would disagree with that statement. However, I would stress that hydration must never be withheld with the deliberate intention of ending life.

When advance directives become legally binding in the UK, people will be able to opt for death by dehydration simply by signing an advance directive that prohibits the use of artificial hydration under certain circumstances[3]. This happens already in some States in the USA. Competent patients can of course refuse artificial hydration or medical treatment simply by saying "No". Sometimes old people who are tired of life take matters into their own hands and stop eating and drinking.

Difficult quality of life considerations are an important part of medical decision making. It may be acceptable to withhold artificial hydration if the means of administering it is too great a burden for the patient.[4] This could apply to tube feeding or gastrostomy feeding in many clinical situations, including advanced dementia, and some stroke patients. Many very difficult decisions have to be made in younger people with 'learning difficulties'. There are no easy answers to these problems.

The British Medical Association (BMA) recognise that there are "substantial and unresolved issues concerning the withdrawal and withholding of treatment from patients…".[5] Unfortunately, the guidelines that the BMA Medical Ethics Committee published in June 1999 did little to resolve these issues, and caused considerable alarm and concern. The task of the Committee was a difficult one, and they may have been pushed into unwise and hasty decisions by pressure from politicians…. There may well be economic advantages to be gained from the early death of ill or disabled people, as the Federal Government in the USA noted some years ago.[6] This message will not have been lost on those responsible for our cash-strapped Health Service and could well have been part of the covert thinking behind moves to make advance directives legally binding in the UK. The British Government, like that of the USA could stand to gain financially from the early death of patients who might otherwise be a burden on the health service. Few politicians would admit this in so many words, but economic arguments are powerful and the temptation to act must be strong.

Many people were appalled in 1996 when the British Medical Journal (BMJ) published an editorial "Jack Kevorkian: a medical hero", written by the North American Editor of the BMJ and a Professor of Medicine and Bioethics from Canada.[7] Dr Kevorkian, an unemployed pathologist, was killing patients at their request in the back streets and garages of Michigan, and dared the law to stop him. He was convicted of second degree murder in 1999.

One of the key principles of medical ethics, as agreed at an international conference held in Paris in 1987, is set out in Article 2 of Principles of Medical Ethics in Europe.[8] This states that "The doctor may use his professional knowledge only to improve or maintain the health of those who put their trust in him; in no circumstances may he act to their detriment". The conference report was unanimously adopted by all participants, including the General Medical Council representing the United Kingdom. The BMJ editorial flouted Article 2 and undermined professional integrity. It is ominous that there was no public reprimand about this editorial from the BMA or the General Medical Council. Editorial freedom it would seem, is more important than professional morality and respect for the law.

The law on euthanasia was very carefully reviewed by Parliament at the time of the Bland case, and the result of the carefully reasoned debate was that euthanasia remains illegal in the United Kingdom at present. That decision should be respected, but there are constant attempts to undermine the law. Those who break the law are not heroes. The true medical heroes are those who truly care for their patients and support them through pain and distress, until life comes to a natural end.

Many letters of protest were written about the notorious Kevorkian editorial and several were published in the BMJ of July 27th, 1996. Some were from palliative medicine specialists at the forefront of the fight against euthanasia.[9,10] Dr Ilora Finlay and colleagues from the University of Wales College of Medicine stressed many practical reasons why killing a patient, even when problems seem insurmountable, must remain prohibited by law. In summary, they said that the law protects vulnerable patients, it protects doctors from themselves, and it protects doctors from relatives and managers who may stand to benefit from a patient's early death."

A Geriatrician, Dr C A Crowther[11] drew attention to Pope John Paul II, whose letter *Evangelium Vitae* upholds the value of human life and exposes the prevailing "culture of death" in which we are immersed.[12] Robert Balfour, a Consultant Obstetrician[13] quoted Dr Everett Koop, a former Surgeon General in the USA who predicted a euthanasia programme for various categories of citizens and pleaded "Let it never be said by historians .. . that there was no outcry from the medical profession."[14]

Intentional and deliberately planned death should have no place in medicine, yet the concept has been introduced into public debate quite deliberately. The BMJ editorial was a blatant example of this. Others have introduced the issue more subtly and unobtrusively. In recent years, several influencial people have helped to promote euthanasia. One such, John Harris, a Professor of Applied Philosophy who advocates doctor assisted suicide, was chosen by Age Concern to chair a study group that prepared a statement on values and attitudes in an ageing society. Their views, advocating doctor- assisted suicide and euthanasia, were presented to the public in a glossy brochure, and on the internet, as part of the Age Concern Millenium Debate of the Age.[15] This initiative- said to be independent, but rumoured to have government funding aimed to raise awareness about the implications of our changing demography, in particular the increasing number of old people in our society. Another aim was to achieve policy changes, and help to set personal and national priorities through a national programme of events. Those who cooperated and interpreted the theme according to operational policy were allowed to use the 'age speech-bubble logo'! The Debate of the Age was proudly presented as the "Largest, most involving social campaign ever envisaged outside government."[15] Feedback was presented to the Government in Spring 2000, but if there was any publicity I missed it! The organising committee included several representatives from the world of finance and insurance, the editor of the BMJ, Professor John Harris, some media experts, a token Bishop and others. The debate was of course very wide ranging and covered many areas that were unrelated to medical ethics. Nevertheless, the views expressed on euthanasia in the interim papers were sinister and dangerous. Meanwhile the Lord Chancellor and the Government assured the public that there were no plans to legalise euthanasia! However subtly the spin doctors work, the public must not allow themselves to be fooled.

From time to time a General Practitioner, formerly the Chairman of Doctors for Assisted Dying, is invited to speak on radio or television, or writes to *The Times*. He is proud that he has killed terminally ill patients in the course of his medical career. The police have decided not to prosecute him as the crimes were committed many years ago. Yet ageing war criminals are still prosecuted. Why should this doctor have immunity from prosecution? [16]

In 1992 a Consultant Rheumatologist was convicted of attempted murder. Having found himself unable to control his patient's severe pain, he gave her a lethal injection of intravenous potassium chloride, and she died within minutes.[17] Despite the conviction, he was allowed to continue to practice by the General Medical Council (GMC). Yet his action contravened both the law, and Article 2 of Principles of Medical Ethics in Europe to which the GMC had been a signatory. Had they forgotten about this, or did they choose to overlook the fact? Where now is the resolve to see that these ethical principles are put into practice? Where is the resolve to respect the law of the land?

In his book 'A Preface to Paradise Lost', C.S. Lewis commented on Milton's epic poem and was fascinated by mankind's ability to argue ourselves into a course of action that we know to be wrong. Eve, is tempted to eat the forbidden apple. She has dubious reasons for offering to share the apple with Adam in the Garden of Eden.[18]

C.S.Lewis wrote:

"I am not sure that critics always notice the precise sin which Eve is now committing, yet there is no mystery about it. Its name in English is Murder. If the fruit... means death, then he must be made to eat it, in order that he may die.... And hardly has she made this resolve before she is congratulating herself upon it as a singular proof of the tenderness and magnanimity of her love ....

... The whole thing is so quick, each new element of folly, malice and corruption enters so unobtrusively, so naturally, that it is hard to realise that we have been watching the genesis of murder.... Thus, and not otherwise, does the mind turn to embrace evil. No man perhaps ever at first described to himself the act he was about to do as Murder, or Adultery, or Fraud, or Treachery, or Perversion; and when he hears it so described, by other men he is (in a way) sincerely shocked and surprised. Those others "don't understand". If they knew what it had really been like for him, they would not use those crude 'stock' names. With a wink, or a titter, or in a cloud of muddy emotion the thing had slipped into his will as something not very extraordinary, something of which rightly understood and in all his highly peculiar circumstances, he may even feel proud."[19]

How well these thoughts of CS Lewis describe the varied reactions to the hydration debate!

We all have a responsibility to ensure that withholding hydration is not used as a means of ending life. The basic human need for life-sustaining food and water, should be met in a way that is morally acceptable, medically acceptable, and in keeping with the law of the land.

We all have a responsibility to ensure that doctors and health care workers are not permitted to kill their patients or assist patients to kill themselves.

How sad it would be if the celebration of 2000 years of Christianity should coincide with an age when human life became disposable in civilised society!

References

1. C Ben Mitchell, 'When learned doctors murder'. Editorial. *Ethics and Medicine.*1999; **15:1**, p1.
2. Hoefler J M, 'Managing Death' pp 117 & 134, *Westview Press 1997*
3. Craig G M, 'No man is an island. Some thoughts on advance directives'. *Catholic Medical Quarterly* 1999. **XLIX No.3**, 7-14.
4. House of Lords Select Committee. Report on Medical Ethics. London; para. 251-7, *HMSO:* 1994.
5. Wilks M, Letter *The Times* January 9th 1999; p.21, col. 3.
6. Memorandum from R A Derzon, USA Department of Health, Education and Welfare, Health Care Financing Administration, to President Carter. 1997.
7. Roberts J, Kjellstrand C, 'Jack Kevorkian: a medical hero'. *British Medical Journal* 1996; **312:** 1434.
8. "Report of the Conference International des Ordres et des Organismes d'Attributions Similaires", Paris. 1987.
9. Twycross R, Letter. *British Medical Journal* 1996; **313:** 227.
10. Finlay I, Routledge P, et al. Letter. *British Medical Journal* 1996; **313:** 228.
11. Crowther C A, Letter. *British Medical Journal* 1996; **313:** 227.

12. Pope John Paul II. 'Evangelium vitae'. *Catholic Truth Society,* London, 1995.
13. Balfour R, Letter. *British Medical Journal* 1996; **313:** 228.
14. Schneffer P A, Everett Koop C. 'Whatever happened to the human race?' London: *Marshal Morgan and Scott.* 1980.
15. The Millenium Debate of the Age. Coordinated by *Age Concern* England in 1998.
16. Note. The doctor was eventually struck off the medical register in 2005.
17. Dyer C. Rheumatologist convicted of attempted murder. *British Medical Journal* 1992; **305:** 731.
18. Text adapted from BBC Radio 4. "Something Understood" of February 27th 1999, Producer Tasmin Collison for Unique Broadcasting Production of London.
19. Lewis C S. A Preface to Paradise Lost (c) Oxford University Press 1942. Re-issued in *Oxford Paperbacks.* 1960 p.126-127. Quoted with permission.

Respect for Life: a Framework for the Future

Some comments and suggestions from Dr Gillian Craig.

Ethical dilemmas that come to public attention show how difficult medical practice can be. There are no easy answers to the problems raised. Many people over the years have tried to contribute to the process by which ethical decisions are made in medicine, but in general the end result of all this thought has been of little practical value to a busy doctor. New life support techniques have produced new dilemmas for society and the medical profession to solve. We now have a plethora of guidelines.

It is customary for ethicists to talk in terms of four principles of beneficence, non-maleficence, autonomy and justice.[1] The emphasis these days tends to be on autonomy – i.e. the wishes of the individual patient. For the doctor the principle 'First do no harm' is vital. We also need to remember the basic maxim 'Thou shalt not kill'.

It is fashionable at present to consider 'therapeutic decisions' at the end of life in terms of benefits, burdens and best interests. These B words trip off the tongue in discussion, but do not stand up to careful scrutiny, as theologian Peter Jeffery has demonstrated in a closely argued chapter in his recent book *'Going against the stream.'*[2] Jeffery argues that the starting point in any discussion on foregoing treatment must be respect for life. To be of practical value ethical frameworks must be workable, understandable, realistic and universally applicable. This is a tall order, but having ruled out solutions based on substituted judgement, or quality of life assessments Jeffery favours a framework based on the concept of proportionality, which some people may find helpful [2]. Decisions based on substituted judgement, i.e. on the view of a proxy decision maker or other third party, as to what an incapacitated person's wishes might be, are known to be flawed. Decisions made on quality of life judgements by third parties are also inherently flawed, and in America such judgements are not allowed as a legal reason for discontinuing treatment. This

253

means, notes Jeffery 'that health professionals can only make quality of treatment judgements, and not quality of life judgements, otherwise the acts are a disguised form of euthanasia.'[3]. The same danger is apparent when the patient's 'best interest' is invoked as a reason for withdrawing life supportive measures.

Jeffery argues that the concept that a treatment can be withdrawn because it is 'conferring no benefit' is so broad that it could be applied to anyone incurably ill with a fatal condition [4]. There are also objections to the burden argument, for as Jeffery points out 'what is a burden to one person is quite acceptable to the next.' Widening the concept to include the burden on the family, insurance company or state is anathema to most physicians whose prime responsibility is to the individual patient. However such considerations cannot be ignored completely. When resources are finite, the needs of other patients on the waiting list may enter the equation. Thus it is easy to see why some elderly incurable patients may be seen as expendable.

It will be readily apparent that every case will be different, and must be considered carefully and with sensitivity, taking into account the clinical situation and the views and wishes of the patient. When the patient is confused, unconscious or mentally incompetent, the views of their nearest and dearest friends and relatives should be sought. It is the doctor's role to advise and offer appropriate treatment, which a competent patient may accept or refuse. When the patient is mentally incompetent the burden of responsibility is more onerous, and treatment can be given only if it is strictly necessary. Those who look to the law to safeguard the interests of mentally incompetent patients may be sadly disappointed.

When all is said and done, the advice of the House of Lords' Select Committee on Medical Ethics still has much to recommend it. After careful deliberation at the time of the Bland case, they concluded that it should be unnecessary to consider the withdrawal of hydration or nutrition unless the means of administration was in itself a burden to the patient [5]. That eminently sensible conclusion was ignored by the Law Lords in their judgment in the Bland case, for it was their intention to allow Bland, a patient in a permanent vegetative state, to die. I doubt whether their Lordships realised at the time how wide the repercussions of that judgment would be.

Factors that spin on the wheel of fortune to determine the patient's fate:

- Clinical diagnosis
- Treatment available
- Patient's physical condition
- Patient's mental state
- Benefits and burdens of treatment
- Patient's best interest
- Patient's wishes
- Relative's views
- Views of senior clinician and clinical team.
- Views of a Court under some circumstances.

A practical approach

For practical purposes when considering whether artificial hydration or nutrition is appropriate the responsible doctor should consider the following basic points:-

1. Is it necessary?

2. Is it feasible?

3. Can the patient tolerate the procedure?

4. Does the patient wish to undergo the procedure?

5. Is the patient capable of giving informed consent?

6. Beware of making quality of life judgements. Nevertheless consider whether prolonging life will be a boon to the patient or an intolerable burden. Ask yourself and others- What would the patient want?

7. Is the patient mentally incapacitated or lacking in self-awareness? If so obtain a second opinion from an experienced doctor according to BMA guidance if in the UK[6]. If the relatives disagree with a proposal to withhold artificial hydration and nutrition listen carefully to their views, for they could be right. Take into account and respect deeply held religious views. If dissent remains after careful discussion legal advice should be sought.

8. Is the condition reversible or permanent? Have all reversible features been treated? If not, why not?

9. Is the patient in a permanent vegetative state? If so, in the UK, there is a legal obligation to obtain permission from a Court before withholding artificial hydration and nutrition.

10. Is the patient terminally ill and death imminent? If so follow the guidance of the National Council for Hospice and Specialist Palliative Care Services (NCHSPCS), as issued in July/August 1997 [7]. Long term nutrition will not be a priority in this situation but attention should be paid to hydration [8]. Subsequent NCHSPCS guidance for use in the last few days of life plays down the importance of hydration and is not entirely satisfactory [9]. General Medical Council guidance issued in August 2002 should be heeded.[10]

11. If death is not imminent, and there are no clear indications that artificial hydration and feeding would be very distressing, or would have no effect, then give fluids and nutrition by whatever means seem most appropriate, unless there are clear contraindications. If you do not feel this approach is appropriate obtain a second opinion and consider the legal position before treatment is withdrawn[10].

12. Take heed of guidance issued by respected professional organisations, but do not allow yourself to be forced into actions that you consider immoral. Be prepared to justify your conduct and stand firm. Keep in touch with a supportive peer group.

13. Be gentle with relatives and try to ensure that they have appropriate emotional and spiritual support.

14. There comes a time when everything possible has been done, but the patient lingers on in a twilight existence that some see as a fate worse than death. Then it may be appropriate to gently suggest that it might be best to let them go, and hand them with love to God.

Acknowledgement

The above paper was first published in the Catholic Medical Quarterly Volume LIV No.1 (299) p 13-15, in February 2003.

References

1. Beauchamp T, and Childress J.F. Principles of Medical Ethics. First issued in 1978. 4th edition *Oxford University Press* 1994.
2. Jeffery P. Going Against the Stream. Ethical aspects of ageing and care. Chapter 5 Mortal questions. *Gracewing,* 2001.
3. Ibid page 158.
4. Ibid page 159.
5. House of Lords' Select Committee. Report on Medical Ethics. 1994; para 251-7 London, *HSMO.*
6. Withholding and withdrawing life-prolonging medical treatment. Guidance for decision making. *BMJ Books.* 1999.
7. Ethical decision – making in palliative care. Artificial hydration for people who are terminally ill. *National Council for Hospice and Specialist Palliative Care Services.* London July/August 1997.
8. Craig G.M. Palliative care from the perspective of a Consultant Geriatrician: the dangers of withholding hydration. *Ethics and Medicine,* 1999: **15.1**:15-19.
9. Changing Gear – managing the last days of life in adults. *NCHSPCS* London, December 1997.
10. Withholding and withdrawing life-prolonging treatments: good practice for decision making. *General Medical Council,* London. August 2002.

Epilogue

It is time to draw this book to a close. I have said enough to demonstrate that patients are in danger and to give readers a glimpse of the dark side of medical ethics that is normally hidden from view. Some of the information will have been disturbing and painful to read, but the truth must be told, for medical ethics is moving into dangerous and uncharted territory. It is time for men and women of good will to speak out. We must turn away from death-orientated medicine, towards an approach that respects and reveres the divine spark that makes all human life special.

A doctor's role is to be a healer, a giver of life, not a taker of life. Politicians and economists should remember this, and ensure that doctors have the resources they need to carry out their work to a high professional standard. Resources must be shared with justice and with equity, but that should not mean that the weakest go to the wall. Basic sustenance should be provided for all if this is humanely possible.

Doctors and managers in the National Health Service have become pawns in a deadly game of chess, where the basic rules of morality are in danger of being overturned. All players in this saga operate with different motives. Politicians must satisfy the demands of the electorate in order to remain in power. Economists concentrate on wealth creation and aim to balance the books. The medical profession should concentrate on the health and welfare of their patients, and the legal profession should ensure that all keep within the rules. But which rules? The laws laid down by Parliament, the European Convention on Human Rights, the Charters of the United Nations, or the Ten Commandments?

In an increasingly secular world we are in danger of ignoring the great taboo that prohibits intentional killing except in a just war. We ignore the wisdom of ages at our peril!

In years to come we must all decide where our allegiance lies. Doctors and nurses have a responsibility to respect human life and should at all times act in a patient's best interest. Those who believe in God must stand firm and hold fast to that which is good.

> Once to every man and nation
> Comes the moment to decide,
> In the strife of truth with falsehood
> For the good or evil side;
> Some great cause, God's new Messiah,
> Offering each the bloom or blight-
> And that choice goes on for ever
> 'Twixt that darkness and that light..

J.Russell Lowell, 1819-1891.
From The English Hymnal 1933; p729, © Oxford University Press.

257

Bibliography

Austin Baker J. The Foolishness of God. *Collins. Fontana Books* 1975.

Medical Ethics Today: Its Practice and Philosophy. *BMJ Books,*1993.

Brogden M. Geronticide. Killing the elderly. *Jessica Kingsley*, London 2001.

Brown H. and Gibbs K. (eds) Euthanasia. A Christian Perspective. The Church of Scotland Board of Social Responsibility. *Saint Andrew Press* Edinburgh. 1995.

Cameron N. (Ed) Death without Dignity. *Rutherford House*, Edinburgh 1993.

Curran C. Politics, Medicine and Christian Ethics. *Fortress Press*, Philadelphia, 1973.

Goldsmith M. Hearing the Voice of People with Dementia. *Jessica Kingsley*, London 1996.

Gormally L. (Ed.) Euthanasia: Clinical Practice and the Law. *Linacre Centre* London 1993.

Habgood J. Being a Person. *Hodder and Stoughton* 1998.

Hoefler J.M. Managing Death. *Westview Press*, 1997.

Hume B. Searching for God. 1977. Reissued by *Hodder and Stoughton*, 1999.

Jeffery P. Going against the stream. *Gracewing*, 2001.

Jewell A. (Ed) Spirituality and Ageing. *Jessica Kingsley*, London 1999.

Keown J. (Ed) Euthanasia examined: Ethical, Clinical & Legal Perspectives. *Cambridge University Press*. 1995.

Lewis CS. The Problem of Pain. *Collins. Fount Paperbacks* reprint 1977.

Lennard-Jones J.E. Ethical and legal aspects of clinical hydration and nutritional support. *British Association for Parenteral and Enteral Nutrition*. 1998.

Oderberg D. Applied Ethics. *Blackwell*, Oxford 2000.

Paul S.S. and Paul J.A. Humanity Comes of Age. *World Council of Churches Publications*, Geneva 1994.

Siegal B.S. Love, Medicine and Miracles. *Arrow Books Ltd*. 1988.

Sinason V. Mental Handicap and the Human Condition. *Free Association Books*. London 1992.

Smith. Wesley J. Forced Exit. *Spence Publishing*. Second edition. 2003.

Vack P. Facing the Lion. *WinePress Publishing*, PO Box 428, Enumclaw, WA. 98022, USA, 2001.

Wolfensberger W. The New Genocide of Handicapped and Afflicted People. *Syracuse University Division of Special Education and Rehabilitation* 1987.

Wyatt J. Matters of Life and Death. *Inter-varsity Press*, 1998.

Zucker M. and Zucker H.D. (Ed) Medical Futility. *Cambridge University Press*, 1997.

INDEX

For some sources of help or
information see page 205.

Topics addressed in Challenging Medical Ethics Volume 1
"No Water-No Life: Hydration in the Dying." Craig GM (Ed)
Fairway Folio **March 2005. ISBN 0 9545445 3 6**

- Ethical, legal and medical dangers of sedation without hydration in the dying. Key papers from professional journals document a decade of debate from 1994 to 2005 in the words of the main protagonists.
- Case reports illustrate clinical situations encountered.
- The problem of post-traumatic stress in dissenting relatives.
- Addressing the anxieties of relatives.
- Legal issues: double effect and the neglect factor.
- The "Right to Die" debate. Patients who refuse food and water.
- The physiology of thirst. Dehydration and methods of rehydration.
- Some professional guidelines in the UK.
- Comments from palliative carers in the USA, Japan and Australia.

Sales and distribution
Please address orders and enquiries for both books to:
PO Box 341 Enterprise House, Northampton NN3 2WZ (UK).
